D1713899

Successful Aging as a
Contemporary Obsession

Global Perspectives on Aging

Sarah Lamb, Series Editor

This series publishes books that will deepen and expand our understanding of age, aging, ageism, and late life in the United States and beyond. The series focuses on anthropology while being open to ethnographically vivid and theoretically rich scholarship in related fields, including sociology, religion, cultural studies, social medicine, medical humanities, gender and sexuality studies, human development, critical and cultural gerontology, and age studies. Books will be aimed at students, scholars, and occasionally the general public.

Jason Danely, *Aging and Loss: Mourning and Maturity in Contemporary Japan*
Parin Dossa and Cati Coe, eds., *Transnational Aging and Reconfigurations of Kin Work*
Sarah Lamb, ed., *Successful Aging as a Contemporary Obsession: Global Perspectives*
Margaret Morganroth Gullette, *Ending Ageism, or How Not to Shoot Old People*

Successful Aging as a Contemporary Obsession

Global Perspectives

EDITED BY SARAH LAMB

RUTGERS UNIVERSITY PRESS

NEW BRUNSWICK, CAMDEN, AND NEWARK, NEW JERSEY, AND LONDON

Library of Congress Cataloging-in-Publication Data
Names: Lamb, Sarah, 1960– editor.
Title: Successful aging as a contemporary obsession :
global perspectives / edited by Sarah Lamb.
Description: New Brunswick : Rutgers University Press, [2017] | Series: Global
perspectives on aging | Includes bibliographical references and index.
Identifiers: LCCN 2016033721| ISBN 9780813585345 (hardcover : alk. paper) |
ISBN 9780813585338 (pbk. : alk. paper) | ISBN 9780813585352 (e-book (epub)) |
ISBN 9780813585369 (e-book (web pdf))
Subjects: LCSH: Aging—Social aspects—Cross-cultural studies. |
Older people—Cross-cultural studies.
Classification: LCC HQ1061 .S8449 2017 | DDC 305.26—dc23
LC record available at https://lccn.loc.gov/2016033721

A British Cataloging-in-Publication record for this book
is available from the British Library.

∞ The paper used in this publication meets the requirements of the American
National Standard for Information Sciences—Permanence of Paper for Printed Library
Materials, ANSI Z39.48–1992.

www.rutgersuniversitypress.org

Manufactured in the United States of America

One of the privileges given to those who've avoided dying young is the blessed right to grow old. The honor of physical decline is waiting, and you have to get used to that reality.

–Haruki Murakami, *What I Talk About When I Talk About Running*, 2008

CONTENTS

Preface   xi

Acknowledgments   xv

Introduction: Successful Aging as a
Twenty-first-Century Obsession   1
    SARAH LAMB, JESSICA ROBBINS-RUSZKOWSKI,
    AND ANNA I. CORWIN

PART I
Gender, Sexuality, and the
Allure of Anti-Aging

1   Successful Aging, Ageism, and the Maintenance of
    Age and Gender Relations   27
        TONI CALASANTI AND NEAL KING

2   Opting In or Opting Out? North American
    Women Share Strategies for Aging Successfully
    with (and without) Cosmetic Intervention   41
        ABIGAIL T. BROOKS

3   Aging Out: Ageism, Heterosexism, and Racism
    among Aging African American Lesbians and Gay Men   55
        IMANI WOODY

4   Erectile Dysfunction as Successful Aging in Mexico   68
        EMILY WENTZELL

PART II

Ideals of Independence, Interdependence, and Intimate Sociality in Later Life

5   Beyond Independence: Older Chicagoans
        Living Valued Lives   85
        ELANA D. BUCH

6   Growing Old with God: An Alternative Vision
        of Successful Aging among Catholic Nuns   98
        ANNA I. CORWIN

7   Aspiring to Activity: Universities of the
        Third Age, Gardening, and Other Forms of
        Living in Postsocialist Poland   112
        JESSICA ROBBINS-RUSZKOWSKI

8   Should Old Acquaintance Be Forgot? Friendship
        in the Face of Dementia   126
        JANELLE S. TAYLOR

PART III

National Policies and Everyday Practices: Individual and Collective Projects of Aging Well

9   Getting Old and Keeping Going: The Motivation
        Technologies of Active Aging in Denmark   141
        ASKE JUUL LASSEN AND ASTRID PERNILLE JESPERSEN

10   Foolish Vitality: Humor, Risk, and Success in Japan 154
        JASON DANELY

11   Nurturing Life in Contemporary Beijing   168
        JUDITH FARQUHAR AND QICHENG ZHANG

12   Depreciating Age, Disintegrating Ties: On Being
        Old in a Century of Declining Elderhood in Kenya   185
        JANET McINTOSH

PART IV
Medicine, Morality, and Self:
Lessons from Life's Ends

13   Successful Selves? Heroic Tales of Alzheimer's Disease and
        Personhood in Brazil   203
        ANNETTE LEIBING

14   Comfortable Aging: Lessons for Living from
        Eighty-five and Beyond   218
        MEIKA LOE

15   Ageless Aging or Meaningful Decline? Aspirations
        of Aging and Dying in the United States and India   230
        SARAH LAMB

        Epilogue: Successful Aging and Desired Interdependence   243
        SUSAN REYNOLDS WHYTE

        Notes on Contributors   249
        Index   253

PREFACE

This is not another book on how to age successfully. On the face of it, though, the notion of successful aging sounds so inspiring and uplifting: why question it? Since the successful aging movement emerged in North America around the 1980s as a medical, public health, commercial, and popular cultural endeavor,[1] we've seen some obvious benefits. Who doesn't welcome messages of aging as a positive life phase, or medical advances warding off debilitating and life-threatening diseases, or public education about what one can do as an individual to improve one's own health across the life course? Successful aging envisions inspirationally that the negatives of aging can be pushed further and further away, or even made to disappear, by medical technique and individual effort. As one reviewer of this book manuscript put it, who wouldn't want to live healthier and happier through age ninety or one hundred, and then die quickly with no decline and suffering?

Other facets of the successful aging movement, however, are less appealing. In proposing a hyperpositive view of aging, the whole notion of successful aging is, in ways that can be hard to recognize, in some respects profoundly ageist—resting on a deep North American cultural discomfort with aging, old age, and being old. Ageism refers to prejudice or discrimination based on a person's age—akin to prejudice based on a person's race or sex/gender at the root of racism and sexism. Ageism, additionally, goes beyond prejudice against particular older individuals to entail a broader, pervasive aversion to and embarrassment about the condition of old age in general, in oneself and others, and in humankind. This is why it is impolite in North American society, for instance, to call someone "old." This antipathy to oldness can be seen within the successful aging movement, in its attempts to eradicate the kinds of declines, vulnerabilities, and dependencies previously commonly associated with old age.

But it is not as easy to eradicate human frailty as it is to wipe out a disease like polio, and perhaps not as unequivocally desirable as well. What of those of us who don't make it to ninety or one hundred without pain and suffering? If one develops vulnerabilities in later life, does that mean that one has "failed" at aging?

One aim of the book is to ask such questions, not to offer easy answers but to invite critical dialogue on a wider set of possibilities for imagining what it is to live meaningfully in later life. A binary paradigm of aging as good or bad, successful or failed, is too simple a model, and too evaluative, to capture the complexity and ambiguity of life as lived. To help us expand our imaginations, the volume explores the complex and varied ways older people themselves—across a range of cultural, national, religious, class, racial-ethnic, gendered, sexuality, health, and life-experience backgrounds—practice and understand their own aspirations for aging.

The successful aging paradigm is also fascinating to examine as a contemporary social-cultural, political-economic, and medical-philosophical project, prevailing in North America and Western Europe and with diverse instantiations spreading around the globe. A second aim of the book is to explore this intriguing social-cultural phenomenon, a major contemporary movement of our time. The successful aging paradigm rests on certain understandings of individualist, autonomous personhood, featuring a sense of individual control over one's own self and life, as well as values of agelessness and avoiding oldness. In this way, the book's project resonates with one of anthropology's core aims: to make visible that which can seem so ordinary and taken for granted that it can be hard to recognize, and thereby to open our everyday worlds to fuller understanding and cultural critique.

How did I, a US cultural anthropologist who specializes in India, become interested in critically examining my own society's notions of successful aging? For many years I had been studying social-cultural life in India, where I encountered cultural paradigms of aging that seemed quite different from those surrounding me in the United States. In India, for instance, people often speak of the value of learning from the fact of human transience, and of the necessity and pleasure of familial-social interdependencies that persist throughout the life course. According to Hindu Indians, two of the four classical stages of life or *asramas* take place in older age, with their own meaningful transitions and projects. Although people recognize hardships and problems in old age, as throughout life, in general it is not considered impolite or embarrassing to refer to someone as old. In contrast to what gradually became very familiar to me in India, some of our own successful aging notions in the United States— including the paradigm's aspirations for agelessness, individual independence, and eradicating old age—had long struck me as a little weird. At the same time, as an enculturated American, I was very much enjoying the pursuit of health and vitality—inspired by the widespread cultural project around me mandating and celebrating individual responsibility for one's own health, the premise that there are things one can control in one's own life, such as exercise and diet, that might make a difference.

When I was then suddenly struck with a serious case of cancer shortly after turning fifty-one (five years ago at this writing), just days after running the Boston Marathon, I realized in a personal way how vitality and good health may not be a reasonable expectation for all. My surgeon said I likely had just eighteen to twenty-four months to live. Facing chemotherapy, vulnerability, and mortality, I was of course sad to think I may have to die before I could pursue many of the things I had hoped and expected to do in my life, and to contemplate the pain my loved ones would face if I were to pass away so soon. Those feelings of sadness, no matter how sharp, were not surprising to me. But what did puzzle me was to realize that I had been trained by my society to experience this new reality of mine as not only sad but also radically embarrassing. How odd is that? I had somehow failed at maintaining my own good health—at being a healthy, good, successful person and self. This feeling of embarrassment and failure went beyond a sense of specific blame—that I was at fault for getting the disease—to entail a harder-to-pinpoint, more diffuse and morally inflected shame of being vulnerable and weak.[2]

For years I had been wanting to investigate critically the successful aging project through my lens as a cultural anthropologist, and now my own experiences with cancer diagnosis and treatment gave me some new perspective and insight. I began to do fieldwork with US elders and found that many older Americans also seemed unconsciously to feel ashamed when they faced vulnerabilities in later life, such as a cancer or Parkinson's diagnosis, or the need to use a cane or walker.

At the same time, as a lifelong member of US society, I certainly continue to find myself participating in many of its anti-aging and individual-responsibility-for-one's-own-health ideals. I am now very grateful to be in seemingly glorious good health and look forward to many more years. When I recently spoke to a fifties-ish friend about the US successful aging project—and its emphasis on people taking responsibility for their own health, through exercise, eating well, consuming health knowledge, and engaging in productive activities, and about how many of my older US interlocutors are enjoying and finding inspiration in all of this—my friend said eagerly, "I'll do all that! I know I'll do all that!"

So the aim of this volume is not to discard all prevailing projects of successful aging—which many individuals, governments, and public health agencies find inspirational, self-affirming, and fun. (Being healthy at any stage of life tends to feel good and cost less.) Rather, the volume helps us recognize the successful aging movement's both positive and negative elements, and to explore its intriguing nature as a major cultural and public health movement—dare I say obsession?—of our time. The volume highlights the varied perspectives of older persons around the globe as they pursue diverse visions of valued aging—involving body and health, family and friendship, interdependence and independence, spirituality and humor, gratitude and regret, prejudice and respect, and, ultimately, insight on what it is to be human. In so doing, the volume offers rich alternative visions to the contemporary North American emphasis on avoiding oldness.

NOTES

1. See chapter 1 for a brief history of the successful aging movement.
2. As far back as 1980, Robert Crawford pointed out how good health has become a sign of individual moral character, while bad health is attributed to individual failings ("Healthism and the Medicalization of Everyday Life," *International Journal of Health Services* 10 [3]: 365–388). Note how I felt compelled above, when sharing my story of cancer, to include mention of just having run a marathon, to mitigate the sense of personal failure my news of cancer might convey.

ACKNOWLEDGMENTS

Many people and institutions have contributed to this project, in ways more profound than I can enumerate here. I would like first to express my gratitude to the numerous older people and their communities in India and the United States who have generously shared with me their time, conversations, and insight. From them I have learned so much.

My colleagues Jessica Robbins-Ruszkowski and Anna Corwin helped inspire this project from the outset through our animated discussions over breakfast at the 2013 American Anthropological Association meeting. Together we designed a series of two panels for the 2014 Gerontological Society of America and American Anthropological Association conferences, in which several of this volume's contributors participated. The enthusiastic reception from the audiences at both meetings encouraged us to move forward to publish this book. After I drafted the volume's introduction, Jessica and Anna each offered valuable input, and I am pleased to list them as coauthors. Colleague and contributor Emily Wentzell likewise made very useful interventions into the introduction.

I am grateful for the friendship, editorial advice, and invaluable discussions over the years with Diane Mines, who read drafts of the preface, introduction, and my own chapter for the volume, and who has been instrumental to my development as an anthropologist since our early days together in graduate school at the University of Chicago. I have also gained insight and sustenance from my wonderful group of colleagues at Brandeis in anthropology and in women's, gender, and sexuality studies. I drafted the introduction and preface at two delightfully productive and revitalizing writing retreats with Elizabeth Ferry, Anita Hannig, and Janet McIntosh. My writing group, with my colleagues Elizabeth Ferry, Caitrin Lynch, Cinzia Solari, and Smitha Radhakrishnan, has contributed in important ways to my thinking and prose.

By closely reading each chapter through their lenses as students and scholars of our society, my graduate student research assistants, Laura Broadwater, Paige Henderson, Sasha Martin, and Kaitlin Seegman, benefited the volume immeasurably. I have gained insight from the exceptional and probing undergraduate students I have worked with at Brandeis in my class, Aging in Cross-Cultural Perspective. I have also greatly benefited from conversations with the senior members of the anthropology classes I taught at the Brandeis Osher Lifelong Learning Institute (BOLLI) and NewBridge on the Charles, where we managed to weave in spirited discussions of successful aging notions.

Financial support for fieldwork and the book's publication was gratefully received from the Theodore and Jane Norman Fund for Faculty Research at Brandeis University.

I have been privileged to present some of my work-in-progress on this project to the Stein Institute for Research on Aging at the University of California at San Diego Medical School; the Department of Comparative Human Development at the University of Chicago; the Lyceum Lecture Series at Oxford College of Emory; the Women's, Gender, and Sexuality Studies Distinguished Faculty Lecture Series at Brandeis University; the Center for Healthy Aging at the University of Copenhagen; the University of Heidelberg symposium "New Approaches to Ageing in South Asia and Europe" at the Max Mueller Bhavan in New Delhi; Vidyasagar University in Medinipur, West Bengal; Ramananda College in Bishnupur, West Bengal; the Wellesley Neighbors group for midlife and older adults; and the Kendal Crosslands Retirement Community in Pennsylvania. At each venue, I have learned from very stimulating conversations with colleagues and audience members.

I am grateful to the editors at Rutgers University Press for guiding me through the voyage of producing this book. Marlie Wasserman was the editor first excited about this project and about publishing more books on aging in general. Kimberly Guinta then took over masterfully as editor with her sage guidance. I am grateful also to copyeditor extraordinaire Margery Tippie and to my skilled and perceptive indexer Cynthia Savage. Several anonymous reviewers for the press provided very useful suggestions. I am particularly indebted to the one reviewer who seemed so to like the notion of successful aging that it helped me and other authors sharpen our arguments.

My parents and parents-in-law—Sharon Rowell, Sydney Lamb, Susan Lamb, Doris Black, Robert Black, and Barbara Black—have taught and supported me in countless ways. My two wonderful daughters, Rachel and Lauren Black, have brought me such joy and meaning. I am ever grateful for their discerning, lively conversations that on a daily basis push forward my thinking. My close neighbor families have been beloved friends and like extended kin over many years, including Frida Boyd, who passed away just weeks ago at this writing after living a long and vibrant life, and dying in such a remarkably graceful and mindful way that she awed us all. I have learned so much about life, aging, and humanity from all of you.

My husband, life partner, and best friend, Ed Black, has continued to be an incredible source of support, fun, companionship, love, ambition, and intellectual stimulation throughout my career as an anthropologist, and has made my life and work enjoyable.

These words of appreciation would not be complete without directly thanking the outstanding scholars who have contributed their work to make this volume happen.

Successful Aging as a Contemporary Obsession

Introduction

Successful Aging as a
Twenty-first-Century Obsession

SARAH LAMB, JESSICA ROBBINS-RUSZKOWSKI, AND ANNA I. CORWIN

With the rise in the aging population, we are witnessing a burgeoning discourse on how to age well. According to dominant medical, public health, psychological, and popular cultural narratives prevailing in North America and Europe, we each have the potential—and, indeed, the moral and political obligation—to make our own aging "successful," thereby staving off the impending disabilities and burdens of late life.

This book invites us to think critically about our visions of successful aging. It uses the knowledge of diverse places, people, and perspectives that we have gathered as cultural anthropologists and sociologists to help us realize that the contemporary paradigm of successful aging is not the only way, nor necessarily the best, most humane, or most inspirational way, to imagine aging and what it means to be human.

The term *successful aging* first appeared in Robert Havighurst's 1961 article for the original issue of the journal *The Gerontologist.* Physician John Rowe and psychologist Robert Kahn subsequently published their landmark book *Successful Aging*, presenting results of a major MacArthur Foundation Study of Aging in America—a project seeking to clarify the factors that promote mental and physical vitality in later life (1998). Since the 1980s, successful aging has persisted as the dominant paradigm in gerontological research, appearing also under such related labels as "active aging," "healthy aging," "productive aging," "vital aging," "anti-aging," and "aging well."[1] The World Health Organization devoted World Health Day 2012 to Healthy Ageing, and the European Union designated 2012 as the European Year for Active Ageing.[2] In North America and Western Europe, centers for healthy aging, active aging, and successful aging abound. Popular cultural and self-help books on the topic are flourishing.

Take, for instance, the abundant literature available on Amazon.com, the world's largest online shopping site. A search for texts on successful aging elicits a wealth of alluring titles, including the following, to name only a few:

- *Winning Strategies for Successful Aging*
- *Successful and Healthy Aging: 101 Best Ways to Feel Younger and Live Longer*
- *Live Long, Die Short: A Guide to Authentic Health and Successful Aging*
- *Do Not Go Gentle: Successful Aging for Baby Boomers and All Generations*
- *100 Days to Successful Aging: A Workbook for Living Fully*
- *The Joys of Successful Aging*
- *In Full Bloom: A Brain Education Guide to Successful Aging*
- *Healthy at 100: The Scientifically Proven Secrets of the World's Healthiest and Longest-Lived Peoples*
- *Aging Backwards: Reverse the Aging Process and Look 10 Years Younger in 30 Minutes a Day*
- *Younger Next Year: Live Strong, Fit, and Sexy—Until You're 80 and Beyond*
- *Live Young Forever: 12 Steps to Optimum Health, Fitness and Longevity*
- *Get Healthy for Your Next 100 Years: A Top MD's Guide to Successful Aging*
- *Successful Aging 101*
- *Healthy Aging for Dummies*[3]

Individual agency and choice are perhaps the most salient themes in both the academic and popular literature on successful aging. If aging was previously imagined in North America as a natural process of decline largely beyond the control of the individual, the successful aging paradigm has turned that assumption on its head. It says that *you* can be the crafter of your own successful aging—through diet, exercise, productive activities, attitude, self-control, and choice. Aging well becomes a vital personal and moral project, benefiting not only the individual but also one's broader family, society, and nation.

John W. Rowe and Robert L. Kahn pronounce in their pivotal 1998 *Successful Aging* text, for example: "Our concept of success connotes more than a happy outcome; it implies achievement rather than mere good luck. . . . To succeed in something requires more than falling into it; it means having desired it, planned it, worked for it. All these factors are critical to our view of aging, which, even in this era of human genetics, we regard as largely under the control of the individual. In short, successful aging is dependent on individual choices and behaviors. It can be attained through individual choice and effort" (37). In her *100 Days to Successful Aging*, Barbara Bruce proclaims: "I am talking about simple, but not necessarily easy, things you can *CHOOSE* to do to age successfully."

"YOU can change your prospects for a long and healthy life." "It is never too late to begin. JUST DO IT!"[4] Another text announces, "While we don't have a choice whether or not to age, we DO have a choice on HOW to age. We can, for instance, age helplessly. . . . And, at the same time, we can also choose to age gracefully. Happily. Successfully!"[5] In their top-selling *Younger Next Year: Live Strong, Fit, and Sexy—Until You're 80 and Beyond*, Chris Crowley and Henry Lodge, MD, proclaim inspirationally: "Why, you can choose to live like fifty until you're in your eighties. In your eighties, my man! We mean it. . . . Most of us really do not have to age significantly" (2007, 4). They go on, after portraying a common decline narrative of aging: "But it's a *choice*, not a sentence from on high. You can, just as easily, make up your mind—and tell your body—to live as if you were fifty, maybe even younger, for the rest of your life" (6, emphases original).

Such a bold new vision of aging successfully seems immediately appealing, positive, and inspirational. Who wouldn't want to be healthy, active, fulfilled, and successful? Indeed, each of us—the authors of this introduction and the book's chapters, anthropologists and sociologists who have conducted research across the Americas, Europe, Africa, and Asia—has studied and encountered many people, at times ourselves among them, who are inspired by and quite delightedly embrace the ideals of the successful aging movement. We all also welcome many of the obvious and dramatic benefits of modern medicine's related technologies of prolonging life and extending health.

Yet when one looks deeper and scrutinizes the successful aging paradigm's cultural and moral assumptions, one finds successful aging to be not only a particular cultural and biopolitical project but,[6] despite its inspirational elements, in some ways a counterproductive one, worthy of critical examination. As anthropologists and sociologists who listen to the voices and stories of older people across diverse social and cultural contexts, we find that they have much critical insight to offer.

Why Question Successful Aging? Listening to the Voices of Elders

Meet Dora Koenig, for instance.[7] Dora grew up in Brooklyn, New York, to immigrant Jewish parents, studied art at Columbia University, and eventually settled in a lovely tree-lined neighborhood of Brookline, Massachusetts, where she bought a brown-shingled home that she filled with art—her own and others'—while teaching painting at the Massachusetts College of Art and Design and authoring several books. In many ways, Dora at age seventy-two vividly embodies her society's contemporary vision of successful aging. She values independence, finding the idea of eventually needing to move into assisted living "horrifying," and enjoys living alone, having chosen not to marry or have children. "My quote used to be," she says, "'You're going to have to scrape me off the floor [to get me out of this house]!'" Dora also regards aging well as a purposeful project: "We have such a culture of achievement, and I am a major pursuer of achievement," she professes. As part of her project of aging well, Dora began going regularly to a gym, "because I was determined that my body wouldn't rot." She took up taking and teaching classes at a lifelong learning institute, as she views "real engagement" as key to aging well. She has also been inspired by the Jewish philosopher Baruch Spinoza, whose "idea of successful living is to be joyful and active out of resources inside yourself. You know, not expecting things to come onto you or into you. . . . So I feel very lucky that I feel so rich on the inside. I mean, I don't have enough time in the day!" expressing here also her sense of resonance with her society's perception of the value of productivity, where being busy is a badge of honor at any age.[8] She takes tai chi and yoga classes, both for overall fitness and to help with the balance issues that can impact elders. Dora reflects: "These [activities] give you an example of how I keep looking—I've done everything—tai chi, yoga—from each of these, I've learned how to make my aging better." Dora also expresses an inner sense of agelessness found in broader discourses on successful aging:[9] "I feel exactly the same as when I was a kid." Proud of her upbeat and energetic approach to aging, when asked directly how she might herself define "successful aging," Dora replied with confidence: "I think it's what I'm doing."

At the same time, Dora Koenig questions features of our society's successful aging paradigm. Diagnosed with cancer at age fifty-four, Dora was told that she would "be dead in three years" and "to get [her] affairs in order." A cultural model implying that the individual is in control leaves one open to a sense of personal failure and embarrassment if things don't continue to go well. In Dora's case, she was deeply embarrassed by her cancer: "What happened when I got sick—I come from a very high-achieving family—I was profoundly embarrassed that I was going to die. Nothing short of that. For six months I couldn't tell anybody. That's weird. . . . It was like I had a personal failing." Now she looks back and feels that her brush with mortality, though terrible to experience at the time, actually helped her to grow a lot, but she blames our society for treating illness and death like an embarrassing failure. Dora also believes that we should learn to accept some dependence on others and to ask for help, but we're not taught that this is okay. Her ninety-two-year-old neighbor lives all alone, which makes Dora "very angry—how's that for irrational? since I live alone myself." She recalls a friend asking, "'Why does it make you so angry?' And it's because I see myself as maybe— . . . I can see myself being as stubborn as she is. She's extremely stubborn. She can hardly see. She can't drive. She can't read. And she will not leave that house! I'm very fond of her and I find it very hard to be with her because she's like the ghost of what's coming." When anthropologist Sarah Lamb, while interviewing Dora, mentioned the notion of "permanent personhood" found in our North American visions of successful aging, where models of aging well imply a sense of enduring permanence as a person rather than embracing change through aging,[10] Dora interrupted, "Oh, I believe permanent personhood is an evil idea. Because it is so wrong! It is just not true. And it is like never-never land and princesshood. It just doesn't help you be a person." She reflected that she is striving instead to cultivate "a very rich relationship with *reality*, namely *mortality*, and what do you want to make with the time you have now?"

Another US older adult, Maurice Kleinman, spoke of his painful struggle to accept at age eighty-four that he needs a cane to walk safely without falling. Using a cane can feel stigmatizing, signifying the one stage of life—old age—we are embarrassed by and strive to eliminate. Maurice Kleinman's wife, Elaine Kleinman, seemed more willing to accept changes of age, as she reflected: "I grew up with the illusion that if I did things in a certain way, I could control what the outcome would be. . . . I'd say that probably one of the ways I've changed the most [as I've aged] . . . is the capacity to *accept* your limitations, and not to be in struggle with that: The world changes; you change. . . . This is what I've learned the most in my later years and what I've found the most reassuring." Similarly, anthropologist Anna Corwin has studied the lives of older Catholic nuns in a US convent and finds that their experiences of physical and psychological well-being in late life may be increased precisely because they do *not* uphold the ideals of independence, productivity, and individual control prevailing in popular Western successful aging models (this volume).

Cross-culturally, we find other perspectives on what it is to age well. These perspectives are often tied to alternative forms of personhood.[11] In India, for instance, as in many nations beyond Europe and North America, forms of (inter)dependence, frailty, mortality, and human transience are widely regarded as normal, inevitable, and even in some ways valued parts of personhood and key aspects of the human condition. It is common for Indian elders in the metropolis of Kolkata, for example, to speak freely of their own coming deaths, as Purnima Banerjee reflected casually one morning on her front verandah over tea, while still enjoying robust physical health in her seventies: "I say to God, 'Whenever you are ready, take me.' . . . I am not afraid of death, because it is inevitable. Because I am born, I know I have to die. No one born can escape death," and "We have to accept decay. I have accepted." Further, appropriate dependence on others within an intimate family or (if necessary) institutional setting is generally more highly valued by Kolkatans than individual bodily health (Lamb 2009). Despite the suffering and confusion that can be entailed by a diagnosis of Alzheimer's disease, anthropologist Bianca Brijnath (2014) finds that those with dementia within Indian families are normally regarded as full social persons, enmeshed in loving and reciprocal kin networks of care and *seva*—a core family value defined as respectful service to elder family members. Anthropologist Janet McIntosh in this volume explores how Kenyans envision the problem of aging in contemporary times as not the risk of too little independence but rather too little dependence, or not enough people around on whom to be appropriately dependent.[12] Anthropologist Emily Wentzell finds in Mexico that instead of using drugs such as Viagra to continue youthful sex lives, many older Mexican men collaborate with their wives and physicians to frame erectile difficulty as a prompt to embody age-appropriate, mature masculinities (Wentzell 2013, this volume). At the same time, North American and European models of successful, healthy, and active aging are spreading around the world as part of broad cultural, economic, and biomedical processes of globalization.

The book's contributors bring a critical anthropological and sociological lens and the diverse perspectives of subjects in North America, Latin America, Europe, Africa, and Asia—from Catholic nuns to Hindu ashram dwellers, from women seeking plastic surgery to men forgoing Viagra, from state-sponsored healthy aging programs to individual fitness plans, from lifelong learning aspirants to dementia sufferers—into conversation with the burgeoning medico-public discourse on successful aging. The contributors ask, how does the successful aging project shape current experiences of aging, forms of personhood, and visions of how best to live? How does the dominant successful aging paradigm inspire some, even as it excludes others? How might this particular cultural and biopolitical model reproduce the very forms of inequality and ageism that it is meant to counteract? Might the experiences of older adults who are excluded from "successful aging" reveal other forms of moral personhood in old age? And how might scrutinizing visions and projects of successful aging—as similarly and distinctly fashioned in the Americas, Europe, Asia, and Africa—shed light on unique experiences of modernity? Ultimately, how can we use our lenses as ethnographers and cultural critics to understand this major contemporary obsession?

The remainder of this chapter will first offer a brief history of the successful aging movement and exploration of its underlying cultural assumptions and political-economic contexts. We will then turn to a brief discussion of the book's key aims and what to expect in the chapters to come.

The Successful Aging Movement

The emergence of the successful aging movement can only be understood by examining certain broader cultural-historical processes of the twentieth and early twenty-first centuries.[13] As sociologist Nikolas Rose describes in *The*

Politics of Life Itself: Biomedicine, Power, and Subjectivity in the Twenty-first Century (2007), contemporary medicine has come to foster a notion of health as a personal social-ethical imperative. From official discourses on health promotion, to popular discourses on dieting and exercise, to corporate wellness programs and higher insurance rates for employees not pursuing healthy lifestyles, to public awareness campaigns to promote healthy aging, we see an increasing stress on personal responsibility for one's own health—the maintenance and optimization of the healthy body and self. Anthropologist Susan Greenhalgh reflects, in her analysis of the related American war on fat: "Since around 1900, one of the social responsibilities of the good (bio)citizen has been to maintain a certain kind of body. . . . Managing our own health and ensuring a medically 'normal' weight and fit body are fundamental duties of the good biocitizen today" (2015, 19). In such a context upholding health as a super value, good health is regarded as the moral duty of all individuals, fostering not only a healthy self but also a healthy and productive society, while bad health becomes attributed to individual failings (Crawford 1980, 2006; Greenhalgh 2015, 20).

This emphasis on personal responsibility complements neoliberal ideals about individual freedom, self-governance, and minimizing public support prevalent in North America and in many arenas around the world today. Neoliberal ideals of individual responsibility are especially relevant, given that the United States, like other nations, is facing an unprecedented demographic shift of population aging. As US baby boomers reach sixty-five, the proportion of older persons in relation to those of traditional working ages—often termed the "old-age dependency ratio"—is projected to climb dramatically. The higher the old-age dependency ratio, the greater the potential burden on the state and society. Yet, if healthy, fit, active older citizens can take care of themselves by pursuing the ideals of health and life, then they can supposedly avoid becoming burdens. In other words, older adults who do not engage in these pursuits are assumed to be burdensome. The good citizen becomes "one who reduces health-care costs to the body politic by taking responsibility for his or her own health through lifestyle modifications" (Greenhalgh 2015, 21). In such ways, the successful aging movement is flourishing in a particular cultural-historical context.

Among the cultural-historical values upon which the successful aging paradigm rests are those surrounding individualist personhood and ideologies of the life course. Several common themes here stand out as worthy of scrutiny. These include (1) individual agency and control; (2) the value of maintaining independence and avoiding dependence; (3) the merit of productive activity; and (4) a vision of permanent personhood or not aging at all, while pursuing the goals of agelessness and avoiding oldness.

How We Age Is Up to Us: Visions of Individual Agency and Control

The most prominent theme underlying the successful aging movement is the notion of individual agency and control. As introduced above, the central premise of successful aging from its inception is the argument that how we age is mostly up to us.[14] Widely regarded as "revolutionary" and "changing our understanding of aging forever" (Landry 2014, 31), the successful aging movement argues seductively that the way you live—what you can do as an individual—is more important than genes or fate or an inevitable biological unfolding of age-related declines.

To Rowe and Kahn, three individual-centered actions are core to the successful aging project: (1) doing what one can to avoid disease and disability, (2) maintaining high physical and cognitive function, and (3) continuing active engagement with life (1997, 438; 1998, 38–39; see also Landry 2014, 35).[15] The plethora of self-help books on successful, healthy, and active aging also celebrate the theme of aging as an individual project. Richard Kownacki proclaims motivationally, in his *Do Not Go Gentle: Successful Aging for Baby Boomers and All Generations*, the front cover adorned with two grandmothers gleefully skydiving: "The good news is that you can regain control of your life and well-being by practicing the principles of successful aging. Each of us individually has the ultimate responsibility of our own health and well-being. If we rely exclusively on the government, our doctors, the professionals or anybody else to do it for us, it's easy to become complacent. Rebel against complacency and denial. In short, become the hero of your own life story" (2010, 76). Physician Henry Lodge elaborates in *Younger Next Year*: "The more I looked at the science, the more it became clear that such ailments and deterioration [heart attacks, strokes, cancer, diabetes, falls, fractures, and serious injuries] are *not* a normal part of growing old. They are an outrage. . . . 'Normal aging' is intolerable and avoidable" (Crowley and Lodge 2007, 29). He goes on: "The good news on this front is that you do not need to wait for a presidential commission or a national health initiative to do something. This fight can be led, fought and won one person at a time. Starting with you" (30). The *New York Times* reports on a recent study of the effects of exercise on aging: "The findings suggest that many of our expectations about the inevitability of physical decline with advancing years may be incorrect and that how we age is, to a large degree, up to us" (Reynolds 2015).

We see here a vision of aging that emphasizes the power of individual agency and the individual self as a project. Such a vision resonates with individualist notions of personhood favored in the United States and with broader American myths of self-control. Anthropologist Arthur Kleinman comments: "It is our assiduous denial of existential vulnerability and limits that is extraordinary in American culture." He goes on to reflect: "Much of our society, of course, is founded on a myth of self-control (Jefferson's perfectibility of man), mastery of the environment (taming the frontier), . . . and denial of human limits, including the ultimate one, death itself" (2006, 7). Our contemporary obsession with successful aging is one new instantiation of this powerful American myth.

Taking Care of Yourself: The Ideal of Independence

A second central theme in the successful aging paradigm resonating with broader North American cultural ideals is that of independence. In their landmark text *Successful Aging*, Rowe and Kahn report: "Older people, like younger ones, want to be independent. This is the principal goal of many elders, and few issues strike greater fear than the prospect of depending on others" (1998, 42). They define independence as "continuing to live in one's own home, taking care of oneself" (1998, 42, 125), while characterizing independence as a "positive" condition and dependence as a "bleak" one (14). The Centers for Disease Control and Prevention's Healthy Aging Program presents independence as synonymous with well-being on its landing page: "Our materials are designed to assist health professionals in learning about and engaging in activities . . . to promote independence and wellbeing."[16] Popular self-help books on successful aging also highlight the theme of independence, such as in Eric Pfeiffer's *Winning Strategies for Successful Aging*: "The important thing at this stage is to *maintain a sense of independence*" (2013, 180, emphasis original).[17]

This ideal of maintaining independence in late life may seem obvious and taken-for-granted to many in the United States, but it is worthwhile to take a moment to reflect critically upon the vision of appropriate in/dependence over the life course underlying this independence-successful aging nexus. Americans do not envision all forms of dependence as bad: children who depend on their parents—for material and emotional support, meal preparation, toileting, and so on—are not normally envisioned as in a "bleak" condition. In India—where more than 80 percent of those sixty-five and over live in households with adult children and grandchildren—few consider it inappropriate, demeaning, or bleak to receive material and emotional support, respectful care (*seva*), and help with daily activities including toileting from their junior kin. Assistance with toileting, in fact, is often presented as a paradigmatic act that Indian parents first naturally provide for their young children and then naturally receive from these same children in a relationship of lifelong intergenerational reciprocity.[18]

Yet American forms of individualist personhood valorize autonomy and self-sufficiency throughout the life course. Living alone at all ages is at unprecedented levels in North America, as Eric Klinenberg examines in his 2012 book, *Going Solo: The Extraordinary Rise and Surprising Appeal of Living Alone*. Older Americans report doing whatever they can to avoid moving in with others, even—perhaps especially—their children. In reality, frail elders in Western contexts do receive much help from family members, but they tend to shun receiving full financial support, co-residence, and intimate bodily care (such as toileting and bathing) from kin. Anthropologists have long found that Americans tend to think of depending on younger relatives for support in old age destructive to their sense of dignity and value as a responsible person (Clark 1972). Andrei Simic observes: "What the American elderly seem to fear most is 'demeaning dependence' on their children or other kin" (1990, 94). However, this focus on independence obscures the actual interdependence that exists throughout the life course. The successful aging movement extends our society's individualist ideals into a seductive promise of eternal independence.

No, You Can't Just Dodder: Active Aging for a Healthy Self and Society

A third key theme of the successful aging movement is that of maintaining productive activity. The fact that many models of successful aging are termed "active aging" highlights the prevailing emphasis on the value of activity. Productive activity ties together all three components of Rowe and Kahn's successful aging model: avoiding disease and disability, maintaining high cognitive and physical function, and engaging with life (1998, 39, fig. 3). Rowe and Kahn remark: "Successful aging goes beyond potential; it involves activity, which we have labeled 'engagement with life.' Active engagement with life takes many forms, but successful aging is most concerned with two—relationships with other people, and behavior that is productive" (40).

In Europe since the early 2000s, active aging policies have promoted healthy activity in contrast to unhealthy passivity (Lassen and Moreira 2014, 39, 43). EU active aging policies advocate for pension reforms to extend working lives, activity centers for the elderly, and new paradigms of self-care, with catchphrases such as "Living longer, working better—Working longer, living better,"[19] framing productive activity as important not only for the health of the individual but for the economic viability of the society as a whole.[20] Active aging is also a central policy framework of the World Health Organization, where activity is connected to health, autonomy, independence, and social, economic, cultural, spiritual, and civic productivity. The WHO articulates clearly: "Maintaining autonomy and independence for the older people is a key goal in the policy framework for active ageing" (though it also acknowledges in the next lines broader family and community connections: "This is why interdependence as well as intergenerational solidarity are important tenets of active ageing"). The WHO also argues for the value of elders "remaining active contributors to their families, peers, communities, and nations."[21]

Across North America, Europe, and Australia, the flourishing of lifelong learning institutes and Universities of the Third Age,[22] senior exercise classes, the postponement of retirement, postretirement work opportunities, and an ethic of busy-ness in retirement support such an active aging motto. Sociologist Stephen Katz, critically examining "the gerontological nexus of activity, health, and successful aging" (2000, 136), remarks: "The association of activity with well-being in old age seems so obvious and indisputable that questioning it within gerontological circles would be considered unprofessional, if not heretical" (135). While some past gerontological theories advocated for disengagement from activity as a sign of healthy, normal aging,[23] a *New York Times* piece titled "No, You Can't Just Dodder" remarks: "These days, older people are not supposed to be sitting in a rocking chair, but . . . studying Italian in Florence, say, or learning the difference between a demi-glace and a velouté at the Cordon Bleu, jetting off to an archaeological dig in Timbuktu or a trek in Nepal or even skydiving, as former President George H. W. Bush did . . . on his 80th birthday." The piece goes on: "It's not just that people have the option of keeping busy. In some ways society is demanding that they do so—to be less of a drain on resources, to remain physically and mentally fit, and as a source of support for the pharmaceutical and other aging-related industries" (Fountain 2005).

We see again broader social values reflected in images of successful, appropriate aging. Activity becomes a means to be successful in aging and maintain oneself as a valued biocitizen, pursuing busy, healthy productivity while avoiding dependence.

You Don't Have to Act or Feel Old: Aspirations of Agelessness and Permanent Personhood

A final theme in successful aging discourse is that of an ageless permanent personhood—a vision of the ideal person as not really aging at all in later life, but rather maintaining the self of one's earlier years, while avoiding or denying processes of decline and conditions of oldness.[24] Anthropologist Janet McIntosh (2009) reflects that those who prize the individual may be especially preoccupied with the self's (putatively) stable, enduring qualities—a preoccupation we certainly find in the anti-aging, antidecline aspirations of successful aging. Some Buddhist, Hindu, and Catholic models of personhood instead highlight transience as a fundamental part of being human.[25]

The theme of ageless permanent personhood is highlighted in various successful aging discourses. The most basic notion of successful aging used in research involves minimal debility past the age of sixty-five or so, or "older adults whose health status is similar to that of younger people" (Depp and Jeste 2006, 18). In *Healthy Aging for Dummies*, part I is titled "So You Want to Look and Feel Young Forever," with chapter I promising "The Fountain of Youth, at Your Fingertips" (Agin and Perkins 2008). Jack LaLanne, in *Live Young Forever*, argues that "We must grow younger, not older" (2009, III) and offers secrets for how to "achieve an amazing level of lifelong health and fitness," "become the most physically attractive person possible," and "have boundless energy every day for the rest of your days, months, years" (back cover). In a section boldly titled "Decay Is Optional," Crowley and Lodge proclaim: "You do not have to *act* old or *feel* old" (2007, 33, emphases original). The natural "default signals" of our bodies turn toward decay after the forties and fifties when "the free ride of youth is over"; but "what we can do, with surprising ease, is override those default signals . . . and change decay back into growth" (34). Anti-aging medicine has emerged as a robust, organized field, with a professional association, annual meetings, and lucrative business opportunities. Anti-aging products such as Jeunesse's Instantly Ageless dominate the cosmetics industry. Today's life-prolonging medicine also shapes nearly every American's experience of growing older—with some obvious benefits but not enough dialogue, making it difficult to know "when that line between life-giving therapies and too much treatment is about to be crossed" (Kaufman 2015, 2). Physician Muriel Gillick comments critically in *The Denial of Aging: Perpetual Youth, Eternal Life, and Other Dangerous Fantasies*: "The ultimate way to ensure that the baby boomers won't have to worry about the perils of old age is to eradicate aging entirely" (2006, 195).

To be sure, some successful aging texts do articulate the value of adapting to and coping with age-associated changes rather than denying them.[26] Even Rowe and Kahn acknowledge that "successful aging means just what it says—aging well, which is very different from not aging at all" (1998, 49). Additionally, some authors underscore special opportunities for positive change in late life, such as increasing wisdom, depth, and spirituality, rather than emphasizing merely staying the same (e.g., Weil 2007). Nonetheless, the dominant impression one gains from perusing the vast contemporary discourse on successful (healthy, active, productive, vital) aging is that of a vision of agelessness. The aging self is, ideally, an ageless self. Idealized images of an ageless self resonate with broader cultural visions prevailing in North America, in which the frailty, fragility, vulnerability, and declines of so-called real old age and agedness (that which cannot be named in polite conversation, in fact[27]) are segregated from successful (anti-) aging.

The successful aging movement has emerged as part of a broad political-medical and cultural enterprise aimed at fostering healthy, independent subjects to meet the demands of population aging—what could be called a contemporary biopolitics of aging—remaking potentially frail, dependent elders into active, fit, productive, ageless adults. Such a vision also rests on a distinctive cultural model of personhood, featuring individual agency, independence, productivity, and intransience. Like the war on obesity discourse (Greenhalgh 2012, 482), the successful aging movement is at once a morality tale, a medical tale, a governmental tale, and an existential tale, enacting cultural norms for persons as healthy, active, independent, and long-living subjects.

Successful Aging and Cultural Critique

We would like to instigate a public conversation about the successful aging movement. We begin by highlighting some critiques of successful aging from our perspective as cultural anthropologists and sociologists.[28] The project of anthropology and its mission of cultural critique is not necessarily to argue that any institution or movement is "all good" or "all bad" but rather to illuminate and challenge the certainties of taken-for-granted assumptions, thereby making room for possibly new and more enlightened models.[29]

Perhaps our most pressing critique of the prevailing successful aging paradigm is that it is profoundly ageist, growing out of a deep cultural discomfort with what could (or should?) be regarded as the normal human conditions of frailty, (inter)dependence, vulnerability, and transience. This is ironic, since the successful aging movement emerged partly as a counter response to the negative views of old age circulating amid North American society, aiming to promote a positive view of aging (Holstein and Minkler 2003). Indeed, to many, especially younger adults as well as elders doing very well by the model's standards, successful aging can be experienced as wonderfully inspirational and life- and self-affirming. In a way, however, both the binary "ill-derly" and "well-derly" (Moody 2009, 68) models of aging are expressions of the same ageist culture, "arguably two sides of the same judgmental coin" (Martinson and Berridge 2015, 65), signifying that it is not okay to be old.

Those who cannot succeed in avoiding oldness are liable to experience blame and social exclusion. Anthropologist Janelle Taylor, reflecting on reactions to her own mother's dementia, portrays the "processes of 'social death,' social exclusion and abandonment" experienced in the United States by persons with dementia (2008, 325), who are regarded as "the not quite (or no longer) fully human" (322). She asks, "Why is it apparently so difficult for people to 'recognize'—as a friend, as a person, as even being *alive*—someone who, because of dementia, can no longer keep names straight?" (324). Sociologist Julia Twigg, analyzing representations of frail older people in "deep old age," reflects on how in the modern West, "to be incontinent is to have one's fundamental social status questioned, one's personhood as an individual denied" (2004, 66).

Members of a Boston-area retirement community Lamb researched were contemplating excluding those with walkers and in wheelchairs from the main dining room. Resident Joan Kaplan explained the movement, "I find it disturbing [pause]—to see a lot of wheelchairs. . . . Sometimes they come in from the nursing home or from the assisted living or from rehab [pause] in their hospital attire, in their wheelchairs—and it's not very nice. It's supposed to be here—I don't like the intermingling of, of the well and the sick." Her husband Michael agreed: "It's very, very dangerous in a way. 'Independent Living' is supposed to be independent living. . . . If the manager isn't on their toes; if they don't have the right regulations, then within a period of five, six, seven, eight years, you have—what amounts to a nursing home." He continued, "You say to yourself, 'There am I, but I'm not ready yet.' I don't want to be confronted with it yet." Joan concurred: "That's what bothers me. Because when we were in our [own] apartment, we didn't have any of this [pause] *exposure*."

These statements by Joan and Michael Kaplan reflect a particular kind of ageism, in which able-bodied older adults must be protected from the mere sight of persons with visible debilities, for such "exposure" is "disturbing," as it portends the possible future debility of Joan and Michael themselves. Currently enjoying the positive status of the "third age" of active, healthy, productive elderhood, Joan and Michael find pleasure in life and enjoy autonomy—but this pleasure and autonomy relies on the active exclusion of "real" old age and agedness, relegated to a "fourth age" they hope never to reach (Gilleard and Higgs 2010, 122).[30] Sociologist Toni Calasanti notes wryly that old age (and here she means "real" old age) is the only life stage we seek to eradicate (2007, 337).[31]

American antipathy toward old age—with the image of the declining body as representing a failure that the virtuous individual can and should overcome—is not new. Finding new form in the successful aging movement, such a vision can be traced back to at least the Victorian era. Historian Thomas Cole writes of the Victorian morality of the 1800s in the United States: "Old age came to represent . . . an embarrassment to the new morality of self-control. The primary virtues of 'civilized' morality—independence, health, success—required constant control over one's body and physical energies. The declining body in old age, a constant reminder of the limits of physical self-control, came to signify dependence, disease, failure, and sin. The devastating implications of ageism lay not in negative images alone but in the splitting apart of positive and negative aspects of aging, along with the belief that virtuous individuals could achieve one and escape the other" (1992, 91). Joan and Michael's desire to keep people in wheelchairs out of their dining room, to segregate the "third age" from the "fourth age," thus reflects a longstanding tendency in American society to split apart experiences of health and illness—and to assign to them divergent moralities.

It can be a real ordeal, of course, to have limbs that no longer glide as smoothly as they once did, or to be stricken with dementia, or to be handed a cancer diagnosis—but should these conditions be embarrassing? Signs of a loss of social personhood, a failure in appropriate living? The only certainty in the life course is that we each will die—and few will simply drop dead at age one hundred after experiencing no bodily or cognitive impairments, forms of frailty, or other signs of oldness. In this way, successful aging sets us each up for failure, while hindering our capacity to come to terms with and learn from the complexities and vulnerabilities of life as lived.

Some counter discourses and new perspectives are beginning to emerge in recent public, medical, and scholarly discourse, beyond simply a denial of old-ness and human transience—as we see in the huge success of Atul Gawande's *Being Mortal*, and the upsurge of popular films not shying away from depicting old age, such as *Amour* in 2012, *Still Alice* in 2014, the two *Best Exotic Marigold Hotel* films in 2012 and 2015, and *I'll See You in My Dreams* in 2015. Gawande exposes how medicine, in all its glory, can cure illness and save lives—but when doctors give primacy to avoidance of mortality, rather than quality of life, or when fear of death runs the show rather than acceptance of "the inexorability of our life cycle" (2014, 10), medicine can do more harm than good. Gawande reflects:

> The progress of medicine and public health has been an incredible boon—people get to live longer, healthier, more productive lives than ever before. Yet traveling along these altered paths, we regard living in the downhill stretches with a kind of embarrassment. . . . We're always trotting out some story of a ninety-seven-year-old who runs marathons, as if such cases were not miracles of biological luck but reasonable expec-tations for all. Then, when our bodies fail to live up to this fantasy, we feel as if we somehow have something to apologize for. (2014, 28)

Our society is ready for new perspectives.

A second critique we pose is that prevailing successful aging discourse overlooks social inequalities, although is rarely recognized as so doing.[32] Roger Landry's portrait of successful aging, for instance, to introduce the premise of his book *Live Long, Die Short: A Guide to Authentic Health and Successful Aging*, depicts eighty-six-year-old Harold, who, rather than declining, travels through Europe with his wife and granddaughter, writes three history books after his retirement from his accounting business, and rides a bike up and down lovely mountain landscapes in Spain—with no mention of the class, race, or national status (including education, passports, money, etc.) required to pursue such a vision, attainable by only the most elite in global society. Additionally, success-ful aging discourse assumes that people are already healthy, and the challenge is only to maintain this existing status. However, inasmuch as health dispari-ties intersect with other forms of social inequality throughout the life course, this presumption of health is exclusionary. Further, although those with lower socioeconomic status may have trouble achieving the prevailing vision of suc-cessful aging as defined by Rowe and Kahn and popular discourse (entailing exercise, full access to medical care, classes, travel, etc.), do many or some nonetheless aspire to or achieve well-being in late life in other ways? This is a question worthy of scrutiny through ethnographic research spending time and talking with people of diverse backgrounds.

A third critique is that successful aging can perpetuate gender stereotypes. Anti-aging ads and products in North America reinforce white, middle-class, heterosexual norms of male performance and female beauty (Calasanti 2007). US women and men both report worries over their aging bodies while engaging in anti-aging strategies, while women are most worried about loss of attractiveness and men concerned with bodies that perform (Brooks this volume; Calasanti and King this volume; Holstein 2015).

A fourth critique is that successful aging is ethnocentric—tied to dominant US cultural ideals about how people should be—although it is not often recognized as such.[33] Any vision of aging well, even one emerging from science and medicine, is inevitably tied to specific cultural values and visions of personhood, such as assumptions that decline is bad and independence good. Through insights gained via cross-cultural scrutiny, anthropologists aim to draw critical attention to institutions and ideologies that readers take for granted.

Finally, successful aging discourse lacks the voices of older people themselves. In the vast public, medical, and academic talk on successful aging, the voices of those to whom the successful aging project is meant to apply—older persons themselves—are rarely heard.[34] When Sarah Lamb has given talks to groups of elders in the United States and India on the successful aging movement, many comment that they believe the ultrapositive images of aging are completely unrealistic, counterproductive, and probably fashioned by much younger persons fearful of their own future aging. This dissatisfaction may stem from the problem of using a binary model—for after all the category of "success" implies its opposite, "failure"—to understand the complexity and contradictions of people's experiences in late life. It is time for the kinds of intimate ethnographic and interview-based research that anthropologists and sociologists engage in, in diverse social-cultural and national contexts with real people, to add fresh insight and perspectives to the dialogue.

What Lies Ahead

We aim to illuminate a powerful contemporary social-cultural, biopolitical, and medical phenomenon—a major movement and preoccupation of our time. The book's sections focus on gender, sexuality, and the allure of anti-aging (part 1); ideals of independence, interdependence, and intimate sociality in later life (part 2); national policies and everyday practices (part 3); and medicine, morality, and self (part 4). The division into sections may be somewhat arbitrary, and salient themes crosscut the various sections. Common themes include the concerns of human embodiment and experience everywhere; diverse understandings of personhood; how biopolitical projects of managing and optimizing aging reach out of the realm of public, state, and biomedical agendas into the everyday lives of aging individuals; the medicalization of aging, frailty, and dying; inequalities of age, race, class, gender, sexuality, and nation; religion and ontology; visions of modernity; and lessons for living.

Many of the book's contributions focus on North America, and cross-cultural materials are often explored more as a means to shed light on and critique facets of the North American successful aging project than to extend the notion of successful aging into new cultural contexts. It is relatively obvious to argue that Western successful aging notions are ethnocentric and not perfectly replicated around the globe; it is less obvious yet very important to examine the kinds of values and assumptions constituting "our own" successful aging project. That is, the aims of this book are less focused on the anthropological project of "making the strange familiar" (here, exploring how other sheep in other valleys think about aging well) than on the related crucial project of "making the familiar strange"—exposing unexamined North American assumptions and taken-for-granted truths. Because these cultural-biopolitical assumptions at least partially underpin worldwide efforts to promote successful, active, and healthy aging (including anti-aging), this focus on critiquing North American notions is particularly apt. For instance, "successful" aging (foregrounded in North America) and "active" aging (foregrounded in Europe) both value autonomous and independent personhood, as well as neoliberal forms of responsibility. Further, ideals and models of healthy, active, self-focused aging are being taken up—in diverse yet overlapping ways—in Asian and Latin American nations such as China, Japan, India, Brazil, and Mexico, wrapped up in shared global policies and imaginaries, which include ideals of modern personhood as well as narratives of a looming crisis of population aging.

Our goal is to bring together rich perspectives drawn from interviews and ethnographic fieldwork in the Americas, Europe, Africa, and Asia to investigate a major concern of our time. By critically exploring visions, projects, and experiences of successful, healthy, active, and anti-aging, the volume investigates profound contemporary conceptualizations—about the nature of the human condition and what it is to be a person, and of core social-cultural and political-economic values surrounding independence and dependence, agelessness and transience, activity/health/vitality and decline, individual agency and limits to human agency, ageism versus recognizing value and pleasure in growing old, and modern projects of biopolitical governance.

Our very ideas about what it is to be a normal, valued, and successful human being over the life course arise out of and are shaped by powerful cultural-historical, political-economic conditions and discourses. A central aim of this book is to expose and complicate contemporary readings of successful aging, to question and defamiliarize Western visions of the place of old age in the life course. Our society needs and, we believe, desires alternatives, critical scrutiny, and public conversation about aging and dying, change and transience, and the limits of individual autonomy—that is, about the contradictions, ambiguities, and opportunities of later life. It is through such dialogue in this collection that we hope to bring fresh insight and perspectives that expand our collective imagination about what it is to age and, by extension, to live.

NOTES

1. *The Gerontologist* published its February 2015 edition as a special issue on successful aging, reflecting on the concept's past and future. Beyond gerontology proper, see also the Spring 2015 issue *Daedalus: Journal of the American Academy of the Arts and Sciences*, dedicated to the "Successful Aging of Societies." See also Rowe and Kahn 1987, 1997, 2015.
2. The full name is "European Year for Active Ageing and Solidarity between Generations": http://ec.europa.eu/archives/ey2012 (accessed 29 June 2015).
3. In order: Pfeiffer 2013; Johnson 2012; Landry 2014; Kownacki 2010; Bruce 2009; Sweeting 2008; Lee and Jones 2008; Robbins 2007; Esmonde-White 2014; Crowley and Lodge 2007; LaLanne 2009; Scott-Mumby 2008; Mines 2013; and Agin and Perkins 2008.
4. Bruce 2009: "Welcome!" section (caps, bolding, and italics original).
5. Amazon.com blurb for *Successful and Health Aging* (Johnson 2012): http://www.amazon.com/dp/1937918572/ref=rdr_ext_tmb, accessed 20 May 2015.
6. Social thinkers have coined the terms *biopolitical*, *biopolitics*, and *biocitizenship* to refer to the modern style of government that regulates populations through biopower—the application of political power on (biological) life itself (such as through reproduction, demography, health); the obligation of the active citizen to take appropriate steps to maximize health; and/or notions of political belonging or citizenship connected to one's bodily attributes (e.g., Foucault 1978, 1984, 2002; Greenhalgh 2012, 2015; Petryna 2013; Rose 2007).
7. Dora Koenig is a pseudonym for one of Sarah Lamb's research subjects. Throughout the book, authors will refer to their interlocutors or research subjects by pseudonym, unless otherwise specified, and occasionally modify minor identifying characteristics of persons in order to protect their privacy.
8. See Ekerdt 1986; Katz 2000.
9. See, e.g., Kaufman 1985 and below.
10. Lamb 2014, and see more on the theme of permanent personhood below.
11. By "personhood," anthropologists refer to beliefs and ideologies as to what it is to be human, or a person, conceptualizations that vary by society.
12. See also Susan Whyte (this volume), and James Ferguson, who reflects on how "the political anthropology of southern Africa has long recognized relations of social dependence as the very foundation of polities and persons alike" (2013, 223).
13. This section is adapted from Lamb 2014, 43–46.
14. See, for instance, Holstein and Minkler 2003; Landry 2014, 13; Rozanova 2010, 217–219.
15. In their 2015 "Successful Aging 2.0," Rowe and Kahn call for complementing the concept of successful aging of the individual "with a body of theoretical inquiry and empirical research at the level of society" (594).
16. http://www.cdc.gov/aging/index.html (accessed 11 June 2015).

17. Anthropologist Elana Buch explores how older Americans in Chicago who hire paid home care workers to maintain their independence in fact only maintain a *sense* of independence; the ideal of the independent person is achieved through obscuring the labor of paid assistants (2013; this volume).

18. For more on Indian, specifically Bengali, notions and practices of intergenerational reciprocity, see Lamb 2000, 46–53; 2009, 32–36; 2013.

19. Lassen and Moreira 2014, 41. See also Eurofound's "Living Longer, Working Better—Active Ageing in Europe" (http://www.eurofound.europa.eu/resourcepacks/activeageing, accessed 11 June 2015).

20. Lassen and Moreira 2014. See also the European Commission's definition of active ageing: "helping people to stay in charge of their own lives for as long as possible as they age and, where possible, to contribute to the economy and society"—http://ec .europa.eu/social/main.jsp?catId=1062&langId=en, accessed 11 June 2015. In Eastern Europe, active aging is part of a broader attempt to westernize formerly socialist countries (Robbins-Ruszkowski this volume).

21. See WHO's "What Is Active Ageing?" and a link at the page's bottom to "Active Ageing: A Policy Framework," http://www.who.int/ageing/active_ageing/en, accessed 16 June 2015.

22. Originating in France in the 1970s, Universities of the Third Age are later-life learning institutions now found in many parts of the world, varying widely in organizational form and content (Formosa 2012; Robbins-Ruszkowski this volume).

23. The influential "disengagement theory" of aging put forward by Elaine Cumming and William Henry (1961) fell out of fashion in favor of "activity" and "continuity" theories of aging (Moody and Sassen 2012, 9–12).

24. See also Holstein 2015; Kaufman 1985; McHugh 2000; Lamb 2014; and Rudman 2015 for other explorations of North American ideals of agelessness, permanent personhood, and avoiding oldness in later life.

25. Corwin this volume, Lamb this volume, Tilak 1989.

26. E.g., Baltes and Baltes 1990; Martinson and Berridge 2015; Moody 2009; Weil 2007.

27. Terms such as "old" and "elderly" are today widely regarded in the US and UK as ageist and unacceptable in polite conversation (e.g., http://www.theguardian.com/society/ 2015/feb/04/old-ditch-ageist-stereotypes, accessed 11 June 2015).

28. Social gerontologists have also critiqued successful aging from a variety of perspectives, as Martinson and Berridge 2015 review (see also Lamb 2014, 44n4).

29. See, e.g., Marcus and Fischer 1986.

30. In the movement to fragment good and bad stages of old age, a "third age" has been coined to refer to the postretirement years of good health, vitality, and fulfillment, from around ages sixty-five to eighty or (hoped-for) longer. The "fourth age" is understood to be the phase of dependence, decrepitude, and death of "late" or "deep" old age, beginning around age eighty or eighty-five or, ideally, marginalized until the very end of life (Gilleard and Higgs 2010; Laslett 1989).

31. See also Calasanti and King (this volume) and Andrews 2009.

32. See Katz and Calasanti (2015, 29–30) for a critique of the kinds intersecting social inequalities (of class, race, ethnicity, gender, and sexuality) that arguably differentially impact the ability to realize ideals of successful aging, a fact largely overlooked by the successful aging paradigm (see also Calasanti and King this volume; Robbins-Ruszkowski this volume; Woody this volume).

33. Martinson and Berridge (2015, 61–62) review several studies offering a similar critique of successful aging models while calling for diverse cultural perspectives.

34. See also Martinson and Berridge's discussion of "the missing voices" of older adults themselves (2015, 60–62).

REFERENCES

Agin, Brent, and Sharon Perkins. 2008. *Healthy Aging for Dummies*. Hoboken, NJ: Wiley.

American Academy of Arts and Sciences. 2015. "Successful Aging of Societies." *Daedalus: Journal of the American Academy of the Arts and Sciences* 144 (2) (Spring).

Andrews, Molly. 1999. "The Seductiveness of Agelessness." *Ageing and Society* 19 (3): 301–318.

Baltes, Paul B., and Margret M. Baltes. 1990. "Psychosocial Perspectives on Successful Aging: The Model of Selective Optimization with Compensation." In *Successful Aging: Perspectives from Behavioral Sciences*, edited by Paul B. Baltes and Margret M. Baltes, 1–34. New York: Cambridge University Press.

Brijnath, Bianca. 2014. *Unforgotten: Love and the Culture of Dementia Care in India*. New York: Berghahn.

Bruce, Barbara. 2009. *100 Days to Successful Aging: A Workbook*. Rochester, NY: Creativity Publishing, Kindle edition.

Buch, Elana. 2013. "Senses of Care: Embodying Inequality and Sustaining Personhood in the Home Care of Older Adults in Chicago." *American Ethnologist* 40 (4): 637–650.

Calasanti, Toni. 2007. "Bodacious Berry, Potency Wood, and the Aging Monster: Gender and Age Relations in Anti-Aging Ads." *Social Forces* 86 (1): 335–355.

Clark, Margaret. 1972. "Cultural Values and Dependency in Later Life." In *Aging and Modernization*, edited by D. O. Cowgill and L. D. Holmes, 263–274. New York: Appleton Century Crofts.

Cole, Thomas R. 1992. *The Journey of Life: A Cultural History of Aging in America*. New York: Cambridge University Press.

Crawford, Robert. 1980. "Healthism and the Medicalization of Everyday Life." *International Journal of Health Services* 10 (3): 365–388.

———. 2006. "Health as a Meaningful Social Practice." *Health* 10 (4): 401–420.

Crowley, Chris, and Henry S. Lodge. 2007. *Younger Next Year: Live Strong, Fit and Sexy until You're 80 and Beyond*. New York: Workman Publishing.

Cumming, Elaine, and William E. Henry. 1961. *Growing Old: The Process of Disengagement*. New York: Basic Books.

Depp, Colin A., and Dilip V. Jeste. 2006. "Definitions and Predictors of Successful Aging: A Comprehensive Review of Larger Quantitative Studies." *American Journal of Geriatric Psychiatry* 14 (1): 6–20.

Ekerdt, David. 1986. "The Busy Ethic: Moral Continuity between Work and Retirement." *The Gerontologist* 26 (3): 239–244.

Esmonde-White, Miranda. 2014. *Aging Backwards: Reverse the Aging Process and Look 10 Years Younger in 30 Minutes a Day*. New York: HarperCollins.

Ferguson, James. 2013. "Declarations of Dependence: Labour, Personhood, and Welfare in Southern Africa." *Journal of the Royal Anthropological Institute* (n.s.) 19: 223–242.

Formosa, Marvin. 2012. "Four Decades of Universities of the Third Age: Past, Present, Future." *Ageing and Society*: 1–25.

Foucault, Michel. 1978. *The History of Sexuality*. Vol. 1, *An Introduction*. New York: Random House.

———. 1984. "The Politics of Health in the 18th Century." In *The Foucault Reader*, edited by Paul Rabinow, 273–289. New York: Pantheon.

———. 2002. *Society Must Be Defended: Lectures at the College de France, 1975–76*. New York: Picador.

Fountain, Henry. 2005. "No, You Can't Just Dodder." *International New York Times* "Week in Review" section, May 15. http://www.nytimes.com/2005/05/15/weekinreview/no-you-cant-just-dodder.html, accessed 15 June 2015.

Gawande, Atul. 2014. *Being Mortal: Medicine and What Matters in the End*. New York: Metropolitan Books.

Gerontological Society of America. 2015. Special Issue: "Successful Aging." *The Gerontologist.* 55 (1) (February).

Gilleard, Chris, and Paul Higgs. 2010. "Aging without Agency: Theorizing the Fourth Age." *Aging and Mental Health* 14 (2): 121–128.

Gillick, Muriel R. 2006. *The Denial of Aging: Perpetual Youth, Eternal Life, and Other Dangerous Fantasies*. Cambridge, MA: Harvard University Press.

Greenhalgh, Susan. 2012. "Weighty Subjects: The Biopolitics of the U.S. War on Fat." *American Ethnologist* 39 (3): 471–487.

———. 2015. *Fat-Talk Nation: The Human Costs of America's War on Fat*. Ithaca, NY: Cornell University Press.

Havighurst, Robert J. 1961. "Successful Aging." *The Gerontologist* 1 (1): 8–13.

Holstein, Martha. 2015. *Women in Late Life: Critical Perspectives on Gender and Age*. New York: Rowman and Littlefield.

Holstein, Martha B., and Meredith Minkler. 2003. "Self, Society, and the 'New Gerontology.'" *The Gerontologist* 43 (6): 787–796.

Johnson, Lisa J. 2012. *Successful and Healthy Aging: 101 Best Ways to Feel Younger and Live Longer*. Melrose, FL: Laurenzana Press.

Katz, Stephen. 2000. "Busy Bodies: Activity, Aging, and the Management of Everyday Life." *Journal of Aging Studies* 14 (2): 135–152.

Katz, Stephen, and Toni Calasanti. 2015. "Critical Perspectives on Successful Aging: Does It 'Appeal More Than It Illuminates'?" *The Gerontologist* 55 (1): 26–33.

Kaufman, Sharon R. 1985. *The Ageless Self: Sources of Meaning in Late Life*. Madison: University of Wisconsin Press.

———. 2015. *Ordinary Medicine: Extraordinary Treatments, Longer Lives, and Where to Draw the Line*. Durham, NC: Duke University Press.

Kleinman, Arthur. 2006. *What Really Matters: Living a Moral Life amidst Uncertainty and Danger*. New York: Oxford University Press.

Klinenberg, Eric. 2012. *Going Solo: The Extraordinary Rise and Surprising Appeal of Living Alone*. New York: Penguin.

Kownacki, Richard. 2010. *Do Not Go Gentle: Successful Aging for Baby Boomers and All Generations*. Wichita Falls, TX: iagehealthy.com.

LaLanne, Jack. 2009. *Live Young Forever: 12 Steps to Optimum Health, Fitness and Longevity*. Mississauga, ON: Robert Kennedy Publishing.

Lamb, Sarah. 2000. *White Saris and Sweet Mangoes: Aging, Gender, and Body in North India*. Berkeley: University of California Press.

———. 2009. *Aging and the Indian Diaspora: Cosmopolitan Families in India and Abroad*. Bloomington: Indiana University Press.

———. 2013. "Personhood, Appropriate Dependence, and the Rise of Eldercare Institutions in India." In *Transitions and Transformations: Cultural Perspectives on Aging and the Life Course*, edited by Caitrin Lynch and Jason Danely, 171–187. New York: Berghahn.

——. 2014. "Permanent Personhood or Meaningful Decline? Toward a Critical Anthropology of Successful Aging." *Journal of Aging Studies* 29: 41–52.

Landry, Roger. 2014. *Live Long, Die Short: A Guide to Authentic Health and Successful Aging.* Austin, TX: Greenleaf Book Group Press.

Laslett, Peter. 1989. *A Fresh Map of Life: The Emergence of the Third Age.* London: Weidenfeld and Nicolson.

Lassen, Aske Juul, and Tiago Moreira. 2014. "Unmaking Old Age: Political and Cognitive Formats of Active Ageing." *Journal of Aging Studies* 30: 33–46.

Lee, Ilchi, and Jessie Jones. 2008. *In Full Bloom: A Brain Education Guide to Successful Aging.* Sedona, AZ: BEST Life Media.

Marcus, George E., and Michael M. J. Fischer. 1986. *Anthropology as Cultural Critique: An Experimental Moment in the Human Sciences.* Chicago: University of Chicago Press.

Martinson, Marty, and Clara Berridge. 2015. "Successful Aging and Its Discontents: A Systematic Review of the Social Gerontology Literature." *The Gerontologist* 55 (1): 58–69.

Martz, Sandra, ed. 1987. *When I Am an Old Woman I Shall Wear Purple.* Watsonville, CA: Papier-Mache Press.

McHugh, Kevin E. 2000. "The 'Ageless Self'? Emplacement of Identities in Sun Belt Retirement Communities." *Journal of Aging Studies* 14 (1): 103–116.

McIntosh, Janet. 2009. *The Edge of Islam: Power, Personhood, and Ethnoreligious Boundaries on the Kenya Coast.* Durham, NC: Duke University Press.

Mines, Jan. 2013. *Successful Aging 101: Tips for Navigating the Aging Process.* Amazon Digital Services, Kindle edition.

Moody, Harry R. 2009. "From Successful Aging to Conscious Aging." In *The Cultural Context of Aging: Worldwide Perspectives*, 3rd ed., edited by Jay Sokolovsky, 67–76. Westport, CT: Praeger.

Moody, Harry R., and Jennifer R. Sassen. 2012. *Aging: Concepts and Controversies*, 7th ed. Thousand Oaks, CA: Sage Publications.

Petryna, Adriana. 2013. *Life Exposed: Biological Citizens after Chernobyl.* Princeton, NJ: Princeton University Press.

Pfeiffer, Eric. 2013. *Winning Strategies for Successful Aging.* New Haven, CT: Yale University Press.

Reynolds, Gretchen. 2015. "How Exercise Keeps Us Young." *New York Times*, "Well" section, January 7. http://well.blogs.nytimes.com/2015/01/07/how-exercise-keeps-us-young/?_r=0, accessed 19 June 2015.

Robbins, John. 2007. *Healthy at 100: The Scientifically Proven Secrets of the World's Healthiest and Longest-Lived Peoples.* New York: Random House.

Rose, Nikolas. 2007. *The Politics of Life Itself: Biomedicine, Power, and Subjectivity in the Twenty-First Century.* Princeton, NJ: Princeton University Press.

Rowe, John W., and Robert L. Kahn. 1987. "Human Aging: Usual and Successful." *Science* 237 (4811): 143–149.

——. 1997. "Successful Aging." *The Gerontologist* 37: 433–440.

——. 1998. *Successful Aging.* New York: Pantheon Books.

——. 2015. "Successful Aging 2.0: Conceptual Expansions for the 21st Century." *Journals of Gerontology, Series B: Psychological Sciences and Social Sciences* 70 (4): 593–596.

Rozanova, Julia. 2010. "Discourse of Successful Aging in *The Globe and Mail*: Insights from Critical Gerontology." *Journal of Aging Studies* 24: 213–222.

Rudman, Debbie Laliberte. 2015. "Embodying Positive Aging and Neoliberal Rationality: Talking about the Aging Body within Narratives of Retirement." *Journal of Aging Studies* 34: 10–20.

Scott-Mumby, Keith. 2008. *Get Healthy for Your Next 100 Years: A Top MD's Guide to Successful Aging.* Reno, NV: Scott-Mumby Author Services.

Simic, Andrei. 1990. "Aging, World View, and Intergenerational Relations in America and Yugoslavia." In *The Cultural Context of Aging: Worldwide Perspectives*, edited by Jay Sokolovsky, 89–107. New York: Bergin and Garvey.

Sweeting, George. 2008. *The Joys of Successful Aging: Living Your Days to the Fullest.* Chicago: Moody Publishers.

Taylor, Janelle. 2008. "On Recognition, Caring, and Dementia." *Medical Anthropology Quarterly* 22 (4): 313–335.

Tilak, Shrinivas. 1989. *Religion and Aging in the Indian Tradition.* Albany, NY: SUNY Press.

Twigg, Julia. 2004. "The Body, Gender and Age: Feminist Insights in Social Gerontology." *Journal of Aging Studies* 18: 59–73.

Weil, Andrew. 2007. *Healthy Aging: A Lifelong Guide to Your Wellbeing.* New York: Anchor.

Wentzell, Emily. 2013. *Maturing Masculinities: Aging, Chronic Illness, and Viagra in Mexico.* Durham, NC: Duke University Press.

PART I

Gender, Sexuality, and
the Allure of Anti-Aging

1

Successful Aging, Ageism, and the Maintenance of Age and Gender Relations

TONI CALASANTI AND NEAL KING

The notion of successful aging is not new. Robert Havighurst's (1961) early formulation argued that aging can be positive, and it focused on social conditions that would enable life satisfaction without depriving other groups in society (Katz and Calasanti 2015). Today successful aging is most closely aligned with the construct espoused by John Rowe and Robert Kahn, whose views were spread widely by the MacArthur Foundation's distribution of their 1998 *Successful Aging* book to everyone in the Gerontological Society of America, as well as the journalists' attention it received (Holstein and Minkler 2003).

By their own account, Rowe and Kahn (1998) sought to construct their model of successful aging to counter ageism and the negative discourse of decline. They argued that ageism, which results from the focus of "both science and society" (1998, xii) on such issues as frailty and long-term care needs, depicts old people "as a figurative ball and chain holding back an otherwise spry collective society" (12). They have sought to reduce the ageism behind and inspired by this vision of old people as dying weight, by using evidence from a variety of scientific studies to demonstrate that people can, indeed, age successfully (12–13).

According to Rowe and Kahn (1998, 38), successful aging involves (1) the avoidance of disease and disability; (2) maintaining high levels of mental and physical function; and (3) active engagement with life, including "relationships with other people, and behavior that is productive" (40). In turn, *productivity* includes "all activities, paid or unpaid, that create goods or services of value" (47). Key to their framework is their claim that individuals can achieve these dimensions of successful aging through appropriate lifestyle choices: "Our main message is that we can have a dramatic impact on our own success or failure in aging. Far more than is usually assumed, *successful aging is in our own hands*" (18, our emphasis). Aging, they argue, is "largely *under the control of the individual.* In short, successful aging is *dependent upon individual choices and behaviors.* It can be attained through *individual choice* and effort" (37, our emphasis). Thus, successful aging posits individual responsibility for choosing whether to enter a devalued social location or work toward success instead. As such, it represents a positive aging discourse that, within the present neoliberal context, places the "bodily, financial and social risks of aging" firmly on the shoulders of individuals and away from states (Laliberte Rudman 2015, 11).

We argue that successful aging will not eradicate ageism by giving more people greater access to forms of personal discipline and engagement, because this does not challenge the inequities that give rise to ageism, the derogation of old age that leads to the calls for greater success in the first place. It does not confront the notion that old age is worse than middle age, that old people should find ways to be more like their younger selves. It fails to address the age relations that denigrate old age and uphold other life stages as the models against which elders will be assessed.

Successful aging does not address the ageism that ushers all who live long enough into this later life stage. Beginning with the insight that inequities intersect, that the subordination of old people is shaped by relations of gender, sexuality, colonialism, and other inequalities, this chapter focuses on the intersection of age and gender in the United States, to show how people hoping to age successfully accept individual responsibility, per the successful aging framework, and pursue their resistance to their own devaluation in gendered ways.

Age Relations

Relations of age draw invidious distinctions that privilege younger adults at the expense of old people (Calasanti 2003). Old people in the United States frequently are marked as relatively ill, unproductive, and needy. Depending on political stripes, groups may also see old people as unjustly consuming more than their share of resources, robbing younger generations via pensions and entitlement programs. These divisions have been institutionalized in work and retirement policies, long-term care policies, and an anti-aging industry that warns adults of the terrible consequences of growing old. Such organizational and mundane attention to the distinct status of old age and its many downsides keeps age salient and maintains the subordination of old people. Consequences for old people include widespread poverty as income and wealth polarize in old age, loss of rights of citizenship and often control over their bodies, and enduring stigma. Younger people face less competition for resources, such as jobs or intimate partners (Calasanti 2010; King 2006).

Widespread attention to "successful aging" in North America is in fact indicative of the institutionalized nature of ageism. No comparable theory exists for other life stages, with comparable discussions of successful infancy, "teenagehood," or young adulthood. Scholarly theories and popular advice address each life stage, but no other stages are treated as if they had no value unique to them, as if no positives resulted from entry into those stages, or as if we needed to justify their existence by minimizing what is unique to them. In each of the other cases, the negatives are offset by positives that also are seen to accrue. It is only old age that, to paraphrase Molly Andrews (1999), we try to eradicate from the developmental landscape. Only in old age do we feel a need to discover and promote positive content where there apparently is little to none.

The inability of successful aging to address this ageism is suggested by Debbie Laliberte Rudman's (2015) qualitative study of thirty middle-aged and older persons. Looking at the broader rubric of positive aging discourses, she finds that her respondents accept the neoliberal mandate to take personal responsibility for their bodily aging. However, they also find that there is only so much that they can do, and they see themselves as failures when they do not succeed in living up to these mandates. Perhaps more to the point of successful aging, an "aversion to oldness" also remains.

The difficulties of addressing ageism with successful aging have been documented in studies by Toni M. Calasanti (in press) and Sarah Lamb (2014). Calasanti found that her middle-aged US respondents understood the dictate to age successfully and sought to do so. But they also felt that they had limited control over their aging and feared growing old. Their comments indicated that ageism had not been alleviated by their belief in the possibility of successful aging. In Lamb's (2014) recent study of thirty privileged Boston-area persons aged sixty-two to one hundred, some expressed dismay with the focus on individual control, which they felt as a sense of personal failure or embarrassment when faced with physical decline.

The findings of these studies suggest that adherence to the possibility of successful aging, and individual responsibility for so doing, can serve to justify ageism. As people age, they are asked to demonstrate that they are not old, and they do so by approximating what is taken to be middle-aged behaviors and appearances. Less privileged groups lack access to resources that might enhance their ability to age successfully (Holstein and Minkler 2003; Martinson and Berridge 2015). But in addition, it is not just a middle-aged standard; inequalities such as those based on gender also influence how and when one is considered "old" and thus not aging. That is, not only will old age happen, no matter what resources one has at one's disposal, but it will be manifested differently for men and women. We discuss how gender might intersect with age relations below.

Gender Relations

Gender has been particularly salient in political economies that make it difficult for women to contribute to the production of goods and reproduction of people at the same time. That difficulty favors men's control of production and thus wealth, rendering women dependent upon them in relations that require much unpaid labor, an expropriation often sublimated as familial love (Collins et al. 1993). These divisions of labor and entitlement incline men toward regular demonstrations of competence at productive labor (Connell 2005) and women toward regular demonstrations of beauty, as part of the capacity to bond themselves to male partners (Hurd Clarke 2011). Patrimonial relations in which women were reduced to property exchanged between men have given way to widespread individual citizenship for adults in North America and many other advanced industrial contexts (Collins et al. 1993). Still, *masculinity* and *femininity*, the activities by which groups distinguish women from men, remain rooted, to varying extents, in those reciprocal but unequal roles. Affiliation with these kinds of work can become a matter of gender identity, the notion that men are breadwinners on account of productive work, that women are objects of desire on account of beauty. Masculinity and femininity have been shaped accordingly, developing sets of gender ideals to which groups hold women and men accountable (West and Zimmerman 1987).

The intersections of age and gender are such that old women in North America may continue to focus on the maintenance of beauty and old men continue to focus on their capacities to perform—in production, strenuous leisure, and sex—as their younger selves may have done. With this chapter, we use self-reports of middle-aged people to assess whether orientations to successful aging reinforce or challenge intersecting inequalities of gender and age.

The Present Study

The data used to assess the impact of successful aging on the everyday lives and gender identities of middle-aged people were gathered by the first author, who conducted in-depth interviews among nineteen middle-aged men and women (ages forty-two to sixty-one) in the United States in 2006–2007 (one interview was conducted by a graduate student). The goal of the semistructured interviews was to understand how middle-aged men and women viewed their bodily changes and aging. Respondents were asked about a variety of related topics, such as bodily changes and concerns, now and in the future; ageism; age-appropriate behaviors and appearances; the meanings and their thoughts about middle age and old age; successful aging; and knowledge and use of anti-aging products and services.

The sample included nine men and ten women; while it was a relatively economically privileged group, and all were white, there was some diversity by class and sexuality in addition to gender. Sixteen were heterosexual, and three were nonheterosexual; three men had never married, and of the rest, one man and three women were divorced at the time. All were employed, with fifteen located in professional and semiprofessional fields, two were in pink-collar occupations, and two (one man and one woman) engaged in more physical or manual labor.

Interviews were conducted in a quiet location that respondents chose, lasted an average of two hours, and were digitally recorded and professionally transcribed. Coding was done iteratively (Miles and Huberman 1994; Taylor and Bogdan 1984) using QSR NUD*IST 6.0; themes were arrived at collaboratively by the first author and a graduate assistant.

Gendered Strategies for Successful Aging

The strategies that these middle-aged adults undertook, and their motivations for so doing, reflected these gendered concerns surrounding performance, professional and domestic productivity, sexuality, and attractiveness. Interviewees were asked about a wide range of products and services that Maxwell J. Mehlman and colleagues (2004, 305) consider anti-aging, including "cosmetic treatments and surgery; exercise and therapy; food and beverages; vitamins, minerals, and supplements; and cosmetics and cosmeceuticals." For each type, respondents were asked if they employed any of these. If they answered affirmatively, they were asked follow-up questions to discern whether their reasons involved concerns about aging, appearance, health, or a combination of these.

Men and women were equally likely to report about modifying their diets, including taking supplements, and exercising. Throughout his interview, Greg, age sixty-one, talked about exercising as a key to fighting aging, as well as to being healthier and sleeping at night. He commented, "when you get older [there] is this desire for routinization and that's, you know, I want to exercise because my acupuncturist says . . . you have to exercise every day or else you are not going to sleep." But women were far more likely to report using products and services that promised to change how you look. Perhaps most revealing is not just which strategies are used—after all, men and women were equally likely to engage in exercise, diet modification, and vitamin/supplement use—but how respondents talked about them. Men spoke of working hard and physical effort, dietary modification, and exercise. They rejected products and services touted as changing bodily appearance without somehow involving hard work. Men stressed the "fight" against ageism and their avoidance of the use of such beauty products as cosmeceuticals.

For example, Greg was adamant about resisting aging "through what I view as being natural mechanisms," by which he means you must work hard, and not just use products that will change the surface of your body. In talking about the extent to which he feels like he should be trying to fight aging, he says, "Well . . . yeah, I certainly go off and fight the aging process. There's no question that this guy isn't spending, you know, seven hours a week exercising, right? What's he doing? . . . I don't want this slope-off, . . . this slow-down thing. . . . But I subscribe to the fact that it requires work. It is work. . . . It does not come in a bottle or it does not come in a pill." He continues, "I will certainly make an effort, but I will not do anything that isn't natural. . . . I am not paying any nickels for surgery, you know. . . . I am not going to use hair products. . . . I don't want to be accused of dyeing my hair, I don't want to be accused of . . . having surgery or something, nip and tuck. . . . I will do everything I can if it means vitamins and supplement and health and good sleeping and rest and all that kind of thing, fine."

Throughout his interview, Mike, age fifty, expressed admiration for those who were "working at maintaining their bodies." He says that "when you are my age, it doesn't mean you are ready to put yourself on a shelf. You just have to work a little bit harder and do a few things to allow you to continue having good quality of life and doing the things that you enjoy doing. . . . To me that's the whole idea of exercise." To be sure, women also talked about the importance of exercising, eating well, or otherwise monitoring their bodies, but they never talked about it as work.

That physical performance is key to men's anti-aging strategies came up repeatedly, and often in contrast to domination in intimate relationships. Men and women alike mentioned products for sexual performance, especially erectile dysfunction, as part of men's anti-aging arsenal, and this was often in contrast to what they felt women's products should be doing. Greg's comments were succinct in this regard: "Well, I think [for] women it's basically facial appearance, and that's hair, the whole business, makeup and that kind of thing. . . . Obviously cosmetic surgery and things like that. For men, it's all about how big your, ah, other brain is [laughter]. . . . It's all about performance and you know it's all about . . . picking up women."

Gendered expectations were also clearly differentiated when respondents talked about bodily strategies more closely aligned with aesthetics. Men and women alike agreed that women's appearance marks them as old differently, and sooner, and that they should attend to this. Dreama noted that men may get gray quicker, but women better do something about it: "You get that dowdy look, . . . a washed-out look. . . . Men seem to have this charisma when they have some gray." Maggie, age fifty-seven, said that "I think women are expected to make more of an effort to try to look younger than men are." And men agreed with Maggie. In fact, in Darryl's view, concern for how she appears to men is the essence of femininity: "I can tell a difference in women that take pride in being a woman than the ones that don't care and don't have any self-pride. I've seen women that are not the most attractive, but they do the best with what they've got and they worry about it and they doll themselves up—they work with what God gave them. I've seen other women that got the tools to work with and don't care. That disturbs me. . . . It doesn't take a lot for a girl . . . to try to doll themselves up to look like a woman." In discussing these particular strategies, Mike said that men should avoid them but that women could use them, "to let the guys know that they are trying to do something to make themselves younger, to make themselves look better for you."

Mike's comment hints at some of the reasons that respondents were all clear that such anti-aging strategies that are geared at attractiveness were not to be used by men. Not only should men's strategies involve hard work, but they should not look as though they care about being younger or attractive. John, age forty-five, talked about not wanting to use hair color now because people would notice. "Maybe the reason I . . . don't think I will ever color my beard is the idea that people will know I have colored my beard. There's no natural or there's no way to make it seem like it was a natural process. . . . Now, I think a woman can . . . get away with people knowing that she artificially tries to look younger. You know, I think people would look differently at a man when they know he colored his hair than they would a women . . . [I]f he didn't color his hair, he would be treated more forgivingly than if the woman didn't color her hair." Jake concurred. Noting that he feels it is his gray hair that marks his age, he makes it clear that he would change that if he could, but coloring it is out of the question: "I don't find an attractive fifty-year-old someone that I go, 'God, is his hair colored?'"

Women also expressed discomfort with men using anti-aging products for appearance. Sue, age fifty-three, said, "I don't think of men using anti-wrinkle cream." In discussing men who dye their hair, Elizabeth, age fifty-eight, commented, "Sometimes that's pathetic. But me getting my hair dyed is not pathetic, is it? . . . I mean if [my husband] started thinking, 'I am getting a little gray, maybe I should color my hair,' I would think, this is really weird. . . . But most men won't dye their hair, you know it looks terrible. And the ones that do, I can always tell. . . . I think men would be perceived as less masculine if they did." Elizabeth's notion that anti-aging activities are gendered is echoed by John, who hypothesized that perhaps men cannot obviously dye their hair because "it could also be that when a man does it he's taking on, he's doing feminized activities. That is, he's doing something a woman would do and so that you know there could also be that kind of [issue about] what it takes to be an authentic male." The difference, in part, appears to go back to who is dominant in heterosexual relationships, as demonstrated by a self- or other orientation. Mike clarified why he works on his body to fight aging: "I am gonna fight it the best I can just to allow myself to be healthier and have a better quality of life as long as I can. It's not for anybody else. It's for me."

Thus, these middle-aged respondents make clear that they know that aging affects their bodies in gendered ways. They know not only what they should do to age successfully, but also what methods men should avoid. Both women and men say that aging threatens their occupational status. But the men are more likely to respond to the threat in ways consistent with ideals of (youthful) manhood. We interpret these patterns in light of conflict over gender and age inequality, in which men as a group maintain strong interests in their association with valued work and social distance from what women do. In this case, women's aging includes obvious attempts to maintain beauty, which maintenance men do only in ways meant to be hidden or at least subtle. Men's successful aging includes shows of skilled, effortful "work," a valiant if losing "fight," and avoidance of any "unnatural" interventions in or on their bodies. Both age and gender inequalities are thus reaffirmed and reinscribed through this successful aging.

Individuals Can and Should Age Successfully

One theme that emerged from many of the interviews was that respondents viewed the successful aging movement as in line with their desires for their own aging (Calasanti in press). When asked what successful aging meant to them, for the most part, respondents did not hesitate; Tom, a fifty-nine-year-old professional, commented that successful aging involves being active, both mentally and physically. Similarly, Mary, a fifty-nine-year-old professional, said that successful aging meant being "energized. Active. Curious. Not bored." Some respondents also included such dimensions of well-being as "happy," "content," and "adaptable." Further, they felt that these outcomes were both achievable and matters of individual responsibility, regardless of their class backgrounds. For instance, Dreama, a fifty-six-year-old whose work is predominantly physical, said, "I do tremendous amounts of studying on nutrition and health . . . because you have to work harder at it. . . . And now that you are older, . . . you can still get the quality . . . out of what you do . . . to make it better as you get older."

None of that, however, counters their narrative of decline and lack of positive content to old age. For instance, when asked how they felt about growing old, respondents remained generally negative.

MAGGIE (age fifty-six): I am not looking forward to it. . . . All the people who are quite a bit older . . . say growing old is the pits.

JAKE (age fifty-one): I don't like it, I don't like that topic.

DARRYL (age forty-two): Nobody wants to get old.

The negative connotations of old are evident in the difficulties respondents had in pinpointing when old age begins. For instance, the definition of old age for Nora, age fifty-seven, is "very much a physical one, you know, if someone is both older in appearance and debilitated in capacity in a really evident way." But as she talks, and considers her own aging, she shifts to a more mental assessment, of the extent to one can adapt, noting that some people can still have a "bright . . . outlook or demeanor." Ultimately, then, the criterion of old age would be that "if you think you're old, then, you know, it's your mind that matters, not your age." She concludes by saying that "just thinking about defining myself as old, I don't know that I would really feel old or consider myself old, even if I were in [bad physical] shape, if I were still mentally alert and feeling, you know, a measure of satisfaction, enjoyment and peace."

Respondents avoided seeing themselves as old when they could, shifting definitions as they distanced themselves from that social location. In so doing, they seemed to suggest that old age is a status without positive aspects. Rumination over whether old age is chronological, physical, or mental served less to define the location than to distance them from it.

Respondents also spoke of inevitable old age with fear, even as they tell of the pursuit of successful aging. For instance, echoing Nora's response above, Carrie, a fifty-two-year-old professional, defined success as being able to answer the question "Are you content?" in the affirmative. As an example, she referred to someone who might be confined to a wheelchair, noting that "you can be immobile and confined to a wheelchair or whatever and be content." But she also acknowledged that "for me, I fear not being mobile." Indeed, in terms of physical changes, respondents were unanimous in their concerns about functional loss, about becoming "frail," "feeble," or "debilitated"; and they described those conditions in ways that affirm the subordination of people in those circumstances.

As well, respondents expressed concerns about their abilities to age successfully, that is, to control that process. Katherine, age fifty-eight, said, "It doesn't matter how much exercise you do, your body just looks more and more different as you age." And while Jim, a fifty-four-year-old professional at the height of his career, maintained that he put a lot of energy into his work to avoid exclusion (see below), he also said that "I can't work harder to stop a physical decline. . . . It's just there are some things I am not ever going to do again." But, he added, "I still work hard to control things [laughter]!"

Thus, we found that our middle-aged respondents did not change their views of old age as they pursued success but instead seemed to interpret successful aging as not aging—that is, as approximating middle age and holding onto that social location—to the extent that is possible. And they rendered all of these judgments in gendered ways, assigning different goals and means to women and men of that temporary success. We next discuss the concerns that respondents raise about old age, with exclusion resulting from physical change, and show how gender shapes them.

Gendered Concerns about Old Age

Respondents worried over the exclusion, marginality, and invisibility that come from growing old; but the focus of these fears varies by gender. The data suggest that class may also intersect with gender, although the sample is too small to allow a test of that. Specifically, all the men and the professional women discuss concerns about their abilities to maintain status in paid labor; in that sense, being able to produce or compete in the workplace came up for both men and women.

For instance, Jim said, "[I] . . . associate aging with sedentary existence. . . . You are no longer a part, you are no longer the player, you are on the periphery. . . . And maybe that's partly what I resist by working hard and working energetically. I don't want to be seen as being brain dead." Mary expressed similar concerns about her workplace status, noting that "I . . . sometimes think that the closer you get to retirement the more, I feel, that you lose power in a sort of simple way that you have to do more to keep a similar level of power and influence."

Men, regardless of class, also talked about their bodies in terms of "doing," which translated into demonstrating strength in the performance of tasks, and they talked about how losses in these regards would lead to being marginalized. Greg said that "I worry that I can't go out in public because I am not able to protect myself and might become victimized, . . . assaulted. . . . Certainly the loss of freedom and power, if you want to put it that way, [worry me]." Similarly, Jake feared not "being in the middle of things" and associates being able to do so with strength and activity: "My plan of attack is to . . . [age] with . . . an aggressive mental outlook and . . . hopefully be in physically good enough shape."

Men worried about their abilities to perform physically and compete as effectively in the workplace, in recreation, and in intimate relations. Jim recalled an encounter with a younger man while engaged in athletic competition, one that resulted in some physical scuffling: "The whole issue of proving myself was much closer to the surface. And I think it's because the intensity of the issue of masculinity was heightened because of age, that I lost it with this guy." Mike was concerned to "make sure that my strength maintains itself." Along similar lines, and in relation to managing his body to ensure he remains capable at work and in recreation, Greg said, "As you get older, you really try to reduce the number of things you do because you want to really maximize whatever time you have. . . . You can't work twelve-hour days anymore. You physically can't do that." Finally,

Patrick, a fifty-four-year-old man, noted that "the most threatening [time was] where I found myself with next to no libido and a couple of experiences I had being less than stellar."

Women, by contrast, spoke of loss of attractiveness as basis for exclusion, which they described as a kind of invisibility. Elizabeth told of how recently, when she was passed by a car full of young men, she was shocked that their honking did not convey that they saw her as a sexual object but that, instead, they called her "mom." She went on to say that "[a] lot of women my age [are] saying that as a sort of sexual person they will start becoming invisible." Mary clarified gender differences in intimate relations and aging, noting that "for men it's probably [about] desire . . . for women, desirability." She concluded that, in fact, women's sexual invisibility is what designates them as old: "One has to struggle to remain sexual. . . . [T]hat's practically the definition of old age, the absence of that."

Women were thus concerned about changes that could make them seem less attractive. Mary was aware that in some of her work her physical changes matter; she says, "You know that people do respond to your attractiveness and . . . your attractiveness decreases at least in conventional ways as you get older and, you know, in weight, body, shape and all that stuff." She also noted that "I often am more self-critical when I am around men and young men especially. . . . I am very much more conscious of my age." She realized the same is not true of men: "I think men can be sexually attractive all their lives really, but [for] women there's a cutoff point. There's more, one has to do a lot more to maintain the illusion, an illusion than men do." Elizabeth felt that her ability to be attractive has gotten worse over time: "I have always had this feeling that . . . with a little effort . . . I could feel like I looked great. You know, lately I am thinking maybe, you know, it's starting to slide a little bit, which bothers me that I even worry about it." And Carrie said she tries to accept the ways her body has changed but then sometimes thinks, "'I can't stand this, I look so frumpy, I am gonna change. . . . I kind of go back and forth between, you know, denial and then acceptance . . . And then horror, denial, acceptance."

Women also worried about not being able to perform domestic labor, multitask, or care for others as effectively. Barb, age fifty-five, said she realizes her age when she is engaged in "scrubbing the kitchen floor. I don't have the energy I used to have to do it the way I think it ought to be done. I run out of steam before I finish the whole thing." And Shelly, age forty-four, worried that, "I am slowing down. My energy, I have less energy which just drives me nuts because I have been the one that's always been able to get twice as much done in half the time." The notion of a loss of energy came up repeatedly among professional women who also took primary responsibility for their families. Elizabeth, a well-known professional in her field, is bothered by this; she said, "I just took it for granted that people can get up in the morning and keep twenty balls in the air all the time." And Carrie concurred: "I don't have the stamina I used to have. If I had a really hard day at work, I come home and just wanna collapse, whereas before I could still come home and . . . do dinner, take care of the kids, and be more active." Thus, while Elizabeth and Carrie are referring to their abilities to take care of paid work and family, the ways in which they talk about their slowing down at work is very different from how men describe this. Men focused solely on paid labor; domestic labor was never mentioned.

Concluding Reflections

The use of the successful aging paradigm, as an injunction on individuals to take responsibility for the nature of their aging and thus for the stigma resulting from it, maintains intersecting inequities, not just ageism alone. Successful aging is gendered in all of the ways documented above, and also in that women are widely considered to age more quickly than men do, a disparity likely anchored in gender relations. By treating women as though their aging is less successful, because they grow "old" more quickly and in particularly gendered ways, we reinforce both inequalities at the same time. Neither age nor gender inequity are goals of the successful aging framework, of course. The point was to reduce age inequality. But this reinforcement of inequity is built in, because the successful aging paradigm never challenges either the gendered ageism that designates women and men "old" at different points or the stigma attached to being "old" per se.

The recent iteration of successful aging, what has been termed Successful Aging 2.0 (Rowe and Kahn 2015), takes on "the important influence of social factors on the capacity of individuals to age successfully" (593) and notes the importance of "macrosocial influences such as economic conditions, access to high-quality affordable health care, public transportation, and urban design" (593). These are institutional matters, to be sure, and worthy problems to solve; but they are not the age relations that subordinate old people, that make old age a social location in a large-scale inequality. This newer version remains focused on what individuals can decide to do to age successfully, looking to the institutional level only for the sake of ensuring that all can make those choices and pursue success with comparable ease. In this revision, such factors become reduced to "personal characteristics such as race, gender, sexual orientation, and socioeconomic status" (593), rather than social positions constructed by systems of inequality. The paradigm continues to direct attention away from the relations that stigmatize aging, in varying ways for different groups, and which subordinate old people.

Rather than challenge the ageism that permeates popular conceptions of growing old, successful aging presumes that old people will wish to minimize the stigma attached to their own aging through the work of engagement and health care. It presumes that the only inequity to address would be that of access to the means to age successfully. The call to expand successful aging to include "more voices" (see Martinson and Berridge 2015) implicitly recognizes that ageism intersects with gender and other social inequalities. But such an expansion is insufficient. Shall we urge and enable old women to be more attractive to men, to age successfully?

We do not oppose work, engagement, self-care, and medicine for those who desire them; but we dispute that this is the best way to minimize the subordination of old people. The problem of ageism is collective and goes unchallenged by efforts to grant more of us more access to individual means to seem like younger men and women. Challenging ageism involves directly *valuing difference*: validating old age as a different and meaningful time of life (Lamb 2014). To address ageism per se we must first recognize old age as a life stage, and one to which unique value adheres, just as other life stages are seen to include positives and negatives. This, not encouraging people to age successfully, must be the starting point for addressing ageism.

REFERENCES

Andrews, Molly. 1999. "The Seductiveness of Agelessness." *Ageing and Society* 19: 301–318.
Calasanti, Toni M. 2003. "Theorizing Age Relations." In *The Need for Theory: Critical Approaches to Social Gerontology for the 21st Century*, edited by S. Biggs, A. Lowenstein, and J. Hendricks, 199–218. Amityville, NY: Baywood.
———. 2010. "Gender Relations and Applied Research on Aging." *Gerontologist* 50(6): 720–734.
———. In press. "Combating Ageism: How Successful Is Successful Aging?" *Gerontologist*, published online July 16, 2015. doi: 10.1093/geront/gnv076.
Collins, Randall, Janet Saltzman Chafetz, Rae Lesser Blumberg, Scott Coltrane, and Jonathan H. Turner. 1993. "Toward an Integrated Theory of Gender Stratification." *Sociological Perspectives* 36 (3): 185–216.
Connell, R. W. 2005. *Masculinities*. Berkeley: University of California Press.
Havighurst, Robert J. 1961. "Successful Aging." *The Gerontologist* 1 (1): 8–13.
Holstein, Martha B., and Meredith Minkler. 2003. "Self, Society, and the 'New Gerontology.'" *Gerontologist* 43 (6): 787–796.
Hurd Clarke, Laura. 2011. *Facing Age: Women Growing Older in Anti-Aging Culture.* Lanham, MD: Rowman and Littlefield.
Katz, Stephen, and Toni Calasanti. 2015. "Critical Perspectives on Successful Aging: Does It 'Appeal More Than It Illuminates'?" *Gerontologist* 55 (1): 26–33.
King, Neal. 2006. "The Lengthening List: Age Relations and the Feminist Study of Inequality." In *Age Matters: Realigning Feminist Thinking*, edited by T. M. Calasanti and K. F. Slevin, 47–74. New York: Routledge.
Laliberte Rudman, Debbie. 2015. "Embodying Positive Aging and Neoliberal Rationality: Talking About the Aging Body within Narratives of Retirement." *Journal of Aging Studies* 34: 10–20.
Lamb, Sarah. 2014. "Permanent Personhood or Meaningful Decline? Toward a Critical Anthropology of Successful Aging." *Journal of Aging Studies* 29: 41–52.

Martinson, Marty, and Clara Berridge. 2015. "Successful Aging and Its Discontents: A Systematic Review of the Social Gerontology Literature." *Gerontologist* 55 (1): 58–69.

Mehlman, Maxwell J., Robert H Binstock, Eric T. Juengst, Roselle S. Ponsaran, and Peter J. Whitehouse. 2004. "Anti-Aging Medicine: Can Consumers Be Better Protected?" *Gerontologist* 44 (3): 304–310.

Miles, Matthew B., and A. Michael Huberman. 1994. *Qualitative Data Analysis: An Expanded Sourcebook.* Thousand Oaks, CA: Sage.

Rowe, John W., and Robert L. Kahn. 1998. *Successful Aging.* New York: Pantheon Books.

———. 2015. "Successful Aging 2.0: Conceptual Expansions for the 21st Century." *Journals of Gerontology Series B: Psychological Sciences and Social Sciences* 70 (4): 593–596.

Taylor, Steven J., and Robert Bogdan. 1984. *Introduction to Qualitative Research Methods: The Search for Meanings,* 2nd ed. New York: Wiley.

West, Candace, and Don H. Zimmerman. 1987. "Doing Gender." *Gender and Society* 1 (2): 125–151.

2

Opting In or Opting Out?

North American Women Share Strategies for Aging Successfully with (and without) Cosmetic Intervention

ABIGAIL T. BROOKS

The "successful aging" paradigm frames our leading cultural narrative on "what it means to age well" (Lamb 2014, 42) in the United States today.[1] A key tenet of this paradigm—namely that a "successful," or healthy, active, and engaged, old age, is a matter of individual choice, effort, and behavior—has entered the American popular consciousness. Through adopting a youthful, can-do attitude, and a disciplined regime of body practices like healthful diet and exercise, successful agers counter longstanding cultural assumptions about aging as a time of disease and decline. To take aging into your own hands, to redefine it in ways that challenge reductive equations between aging and decay, can be an individually empowering experience, mentally, physically, and emotionally. This individual-responsibility, individual-choice frame finds easy resonance in our contemporary era of conspicuous consumption, wherein individuals are "free" to "improve" their bodies by choosing from a dizzying array of surgical, technological, and pharmaceutical products and procedures for purchase. The individualist imperative that informs successful aging also mirrors an increasingly commercialized system of American medicine that seeks to transform individuals into assertive patient-consumers, who are personally responsible for their own health, and who comfortably question their doctors about whether they might have the condition or syndrome—and get the treatment for it—that they learned about on television or online.

On the one hand, successful aging engenders resistance against the stigmatization, negative stereotyping, and invisibility of old age. For example, by redefining embodied aging as a state of physical activity, strength, and movement—or what Stephen Katz (2000) terms "busy bodies"—successful agers counter widespread associations between the aging body, weakness, slowness,

and decline. On the other hand, because the successful aging paradigm signi-
fies youthfulness in attitude, and in physicality, one can also argue that it leaves
ageism unchallenged or, worse still, contributes to it. Equations between successful aging and "anti-aging," "not aging," and "agelessness" (Andrews 1999;
Bayer 2005; Calasanti, Slevin, and King 2006) may well "intensify existing cultural attitudes about aging" and "devalue old age" more than ever (2001–2002).
Further, the individual-choice, individual-responsibility ethic of successful
aging can give rise to the blaming and shaming of older individuals for simply
being and growing old and for failing to *do anything* about it. As Martha Holstein
explains: "We may be viewed askance—at the simplest level for 'letting ourselves
go' when 'control' is putatively within our grasp—and, more problematically, as
moral failures for being complicit in our own aging" (2006, 316).

In our youth- and fitness-obsessed culture in the United States today,
women and men confront ageism. In a climate where profit-based medicine
merges with technological innovation to produce more and more options for
anti-aging intervention, women and men are the targets of direct-to-consumer
advertising and marketing campaigns. Pharmaceuticals like Viagra, for "erectile dysfunction," and Propetia, for baldness, offer middle-aged and older men
the promise of a youthful sexuality and appearance and reflect a lucrative and
expanding market for products designed to treat age-related "conditions" in
men. Yet women consume the vast majority of cosmetic products and procedures designed to minimize and "correct" age-driven changes in physical
appearance. Since 1997, when the American Society for Aesthetic Plastic Surgery first began keeping statistics on cosmetic procedures, women's consumption of cosmetic surgeries and technologies has consistently surpassed men's
at a rate of approximately ten to one. In 2015, a typical year, women had more
than 11.5 million, or just over 90 percent, of the more than 12 million surgical
and nonsurgical cosmetic procedures performed, and procedures specifically
designed to reduce and minimize aesthetic signs of aging on the face and body
topped the charts.[2]

Just as female consumers provide the lion's share of profit for the American and global beauty industry overall, American women's overwhelming use of
cosmetic anti-aging interventions betrays the stubborn cultural residue of what
Susan Bordo calls the "unbearable weight" of the female body (2003 [1993]).
The question of how successfully a woman conforms to traditional, heterosexual
norms of femininity—is she physically attractive? sexually desirable? reproduc-
tively viable?—remains an influential measure, albeit not the only measure, of a
woman's individual and social value in contemporary American culture. These
gendered statistics also suggest an empirical reality still significantly shaped by
what Susan Sontag identifies as the "double standard of aging" (1997, 19–24).
This double standard manifests in a heavier penalty for women—individually,

socially, culturally, and economically—than for men when evidence of aging appears on the face and body. According to Sontag, this inconsistency is gendered in two ways. First, women are valued more by how they look than men are, and men are valued more by what they do than women are. Second, women are held to more narrow and more stringent standards of physical attractiveness and sexual desirability—namely that of a youthful appearance—than men are.[3] Therefore, women, with age, become less physically attractive and sexually desirable in the eyes of others more quickly than men do. Sandra Bartky summarizes this gendered double standard as follows: "The loss of an admiring gaze falls disproportionately on women. . . . A woman's worth, not only in the eyes of others, but in her own eyes as well, depends, to a significant degree, on her appearance" (1999, 67).

If we begin with the understanding that the process of aging—how individuals make sense of, and experience, growing older—is gendered, it follows that individuals' understandings of what it means to age "successfully" will be gendered as well. In this chapter I explore how two groups of North American women define and embody "successful" approaches to aging. Drawing from forty-four intensive interviews with a spectrum of women between the ages of forty-seven and seventy-six who use, and refuse, cosmetic anti-aging interventions, I aim to illuminate how these women differently construct their own successful aging narratives.[4]

All of the women I interviewed—with the exception of one woman, who is Latina—are white. Their material resources, biographies, and current life circumstances vary widely (single, married, divorced, working, retired, unemployed, economically secure, economically struggling). Most, but not all, of the women live in the northeastern United States. Some live in cities, others in towns near urban centers, and some in small towns in rural areas. All are heterosexual. The ages of my interview subjects isolate them from the youth-centric portrayals of female beauty, sexual desirability, and reproductive viability that saturate American media and popular culture today. Yet their race and sexual identity are privileged in these mainstream portrayals and in the imagery in cosmetic anti-aging advertising, marketing, and media coverage. The palpably absent-presence of race and sexual identity in my interview subjects' narratives highlights the importance of new and emergent research that explicitly investigates how American women's lived realities of aging, and the meanings they attach to it, are differently mediated by race, ethnicity, and sexual orientation.

The women in my sample share a concern for the health of their bodies and a commitment to taking good care of them. Each woman practices bodily movement and activity on a regular basis (e.g., walking, yoga, running, gym workouts, and exercise classes). Many subscribe to a conscious and healthful diet and are engaged in civic activities in their communities. Despite these shared successful aging pursuits, however, my interview subjects respond to the age-driven changes in their appearance in markedly different ways. Women's embrace of cosmetic anti-aging intervention fits easily inside a successful aging model as they point to their procedures as evidence of their individual choice and individual responsibility to rein in and manage changes in appearance with technology. My interview subjects who *refuse* cosmetic anti-aging intervention, on the other hand, employ what they call a "natural" aging approach. Their strategy can be understood as upending conventional and mainstream success-ful aging imperatives as they work hard to accept the age-driven changes in their appearance and to appreciate the new opportunities for self-expression these changes represent. The norms and expectations that connote traditional heterosexual femininity—youth, beauty, and reproductive viability—saturate both groups' feelings about and experiences of growing older. As my interview subjects articulate their different approaches to the age-driven changes in their appearance, they reinforce and challenge not only youth-centric definitions of female beauty but also the traditional feminine imperatives of sex object, nur-turer, and reproducer.

Doing Femininity via Cosmetic Anti-Aging Interventions

Women's reasons for having and using cosmetic anti-aging procedures are var-ied and complex—my interview subjects spoke a lot about self and identity, about the relationship between the self and the body, about self-confidence and self-esteem, about invisibility, and much more, as they shared their feelings about growing older and their motivations for their surgical and nonsurgical interventions. Not all of my interview subjects' talk about their interventions was explicitly gendered (though I argue that gender, whether explicitly or implicitly, and to different degrees and in different ways, informs a great many feelings women have about their aging faces and bodies, and the subsequent approaches to aging they choose to subscribe to). Here, however, I call specific attention to how my interview subjects incorporate cosmetic anti-aging inter-vention into their narratives of what it means to age well—to achieve successful aging—as a heterosexual woman in the United States today.

Several women articulated feelings of pain and loss in response to no longer being perceived as a sexually desirable woman in the eyes of others (namely men). "You're losing that whole piece of you," says Caroline, who is forty-seven. Like Caroline, who feels like she is being "cast aside," forty-nine-year-old Claire tells me that she is enduring a "grieving period" as she confronts the loss of her sexual desirability in the eyes of others, and her newfound invisibility, with age: "Like from walking into a room, knowing that, you know, eyes would at least glance at me, to walking into a room and I'm another middle-aged woman."

Some of my interview subjects who embrace cosmetic anti-aging intervention, like Claire and Caroline, above, and Mary—who, at seventy-two, attributes her facelift to the imperative to look young as a woman in a male-dominated workplace, and to compete effectively with younger women in the heterosexual dating marketplace—are clearly motivated by the desire to conserve an aesthetic of youth-beauty and the value it represents. Others are less forthcoming about their motivations to continue to achieve a body that is "recognizably feminine" and do not overtly identify the invisibility they encounter as gendered. Janet, who is sixty-eight, tells me that before her eyelift, people at work saw her as simply "old" and, therefore, didn't seek out her skills and expertise. Anne, who is sixty-five, shares her feelings of being "dismissed" among her artist friends and colleagues: unless she was able to start a conversation with someone "who wasn't ageist" and unless that person realized, "as we started to talk," that she had interesting things to say, she simply felt ignored. And yet, by having cosmetic anti-aging interventions to conform to normative standards of physical attractiveness for women (i.e., *not looking old*), Janet and Anne feel they are more easily able to express themselves—to be visible, listened to, and respected—as *individuals* with unique minds, voices, skills, and expertise. Janet happily reports that, after her eyelift, she regained visibility in the eyes of her colleagues and reprised her role as someone with expertise whom customers sought out and respected. Anne tells me that after her two facelifts she feels and experiences less invisibility among her artist colleagues and friends: "I don't feel as dismissed as I used to feel. . . . I used to feel dismissed."

For my interview subjects who are having and using cosmetic anti-aging intervention, to age successfully, as a woman, means working hard, and taking personal responsibility, to maintain and achieve a physically attractive appearance. Women often include their cosmetic anti-aging interventions in a list of other bodily practices, like exercise and conscious diet, as examples of their commitment to taking good care of themselves and to staying healthy and fit. Melissa, who is fifty-three, works hard to stay healthy, not only through conscious diet and exercise—"I eat right. I exercise. I do try and take care of myself"— but also by having cosmetic anti-aging interventions. "It just sort of fits in with that somehow," she tells me, referring to her recent jaw lift and to her plans for a facelift in the near future. Wendy, who is also fifty-three, describes her two eyelifts this way: "I wanted to care for myself." When fifty-six-year-old Debra says of herself, post-interventions, "I'm in much better shape now," she reveals a strongly felt interdependence between how she looks—namely the extent to which she achieves a physically attractive, or youthful, appearance—and her own self-value.

My interview subjects' use of the phrase "letting yourself go" also communicates their strong allegiance to the equation between self and appearance for women. To "let yourself go," as a woman, is to demonstrate a lack of care about your physical appearance and a lack of commitment to "keeping it up" over time. This lack of care and commitment to maintaining your physical appearance betrays a lack of self-respect and self-value. As Claire explains, letting yourself go is "a choice you make and I don't understand that choice. . . . I don't get why a woman would want to walk around in sweatpants with gray hair and no make-up."

In and through having and using cosmetic anti-aging interventions, my interview subjects demonstrate a fierce commitment to self-care and self-value: they refuse to let themselves go. "I care what I look like," says Debra. Even further, by choosing intervention, they prove their keen awareness and acceptance of the tight conflation between a woman's appearance and her social value. When my interview subjects say "Looks matter," the looks they refer to are those of youthful beauty, and it is women in particular upon whose worth—both social and individual—looks depend. Mary summarizes this widely shared perspective when she says: "Looks, let's face it, have a lot to do with it, whether you like it or not." Even women who articulated some dissatisfaction and critique of the degree to which a woman's value is equated with her appearance expressed resignation about it simply being the way things are: "It's too bad, it's superficial," says Anne, who has had two facelifts. Anne attributes her preoccupation with how she looks to "my upbringing, and my culture." This culture, Anne tells me, "is a part of me" and has "had a big effect on me. . . . I didn't want to fight it," she says.[5]

Choosing intervention means taking individual responsibility to conform to what is socially expected of you as a woman. "You just have to do what you can with what you have," says Mary, referring to her facelift. Since having her facelift, Mary has given this "speech to a lot of women" and become an "advocate" for cosmetic anti-aging intervention. "It's stupid not to do everything you can," Mary tells me. Over and over again, I listened as women favorably contrasted their interventionist approach to that of women who are growing older without cosmetic anti-aging procedures. Julia, age forty-seven, says: "It amazes me when I see women who do nothing." Debra proclaims: "If a woman can afford to do it, she *should* do it." By choosing intervention, Claire demonstrates her commitment to preserving her own self-respect *and* her social-cultural value as a woman: "I care. I care for myself. I care for my husband. I care for the way I am going to be viewed in the world." Mary puts it succinctly when she says: "Looking good" [read "youthful"] is about being "socially acceptable."

For my interview subjects who embrace cosmetic anti-aging intervention, to age "successfully" means fighting back against age-driven changes in physical appearance with technology. To age successfully means continuing to "do femininity" well—and maintaining a body that is "recognizably feminine"—at an older age (Bartky 1999, 27; Smith 1990). In these respects, my interview subjects' embrace of cosmetic anti-aging intervention is not only about the successful achievement of a more youthful appearance but also about a demonstrated willingness *to do the required work*—incorporative of pain, time, and money—to maintain that youthful appearance.

Resisting Feminine Mandates by Aging "Naturally"

Women who choose cosmetic anti-aging intervention seek to minimize aesthetic signs of aging on the face and body with technology. My interview subjects who describe themselves as aging "naturally," on the other hand, work hard to accept the age-driven changes in their faces and bodies and to recognize the potential freedom from traditional feminine expectations these changes represent. Instead of choosing to reject aesthetic, age-driven changes in appearance with cosmetic intervention, these women choose to practice what Susan Wendell calls the "demanding art of acceptance, adjustment and appreciation" (1999, 146) in response to their aging exteriors.

Like the women who embrace intervention, my interview subjects who refuse it are not immune to feelings of alienation from, and discomfort with, the age-driven changes in their physical appearance. Nina, who is fifty-seven, speaks for many when she says: "You think, 'Who is that person? What happened to my hair? What happened to my skin?'" But Nina doesn't turn to cosmetic intervention to manage these feelings. She aspires to a "more democratic aesthetics of the body" (Bartky 1999, 72) instead. Nina tells me that she is "working on accepting" and "trying to appreciate" the age-driven changes in her face, like "wrinkles" and "bumps and discolorations." Others express a growing appreciation of how years of lived experience, and deepening character, are reflected in, and emanate through, the faces of older individuals. Elizabeth, an artist, age sixty-one, finds beauty in the age-driven changes in the appearance of a close female friend because "so much of her integrity, and her character, all those things come through." Rebecca, a flute maker, age fifty-eight, appreciates the complexity in old beauty and the ways in which old beauty differs from young beauty. She draws from her young grandson and the snapdragons from her garden as examples: "It might not be the same kind of beauty. Obviously, it's not like looking at my three-year-old grandson, who's just like this gorgeous little critter. You know, like these snapdragons are drying out, but the shapes and the way they're transforming is still beautiful. And they're not, like, standing up straight and perfect."

My naturally aging interview subjects also frequently articulate a lessening interest and focus on physical appearance, and an increasing interest and focus on inner qualities, both pertaining to themselves, and to others, with age. "Find out about *me*, who I *am*, my insides," fifty-five-year-old Alison tells me. Nancy, a clinical social worker, age fifty-nine, explains that she is "too busy living life from the inside out" to "dwell" on her physical appearance. Catherine, a retired career counselor, age sixty-one, increasingly focuses on "my energy," and "my own spirit," instead of on her physical appearance, as a source of self and social value with age.

The women I spoke with who describe themselves as aging "naturally," like those who choose cosmetic anti-aging intervention, encounter age-induced invisibility as the result of no longer being perceived as a physically attractive, sexually desirable, woman in the eyes of others. As Catherine puts it: "I remember a time where I'd walk down the street and I could get a look. Well, you get to a certain age—and, you know, good-bye to all that." Catherine confides that this lessening in "perceived attractiveness" is a "shift that is hard for all of us as women to make." And yet, however unjust it is, Catherine tells me that she is working to accept this shift—or her new reality—one wherein older women are not looked at as admiringly, and do not receive the same attention for how they look, as younger women do. Like many of her naturally aging counterparts, Catherine articulates her acceptance of this age-induced invisibility by chalking it up to human nature and biology. Because Catherine understands this shift as "probably pretty biological"—she attributes her lessening of sexual desirability in the eyes of others (namely men) to being "noticeably no longer childbearing age"—she feels she has no choice but to accept it. A number of women also equated their increasing invisibility with simply the ways things are—as part of the natural life cycle of things. Alison takes comfort in the universality of her own experience of first being a young woman who received attention for how she looked and then becoming an older woman who does not: "When I was, you know, twenty-five years old I *had* my day. You know, I looked pretty good and I thought I looked pretty good. And I loved to get dressed to go out, you know, I enjoyed it! . . . But that's *past*." Similarly, Sarah, a writer, also fifty-five, uses a life-cycle narrative to bring comfort to a friend who is struggling with her own invisibility, particularly in contrast to the attention her daughter is receiving for how she looks. Sarah recounts what she said to her friend: "I said, 'Well, you know, it's her turn, it's not your turn. You've had your turn, so move on, you know, get into your own things, you're not competing with your daughter to be that.'"

Witnessing age-driven changes in appearance, and experiencing a lessening of sexual desirability in the eyes of others with age, can certainly invoke painful feelings of sadness and loss in my naturally aging interview subjects. However, for the women I spoke with who opt out of cosmetic anti-aging intervention, this shift also marks a new phase of freedom and opportunity to explore, develop, and express themselves outside of the traditional feminine roles of sex object, nurturer, and reproducer—"to get your own things" to repeat Sarah's phrase. From Elizabeth's perspective, it's a "mistake" for women to think that a youthful aesthetic is the "prize": instead, it's something "we all get for a little while" but then "it moves along and we're getting into new things."

Over and over again, my naturally aging interview subjects positively equated aging with worrying less about how their bodies look, whether or not their bodies measure up, and whether or not they are attracting the male gaze. Elizabeth tells me that when she was young, she felt "this sense of inadequacy" because she was being "measured constantly by this label of beauty." For Elizabeth, aging brings a welcome freedom from these insecurities about how her body looks, and whether it looks good enough: "It's a very liberating thing for me. I don't have a lot of the inhibitions and focuses on the exterior that I used to have." Like Elizabeth, Sarah also now enjoys a lessening of preoccupation with her appearance and a lessening of worry about whether she is "beautiful enough" to attract male interest and attention: "I used to worry about, you know, was my mascara all right, you know, or did I look OK? . . . Just that terrible time you go through of, you know, 'Are you beautiful enough? Will this guy love me? Do I look hot enough?' I'm so happy to be out of that life! I'm just so happy that it's gone."

In addition to enjoying the freedom from worrying about being sexually desirable enough to attract male attention, I also heard a lot from my interview subjects about the comfort and relaxation they felt as the result of no longer being the object of the male gaze. Knowing that she is no longer a target of male desire enables Rebecca to feel "less self-conscious" about her body, to come out of her shell, and to enjoy her interactions with others more fully: "I'm not so self-conscious about my looks anymore, which is really good. It makes me more open, I think, to people in general. I have a better time with people." Being caught in the male gaze made Rebecca feel uncomfortable and increased her anxiety about how she looked. Now, at fifty-eight, the male gaze has eroded, and she feels more relaxed about her appearance: "I figure, you know, I'm fifty-eight, and people aren't looking at me like they did when I was twenty, obviously. And I find that really comfortable. I always felt: 'Somebody's looking at me and I should look good.' And now I feel like, 'Oh, you know what, no one's really going to look if I've got this little piece of hair falling down.' And they're not really looking at me that much anymore, which is nice. So it's a relief." It is also a relief for Rebecca to feel that people's interactions with her are not motivated by wanting to "hit" on her or "pick her up"—instead, they are characterized by a genuine interest in who she is as a person, in her personality, and in what she has to say. As she puts it: "When I'm working in the garden people always stop to talk. And I don't feel it's because they want to hit on me anymore. It's just nicer. It's really nicer for me."

My naturally aging interview subjects discover new freedoms as they leave behind them the youth-beauty imperative—and the sex-object identity—of traditional heterosexual femininity. Some also articulate their enthusiasm about reclaiming their bodies for themselves and away from female biology and the reductive social roles and expectations of pregnancy and motherhood that accompany it. Others speak about enjoying newfound freedom, independence, and time for themselves as the intensive emotional, physical, and mental labor of mothering recedes with age.

Now that she is not of childbearing age, Rebecca enjoys having her body all to herself: "It's mine now," she tells me. Rebecca doesn't have to worry about getting her period, and buying menstrual products, and staining her clothes. Because she won't be pregnant again, and she doesn't have to be "responsible for another being in there and nurturing it," she can drink tea and "some alcohol if I want to." As she puts it: "My body's not a temple for another human being at this point. That's a big responsibility gone." Several others also talked about menopause as marking the beginning of a new and exciting phase of life that is centered less on nurturing others and more on nurturing the self. Elizabeth tells me that menopause "definitely changes one's focus," and Nina describes menopause as "a reminder that you can nurture yourself and that this is your time to do whatever feels really important and really right." Nina explicitly connects the end of menstruation to the ebbing of the "physical nurturing" demands of pregnancy and motherhood: "With the idea of menses stopping, and not ovulating, and not thinking that you're kind of there for nurturing in a physical way, the job you have is to figure out your importance in a bigger way." As Nina's children leave the house to begin lives of their own, this shift also opens up room for her to grow in new ways: "You can celebrate *their* going off and being their own selves in a full way, and making their own decisions, and appreciating that but not feeling that responsibility. And then you have all this energy for *whatever else.*"

This newly found "energy for whatever else," to steal Nina's language, manifests in more time for my interview subjects to relax in the mornings before work, to do yoga, and to focus more on what Elizabeth simply calls her "interior work." Nina has gotten more involved in working on political, environmental, and social justice issues in her community, which, she says, have given her a new "sense of purpose." She has also created a new room in her home for weaving, which she equates with "my own creativity" and "what I love to do": "So now I'm going to have a space for weaving that's really *perfect* and right. And it's a kind of a symbol, making space for what I love and what I want to do. For my own creativity, so that's good. And that feels like a good part of *aging*, really."

Concluding Thoughts

My interview subjects choose to have cosmetic anti-aging interventions to lessen the dismissal, negative stereotyping, and invisibility they encounter when they no longer meet the criterion of youthfulness that overwhelmingly informs contemporary cultural understandings of female attractiveness and sexual desirability in the United States today. Saying "yes" to intervention, and achieving a younger appearance as a result, can be an empowering experience for women. Receiving positive feedback and attention for how you look, looking better in clothes, securing a new husband, achieving greater success at work, overcoming invisibility, and regaining the interest of others in you, as a person, with worthy ideas and perspectives to share—these are some, though not all, of the positive outcomes my interview subjects attribute to their cosmetic anti-aging interventions. For women who choose intervention, to take good care of yourself means caring about your physical appearance. Successful aging means accepting that that how you look (i.e., having a youthful appearance) *matters*. Making the choice to age successfully, as a woman, requires not only taking personal responsibility to maintain your physical health and fitness but also working hard to maintain your physical appearance.

My interview subjects who embrace cosmetic anti-aging interventions practice what Martha Holstein calls "age avoidance" as they "take advantage" of an ever-growing stockpile of new cosmetic anti-aging products and procedures in "pursuit of youthfulness" (2015, 101). "Keep working in your labs!" and "There's a whole arsenal out there!" were typical sentiments expressed. Julia speaks for many when she says: "I find it comforting that if I don't like something, I can go fix it."

Women who choose cosmetic anti-aging intervention find ample support for their youth-maintenance approach in what has become a "normative model" for aging well in the United States today (Lamb 2014, 41). Yet for my interview subjects who choose to grow older without intervention, the booming cosmetic anti-aging industry inspires new anxieties in them about their aging faces and bodies.[6] The plethora of advertising and options for cosmetic anti-aging intervention can make these women feel bad about looking old and guilty for not *doing something* about it. For Mia, who is fifty-nine and a real estate agent, the advertising for cosmetic anti-aging products and procedures makes her feel "worse" about her aging face and body: it definitely "increases my anxiety," and "doesn't help my self-esteem," she says. Laura, who is fifty-one and an education adviser, knows that the age-driven changes in her appearance are "normal," and what the body "naturally does at my age." But the plethora of options for cosmetic anti-aging intervention make her feel that fighting these changes is her individual responsibility: "Modern science tells me 'no, that's not true, it could be otherwise.'" Like Mia, who has to make a "conscious choice not to use them," Laura tells me that it's hard to look old, as a woman, when you can choose not to: "If you look the way you do, it's because you've made a choice. You have to feel hard on yourself because you have no one but yourself to blame."

But my naturally aging interview subjects push back even as they describe our culture as one that "doesn't allow aging."[7] They resist the compulsion to conserve the mainstream feminine aesthetic of youthfulness and the value it represents. The strategies they employ in response to the age-driven changes in their faces and bodies are not motivated by the goal of looking young. Instead, they fight back against what Margaret Cruikshank calls the "almost inescapable" judgment that older women's bodies are unattractive (2003, 147). They also work hard to recognize, and to take advantage of, new opportunities for self-growth and self-expression—new sources of agency and empowerment—*outside* of the traditional codes of heterosexual femininity. Unlike their pro-intervention counterparts, whose narratives about their aging faces and bodies commonly center on descriptions of "identity stripping" and "losing what we had" (Gullette 2004, 130), my naturally aging interview subjects are more likely to make sense of their aging exteriors as a compilation of "changeable and continuous selves together" and to see "multiple identities" and "multiple selves" reflected back at them (Gullette 2004, 124–125, 127). For the women I interviewed who describe themselves as aging "naturally," to age well is not about "trying to take control" of the aging body to make it look younger. Instead, they work hard, and reap rewards, as they forge new relationships to their aging bodies and as they realize new avenues for self-expression outside of the body altogether.

NOTES

1. Sarah Lamb usefully summarizes what she calls the "North American successful aging movement"—the key tenets of which she draws from Rowe and Kahn (1998; 1987)—as centered on the following: "independence, productivity, self-maintenance, and the individual as self-project" (Lamb 2014, 41).
2. American Society for Aesthetic Plastic Surgery, Statistics, 2015.
3. Sontag's "double standard of aging" is useful as a model that applies to heterosexual aging in the North American context, and in the case of my interview subjects, heterosexual women specifically. It does not incorporate an analysis of how aesthetic aging varies for women across race, culture, ethnicity, and sexual orientation, nor take into account the current and recent trend among some American men, particularly young men, who are increasingly concerned about physical appearance and body image and who are spending more time and money on activities designed to "improve" how they look. Finally, Sontag's double standard does not incorporate current, recent, and compelling evidence that shows that not only aging women, but aging men, and aging gay men in particular, are experiencing anxiety about looking older and confront comparable pressures to maintain a youthful appearance. See, for example, Lodge and Umberson 2013.
4. For the purposes of my research, cosmetic anti-aging interventions include surgical procedures, like neck lifts, facelifts, and eyelifts and nonsurgical procedures (also known as "injectables," or "fillers") like Botox, Juvaderm, and Perlane. See Brooks 2017, *The Ways Women Age: Using and Refusing Cosmetic Intervention*, for more discussion and analysis of these interviews with North American women, inclusive of the following themes: the self-body relationship; identity; social circles; the decision to

have cosmetic anti-aging intervention and to grow older without it; anti-aging culture; commercialized medicine.

5. When I first introduced Anne in this chapter, she framed her facelifts as a response to the invisibility she felt and experienced as the result of looking old. Here, however, Anne highlights the importance of an attractive physical appearance (i.e., looking young), particularly to her own sense of value and identity, both individually and culturally, as a *woman*. To Anne, both responses are connected, as a woman must be physically attractive to be visible.

6. For more discussion and analysis of how the growing normalization of cosmetic anti-aging intervention in the United States today interacts with women's attitudes and lived experiences of aging, see Brooks 2010.

7. This phrase is Laura's (who is fifty-one and an education adviser), and her sentiment resonates with the findings of age-studies scholar Laura Hurd Clarke, who, in her interviews with older women, uncovered shared feelings of cultural pressure—or what she terms a "moral imperative"—to modify the aging face (2011, 69).

REFERENCES

Andrews, Molly. 1999. "The Seductiveness of Agelessness." *Ageing and Society* 19: 301–318.

Bartky, Sandra Lee. 1999. "Unplanned Obsolescence: Some Reflections on Aging." In *Mother Time: Women, Aging, and Ethics*, edited by Margaret Urban Walker, 61–74. Lanham, MD: Rowman and Littlefield.

Bayer, Katherine. 2005. "Cosmetic Surgery and Cosmetics: Redefining the Appearance of Age." *Generations* (Fall): 13–18.

Bordo, Susan. 2003 [1993]. *Unbearable Weight: Feminism, Western Culture, and the Body.* Berkeley: University of California Press.

Brooks, Abigail. 2010. "Aesthetic Anti-Aging Surgery and Technology: Women's Friend or Foe?" *The Sociology of Health and Illness* 32 (2): 238–257.

———. 2017. *The Ways Women Age: Using and Refusing Cosmetic Intervention.* New York: New York University Press.

Calasanti, Toni M., Kathleen F. Slevin, and Neal King. 2006. "Ageism and Feminism: From 'Et Cetera' to Center." *NWSA Journal* 18 (1): 13–30.

Cruikshank, Margaret. 2003. *Learning to be Old: Gender, Culture and Aging.* Lanham, MD: Rowman and Littlefield.

Gullette, Margaret Morganroth. 2004. *Aged by Culture.* Chicago: University of Chicago Press.

Holstein, Martha. 2015. *Women in Late Life: Critical Perspectives on Gender and Age.* Lanham, MD: Rowman and Littlefield.

———. 2006. "On Being an Aging Woman." In *Age Matters: Realigning Feminist Thinking*, edited by Toni M. Calasanti and Kathleen F. Slevin, 313–334. New York: Routledge.

Hurd Clarke, Laura. 2011. *Facing Age: Women Growing Older in an Anti-Aging Culture.* Lanham, MD: Rowman and Littlefield.

Katz, Stephen. 2000. "Busy Bodies: Activity, Aging, and the Management of Everyday Life." *Journal of Aging Studies* 14 (2): 135–152.

Lamb, Sarah. 2014. "Permanent Personhood or Meaningful Decline? Toward a Critical Anthropology of Successful Aging." *Journal of Aging Studies* 29: 41–52.

Lodge, Amy C., and Debra Umberson. 2013. "Age and Embodied Masculinities: Mid Life Gay and Heterosexual Men Talk About Their Bodies." *Journal of Aging Studies* 27 (3): 225–232.

Smith, Dorothy E. 1990. *Texts, Facts, and Femininity: Exploring the Relations of Ruling.* London: Routledge.

Sontag, Susan. 1997. "The Double Standard of Aging." In *The Other Within Us: Feminist Explorations of Women and Aging*, edited by Marilyn Pearsall, 19–24. Boulder, CO: Westview Press.

Wendell, Susan. 1999. "Old Women Out of Control: Some Thoughts on Aging, Ethics, and Psychosomatic Medicine." In *Mother Time: Women, Aging, and Ethics*, edited by Margaret Urban Walker, 133–149. Lanham, MD: Rowman and Littlefield.

3

Aging Out

Ageism, Heterosexism, and Racism among Aging African American Lesbians and Gay Men

IMANI WOODY

In mainstream US culture, successful aging is often defined as being without disease and disability, with the ability to maintain remarkable physical well-being and high cognitive function while being an engaged and productive member of society.[1] However, this description often excludes intersecting identities of race, class, gender expression, and sexual orientation. These unfortunate exclusions can include African Americans,[2] who are projected to constitute more than 12 percent of the US elderly population by 2050—the largest group of minority elders (Strom, Carter, and Schmidt 2004). These exclusions also include the older lesbian, gay, and bisexual (LGB) population, a group largely left out of the vast successful aging literature, and identified by the Centers for Disease Control and Prevention and HealthyPeople.gov as one of the main gaps in current health research.[3] Compared to the overall older adult population, older LGB people are more likely to age without a partner or close relationships with children, as they are twice as likely to be single, two times more likely to live alone, and three to four times less likely to have children.[4]

Older black LGB people have endured stigma, prejudice, and discrimination as people of color in a white male-dominated culture, as LGB in a heteronormative environment and now as elders in a youth-oriented society—frequently experiencing double, triple, and quadruple oppressions based on age, gender, sexual orientation, and race (Grant 2010). Within the African American community itself, black LGB elders may experience additional intolerance based on their gender identity and sexual orientation, for although a reverence for elders often permeates African American culture, gay and lesbian sexual identities tend not to be widely supported (Strom, Carter, and Schmidt 2004). These factors can keep older black LGB persons from making use of community and social services available to their heterosexual counterparts, while creating forms of exclusion and stress that hinder their quality of life and sense of ability to achieve successful aging.

For black LGB persons, like for their mainstream compatriots, new life questions emerge in older age: When did I change? When did I get old? What will happen now? Will I have enough resources in my old age? Will I become physically or financially dependent? Are elders treated well here? Who will care for me? These more exacting questions also arise: Am I safe to share who I am? Because of my race or ethnicity, will I be treated fairly? Will I be treated well once my sexual identity and gender expression are realized? Are they accepting, or just tolerant, of LGB elders? Am I able to bring my whole self to this environment? For those of us who are older and also LGB, facing the challenges of homophobia and heteronormativity can send us running back to the very closets we fought so hard to leave. This was personified by a black lesbian activist I worked with in the 1980s, who told me years later, regarding identifying as a lesbian, "I don't do that stuff anymore!" She currently works on issues affecting African Americans but minus LGBT matters, perhaps in an effort to remain safe from discrimination.

This chapter examines notions and experiences of aging from the voices of LGB people of African descent living in an urban environment in the United States.[5] It examines the lived experiences of older LBG African Americans who face subtle and blatant racism, homophobia, and ageism—within black communities; within lesbian, bisexual, and gay communities; and within broader American society. As members of multiple minority groups, older lesbian, gay, and bisexual Americans of African descent have survived racism, heterosexism, homophobia, and now ageism, as they face growing older in a hostile environment.

Methodology: Listening to Older Black Lesbian Women and Gay Men in Washington, DC

To explore the experiences of older black LGB persons—perspectives strikingly left out of the broader public and gerontological discourse on successful aging—I used a purposeful sample of fifteen participants in the hopes of offering a microcosm of the wider black LGB older population under consideration. The participants were fifteen self-identified lesbian, gay, and bisexual people of African descent who were fifty-seven years of age and older living in the Washington, DC, metropolitan area. They were identified for inclusion in the study from a church, from a community service organization, and through word of mouth. Of the fifteen people, four self-identified their race and ethnicity as black and eight self-identified their heritage as African American. One participant self-identified as a person of Caribbean African American ancestry, another self-identified as biracial (of Caucasian and African American heritage), and one participant self-identified her ancestry as multiracial (Native American, black American, and Caucasian). The median age of the participants was sixty-four, and each self-identified their current socioeconomic status as middle class. Twelve participants were retired, one was semi-retired, and two worked full time. The group as a whole was highly educated: two participants had doctoral degrees, five had master's degrees (one participant had two master's degrees), one participant had a graduate degree, and seven had received advanced technical training or had some college beyond high school. The participants' religious affiliations included Baptist, Unitarian, and Pentecostal, with more than half considering themselves Christian, and thirteen stating that they had relinquished traditional religion to focus instead on being spiritual and having a personal connection with God of their understanding.

The research explored whether older black LGB experiences included perceived discrimination based on age, heterosexism, and/or sexual orientation and included interview questions such as: Have you ever felt discriminated against because you are lesbian/gay/same-gender loving? Have you ever felt discriminated against in the LGBT community because you are older? Have you ever felt discrimination in the African American community because you were lesbian/gay/same-gender loving and older? Other questions probed included: Is your church or religious institution welcoming and affirming of gay people? Do you feel your doctors and other health care professionals are welcoming and affirming of gay people? Do you feel that there are any barriers for you in participating in social and community programs because of being lesbian or gay? The participants spoke frankly and openly about topics and experiences that were at times very personal and included painful disclosures in interviews averaging two hours in length.

Several major themes emerged from the interviews, including the respondents' sense of alienation in the black community, perceived discrimination and alienation from organized religion, concerns over safety and acceptance, and the need to develop coping strategies in an attempt to ameliorate these forms of exclusion. I labeled several major themes appearing throughout the research, listed here in descending order of prevalence: (1) sense of alienation in the African American community; (2) deliberate concealment of sexual identity and orientation; (3) aversion to LGBT labels; (4) perceived discrimination and alienation from organized religion; (5) feelings of grief and loss related to aging; (6) isolation; and (7) fear of financial and physical dependence.

Intersections of Identity—Black and LGB

Black elders, like their non–African American counterparts, are not a monolithic group; however, a characteristic placed upon all African Americans is their shared early history in the United States. Maltreatment of African Americans has included systematic genocide, annihilation of family, legal life enslavement, and Jim Crow government-sanctioned racial oppression and segregation. Recent events around race in this country, including ongoing police brutality, have underscored how violence and discrimination against black Americans persist. Moreover, black Americans who are also lesbian, gay, or bisexual face discrimination and exclusion due to their sexuality. In the 1940s and 1950s, witch-hunts of LGB people working as teachers and in the government (including the military) were the norm. Lillian Faderman, distinguished scholar of lesbian and gay issues, has asserted that "the 1950's were probably the worst time ever to be a lesbian in the United States" (McLoughlin and Faderman 2009). If one were discovered as a lesbian woman or gay man, one would be fired on the grounds of immorality. For many of today's LGB elders, who came of age in the 1940s and 1950s, these discriminatory activities continue to color every aspect of their lives. Rose,[6] a black lesbian, age sixty-five and retired, shared her experiences: "Never came out at work, even to this day. . . . And being in white corporate America you know it is 'fire at will,' that sort of thing. So I have a friend . . . who is gay and was in the government and we would attend functions together and help each other. We were known as boyfriend and girlfriend . . . which was very safe."

In addition, black LGB older adults live at the intersections of multiple identities, and experience a lifetime inundated by a culture steeped in racism, sexism, ageism, heterosexism, homophobia, and biphobia. Black LGB elders' experiences are impacted by a minimum of two and often four hostile environments: (1) being a person of color in a racist culture; (2) being lesbian, gay, or bisexual in a homophobic and biphobic society; (3) being a woman in a sexist culture; and (4) being an older adult in an ageist culture. For some, the losses and the fear ensuing from so many intersecting forms of hostility resulted in isolation. Many of the participants had been closeted for most of their lives. Some had served in the military. One participant shared that her partner was with her for most of her enlistment. She revealed, "To be in isolation that long, for eighteen years and not be out to anybody other than our best friends, it's just horrible. It created a lot of anxiety in us." Another participant, Astor, a sixty-nine-year-old African Caribbean gay male, related: "Again, it comes down to 'Do I disclose that I am a same-gender loving person?' They can see I'm black. What happens sometimes is again a feeling of isolation and loneliness of . . . if I feel like . . . Clearly being the only black sometimes in a group is not always comfortable. For example, I've been going to [community] meetings, and sometimes I'm the only black person there. It feels weird because whenever they want diversity, it's me, or they expect me to identify some others for them. I [am] . . .

a token black person." The visibility of blackness to Astor contrasts the invisibility of queerness. Although he resents being called upon to be a "token black person," he feels even more isolated by not feeling free to go public with his same-gender-loving identity, an identity that he keeps largely invisible.

Further, participants spoke of how African Americans are exposed to heterosexism not only from mainstream culture but also from the African American heterosexual community. Although many LGB African Americans feel very closely connected psychologically and culturally with their racial and ethnic communities, they are often reluctant to share their sexual minority status because it is outside the norm and mostly unsupported (Szymanski and Gupta 2009). Walter, a black gay male, age sixty-three, described how his mother received him when he was thirteen years old, after being raised by his aunts: "I grew up in North Carolina and moved to Washington when I was thirteen. . . . And that was a whole cultural adjustment for me because my mother was expecting this little boy who played baseball and knew how to fix cars and so forth, and what she got was a queen who knew Shakespeare and theater and could sew a button . . . and cook better than she could. . . . So I had to try to fit into her concept of what a little boy should be. . . . And my mother was homophobic big time."

Other research has found that the sexual values of twenty-six self-identified black lesbian women were rooted in African American culture, as evident in a commitment to a cohesive family unit that included children and the primacy of a spiritual self (Wilson 2005). However, the women in my study commonly voiced feeling isolated from the black community because of their sexual identity and orientation. Darlene, a sixty-year-old black lesbian, recalled:

> Oh my goodness! I had to leave my mother's church. I used to take her to church; she belongs to a Baptist church, and not all Baptist are homophobic. But hers is just—they are one of the ones when everything— . . . like marriage laws, the same-sex marriage laws, or anything to do with gay and lesbian community, they rally [against it]. And my mother's eighty-six and frail, so I was trying to—never liked her church, but I was trying. They don't allow women in the pulpit, I mean for nothing. I mean, when they have a program, the women are relegated to the floor and down below. But the women cannot go up there and that's really hard. I had told my mom that I'm not going back to your church. [Once] the preacher took Mother's Day to talk all about the abomination of gays and lesbians in the church . . . and how they were gonna rally against this and rally against that.

This sense of alienation as a lesbian or gay person in the black community can happen in one's youth, and the pain of loss is thus carried through the years. Clara, a sixty-seven-year-old lesbian who identifies herself as multiracial, recalled:

> My best friend, and she was my best friend for years and years and years. Even though I was doing gay things, nobody knew it. I wasn't out; I was doing it in the closet. And when she found out—I didn't tell her, a guy that I worked with saw me down at some gay club and he came back and told everybody. But everybody knew he was gay because he was real flamboyant, so he came back and told everyone at work that I was at the gay club, so she came back and asked me why I didn't tell her. She went and told her boyfriend . . . who beat her up because she was associating with me and told her never to talk to me anymore. I just had to put this out of my mind. It hurt for a long time.

Doris, a sixty-seven-year-old black lesbian woman, told her mother she was gay after age thirty-five and described her mother's reaction: "Mother always wanted me to get married and that was the big push for her. And so I finally said to her, 'Mother, it won't happen because I'm gay.' And she was, like, that's against God. I said, 'Mother, don't go there, because you know I am a better Bible scholar than you will ever be, so the only issue is, do you still want me to come home.' I had just had surgery. . . . And she said, 'What? What's that got to do with anything? Of course you're coming home.'"

One study found that many of the values held by African Americans stem from their shared African heritage and include communal sharing, spiritual connectedness, family closeness, and respect for one's elders (Strom, Carter, and Schmidt 2004). It is no wonder that all of the participants spoke about being conflicted in telling their family members their sexual identity, fearing rejection and abandonment. Only nine of the fifteen participants advised their families of their sexual orientation. A majority of these told their families after they were thirty-five years old. Three of the nine had been in heterosexual marriages or relationships, with two unions producing offspring. Several of the participants commented that family members stopped speaking for a time; some of the participants are currently estranged from their families. However, many of the participants were firm in their commitment to live their lives fully regardless of the reactions of their family members.

Cheryl, a black lesbian woman, age sixty, explains the reaction she received after she shared her sexual orientation and identity with her parents when she was thirty-nine years old: "I knew I was going to tell my parents. My father was the first one [I came out to]. I thought I'd have more problems with him, but it turned out that my mother was ballistic. She didn't want to hear nothing. I was trying to tell her, and she just didn't want to hear it. [She] didn't want to get it—'I don't wanna hear it.' So she played that game; but I didn't back down." Cheryl went on to share an incident with her wife's family, which was somewhat supportive but only within limits: "They didn't even want to stay in our house when we had a big Thanksgiving celebration, because they had two young daughters, and I guess they thought we were going to jump them. That's all I can figure." She shook her head slowly from left to right.

Warren, the sixty-three-year-old African American gay male, shared:

> I know I have an androgynous look; it was even more so when I was younger. So therefore, there was some discrimination against me by assumption rather than fact, because they would look at me, and because I am androgynous looking they would assume. . . . One of my issues being African American and looking like this was really when I came out in college in the late sixties at the height of the Black Power Movement, and I was distinctly told by a couple of black organizations at the time, "We don't want your kind here." So that is one of the most blatant [examples of discrimination]: "We don't want your kind here," and I knew exactly what they meant.

And Astor described his sense of what was considered appropriate behavior within his family and community:

> I think . . . I just in my head I knew I was. At age five, it's not that I intellectually said, "Oh, I like men." It was just always so curious—so if I sat in a man's lap, I was always bouncing around, and the guy would be trying to keep me still, or at age five I would be doing inappropriate things like trying to open his fly or something. I remember my uncle said, "Something's not right with that boy." . . . I was sexually active as a teenager, but very much closeted about it. What today [one] would say "on the down-low" about it. At the same time, I had a curiosity about women, too, but it was much more passive. If a female approached me I would . . . tend to respond, and it still is that way today.

Doris shared her experience of silencing her sexual identity within her African American community:

> As I was growing up, I knew enough that you shouldn't speak of [being LGB]; even if you thought it, you didn't speak of it. And you assimilate as much as you can. And assimilation meant that you made sure your behavior was above suspicion. As I said, a lot of people suspect, and a lot of people know, but since they've never asked the question [participant raises her eyebrows and shrugs her shoulders], because I would never deny it. See, in the African American community, at least in my experience, that's not something you ask or something you act upon unless the person has done something to you.

The risk of losing the support of the black community because of perceived LGB identities can be devastating and can lead to isolation and depression (Wilson and Miller 2002). This fear of rejection, abandonment, or worse led several participants to state that they did not feel a need to come out to everyone. As a result, many were out only to a select number of people, who included very close friends and close family members. They were out to others only on a need-to-know basis. One participant stated that you have to almost be ready to come out to someone every day. Clarisse, a black lesbian, sixty-seven years old, looked at it this way: "I'm a counselor, so I'm not going to have pictures of my family around because people . . . talk about your family . . . and ask you some personal questions that are not necessary. But if I have [a client] who is gay or lesbian and has some issues of discrimination, I may come out to them." Donald, a black gay male, age sixty-four, had not discussed his orientation with anyone in his family except his sister. He recently retired but was not out at work or out in his neighborhood; however, he was out to some people at the church he attends.

Many participants perceived that this selective showing of oneself is simply the way it is in the African American community. It is a way of life for many in the black LGB community and can cause psychological distress.

Intersections of Identity: Black and Old

Not only did participants in this study face difficulties being black and LGB in a heterosexist and racist society, they also expressed experiencing subtle and overt forms of discrimination and exclusion based on age. Older age could offer more positively, however, a sense of empowerment, and some felt that dealing with racial and gendered oppressions earlier in life had prepared them somewhat to tackle discrimination based on age.

Expressions of ageism permeate US society: by being perceived as old in the United States, one is often devalued and stripped of one's sexuality, beauty, and usefulness (Butler 2005; Calasanti 2005). Doris articulated it this way: "Well, I would say that getting older in this country is difficult because we have no reverence for the elderly, which is not true in a lot of cultures. So when you add another . . . stigma to it now: not only am I old, I'm an old African American female. And females in this country—at least my experience has been that you don't enjoy the same reverence as males do, and then when you add African American to that, then it's even less. So now, I'm already down pretty far, and then when you add being a lesbian to that, that puts you in the toilet."

Many participants saw more egregious forms of ageism in the United States as they got older and lamented that the problem was not getting any better. Warren summed it up this way: "[In] American culture there is so little respect for the elderly. In Japan and China and even in a lot of other European countries there is a much higher level of respect for the elderly, and it seems to me to be getting worse [here]. If you are over fifty you are in the throwaway generation by younger people's standards, and it doesn't seem to be getting any better. The more technologically advanced we get, it gets worse."

In fact, all of the participants stated they had experienced ageism. Their perceptions included feeling as if they no longer had any valuable knowledge to convey; an inability to participate at the same level as they had formerly; and being treated in a condescending manner. These reactions were met with both humor and frustration. One participant shared that his children would always want to drive; one stated that people became oversolicitous; another participant revealed that her cousins would not let her pick up a forty-pound bag—something she has been doing for a great part of her life and can still do. Clara shared her experience with aging and ageism:

> What I find is like being placated because you are older. I have to say things two and three times, not because they don't hear me, but because they don't see me. It's like I've become invisible or something. When I was younger, like even ten . . . years ago, I would say what I needed to say and people would hear me. And now I have to raise myself and my voice to be heard [she sits straight in her chair to demonstrate] to bring back whatever they used to know. Because they see my gray hair or see me walking slowly and want to take my arm, because it's like I don't know anything.

Being a LGB elder who grew up during the AIDS/HIV epidemic brings a particular set of feelings of age. A participant said:

> Here's the really hard part for me: Between 1990 and 2000, I lost a hundred friends to HIV. My entire social circle is [populated with] people I would have grown old with and be socializing with who now are dead. I stopped counting after [the year] 2000. I stopped checking the obits because it just got too overwhelming. My best buddy that I actually hung out with . . . and who came out to me after being married for ten or fifteen years, he died of a heart attack, not HIV [participant begins to cry]. I have three other friends who died of heart attacks again who I would have grown old with. And I have had three suicides.

Some participants expressed a sense of grief and loss because they did not share their sexual orientation at an earlier age and because of the ways they had internalized homophobia now and then. Doris reflected:

> As I get older, what I regret is that I didn't feel safe enough to tell some of the folks who know me and knew me, you know, early on. . . . As you get

older you always think back because there was still some shame to it. And I
wish I hadn't bought into it. If I had to give advice to someone at this stage,
I would say, "Tell somebody, tell several somebody's," because that's the only
way to erase the fact that you have to look around the corner and be careful
who you are seen with and how you are seen. I mean, because it's a bunch of
garbage. It really is, but nevertheless—. . . . I used to tell myself that two strikes
are bad enough.

Despite her feelings of frustration, Doris's comments also highlight a more
positive shared theme of many in this cohort—the ability with increasing age
to shrug off a lot of oppressive behavior, or stand up to it, depending on the
situation. Challenging ageist stereotypes, in fact, seemed to be a regular experience among participants. Doris explained:

When people see you with gray hair, they do one of two things. They either
begin to say "Yes, ma'am," being respectful, or they assume you have no idea
how to do anything. Now most people don't make that mistake about me
because they hear me speak and that's where the PhD comes in. So anyway,
the PhD allows me to carry myself in a certain way, so therefore people that
are younger than I am, even if they think they wanted to. . . . I mean age forty
and a PhD allowed me to say no to a number of things. As I became fifty it
allowed me to say no to people, and at sixty I am free to do all or none of it.

One participant declared, "I know my rights. I know how to sue; I know
about defamation of character. I know the law." Another participant recounted
that in a Bible study class she attended with her wife, the minister started making comments about "those funny women." She told the minister, "You will not
get another check from me to support a ministry that is so mean-spirited." Still
other participants talked about becoming older and wiser. Clara summarized:
"Getting older for me helps me deal with . . . other oppressions and things;
because I am wiser, I pray more. . . . It doesn't bother me as much as it did when
I was younger, angrier, and had a fast temper and stuff like that and would fight
back. . . . Some things still hurt, but I don't have to linger over it, carry it around
with me all the time and cause myself internal harm because of something
someone says or does to me. . . . But when I was young, I didn't think like that."

Further, some research has suggested that older lesbian women who have
been subjected to sexism or racism throughout their lives may have obtained
the skills to cope with the experience of ageism later in life (Moradi et al. 2010).
Specifically, the cultural marginalization of being female and being lesbian may
have created "adaptive strategies" that assist some older lesbians in meeting the challenges of becoming older (Gabbay and Wahler 2002). Several of

this study's participants agreed that challenges based on racial, gender, and sexual-identity oppression earlier in life made it easier to deal with later forms of oppression based on age. Many study participants, further, considered their racial identity to be even more important than their identities of either age or sexuality, as they had experienced forms of bigotry and a pervasive sense of "otherness" throughout their lives, as people of color in a white-dominated society.

Conclusion

Like those of their heterosexual and dominant majority counterparts, older black lesbian women's and gay men's attitudes toward aging are influenced by broader societal norms. Their experiences of aging are also shaped by their parallel experiences as people of African descent and members of a black community. Many have lived through Jim Crow and the civil rights era. Most, in fact, consider their racial identity to be even more significant than their other identities, including identities of gender and sexual orientation. Nonetheless, they find challenging and painful the forms of exclusion they face within their own African American community for having lesbian, gay, or bisexual sexual identities.

As a group, older black lesbian women and gay males face constant stigma and systemic bigotry that in turn can create challenges for integrating their lesbian or gay selves into society, impacting their ability to achieve a sense of successful aging. All of the participants in this study have developed strategies to live less encumbered lives. However, it is important for those who work with or serve this population to consider that many members of this cohort have experienced injurious events and rejection (Kertzner et al. 2009; Moradi et al. 2010) and may find it difficult to access social and community-based services. Barriers to participation in mainstream environments include assumed heterosexuality, lack of respect for one's personhood, fear of being harassed or discriminated against by the staff or others, fear of being outed, and the lack of LGBT and African American cultural sensitivity markers in the physical environment (Pope et al. 2007; Woody 2011). Consequently, this group of older, black, LGB individuals may need cultural markers to access services.

Through talking with this study's participants, this research has found that in African American communities, the most common indicators people use to ascertain the LGB, racial-ethnic, and aging friendliness of organizations—including churches, community centers, health-care facilities, and senior housing—is word-of-mouth corroboration and the organization's external markers of inclusivity. Such markers could include positive messaging regarding age, race, and sexual orientation in mission statements and advertisements, staff attitudes, and the nature of the physical environment (such as images and artwork, material objects, foods, layout, etc.).

Equally important to remember is that this cohort of older black LGB individuals has proven resilient. Several participants remarked on how getting older freed them up to be able to say yes or no, and to do things they had been hesitant to do in their youth. All agreed that challenges based on racial or gender oppression had made it easier later to deal with oppressions based on age. Many have a highly developed network of people whom they call their family of choice. Their worldview of successful aging seemed to focus less on physical activity, enhanced cognitive ability, and individual health, and more on community and the ability to be connected to family, friends, and each other. This view of aging successfully has allowed many of these elders the freedom to "be themselves," and the capacity to share whole parts of themselves, in their later years.

NOTES

1. See, for instance, Rowe and Kahn 1997 and the introduction to this volume.
2. This chapter uses the words black and African American, and elder and older adult interchangeably.
3. See, for instance, Fredriksen-Goldsen et al. 2013; Ward et al. 2014; http://www.healthy people.gov/2020/proposed-objective-landing-page/lesbian-gay-bisexual-and-transgender -health, accessed 3 February 2016; and http://www.cdc.gov/nchs/ppt/hp2020/hp2020_LGBT _SDOH_progress_review_presentation.pdf, accessed 3 February 2016.
4. "Improving the Lives of LGBT Older Adults." http://www.lgbtmap.org/file/improving -the-lives-of-lgbt-older-adults.pdf, accessed 3 August 2015.
5. The chapter draws on my earlier work in Woody 2011, 2014.
6. To protect the confidentiality of all participants, pseudonyms are used.

REFERENCES

Butler, Robert. 2005. "Ageism: Looking Back Over My Shoulder." *Generations* 24 (3): 84–86.
Calasanti, Toni. 2005. "Ageism, Gravity, and Gender: Experiences of Aging Bodies." *Generations* 24 (3): 8–12.
Fredriksen-Goldsen, Karen I., Hyun-Jun Kim, Susan E. Barkan, Anna Muraco, and Charles P. Hoy-Ellis. 2013. "Health Disparities among Lesbian, Gay, and Bisexual Older Adults: Results from a Population-Based Study." *American Journal of Public Health* 103 (10): 1802–1809.
Gabbay, Sarah, and James Wahler. 2002. "Lesbian Aging: Review of a Growing Literature." *Journal of Gay and Lesbian Social Services* 14 (3): 1–21.
Grant, Jaime M. (with Gerard Koskovich, M. Somjen Frazer, Sunny Bjerk, and Lead Collaborator, Services and Advocacy for GLBT Elders: SAGE). 2010. "Outing Age 2010: Public Policy Issues Affecting Lesbian, Gay, Bisexual, and Transgender Elders." National Gay and Lesbian Task Force Policy Institute. http://www.lgbtagingcenter.org/resources/ pdfs/OutingAge2010.pdf, accessed August 3, 2015.
Kertzner, Robert M., Ilan H. Meyer, David M. Frost, and Michael J. Stirratt. 2009. "Social and Psychological Well-Being in Lesbians, Gay Men, and Bisexuals: The Effects of Race, Gender, Age, and Sexual Identity." *American Journal of Orthopsychiatry* 79 (4): 500–510.

McLoughlin, Rita, and Lillian Faderman. 2009. "Interview with Lillian Faderman: Chronicles of LGBT Struggles." *Socialist Review*, no. 333 (February). http://socialistreview.org .uk/333/interview-lillian-faderman-chronicles-lgbt-struggles, accessed February 8, 2016.

Moradi, Bonnie, Marcie Wiseman, Cirleen DeBlaere, Anthony Sarkees, Melinda Goodman, Melanie Brewster, and Yu-Ping Huang. 2010. "LGB of Color and White Individuals' Perception of Heterosexist Stigma, Internalized Homophobia and Outness: Comparison of Levels and Links." *Counseling Psychologist* 38 (3): 397–424.

Pope, Mark, Edward Wierzalia, Bob Barret, and Michael Rankin. 2007. "Sexual Intimacy Issues for Aging Gay Men." *Adultspan Journal* 6 (2): 68–82.

Rowe, John W., and Robert L. Kahn. 1997. "Successful Aging." *Gerontologist* 37 (4): 433–440.

Strom, Robert, Theodora Carter, and Katherine Schmidt. 2004. "African Americans in Senior Settings: On the Need for Educating Grandparents." *Educational Gerontology* 30: 287–303.

Szymanski, Dawn, and Arpana Gupta. 2009. "Examining the Relationship between Multiple Internalized Oppressions and African American, Lesbian, Gay, Bisexual, and Questioning Persons' Self-Esteem and Psychological Distress." *Journal of Counseling Psychology* 56 (1): 110–118.

Ward, Brian W., James M. Dahlhamer, Adena M. Galinsky, and Sarah Joestl. 2014. "Sexual Orientation and Health among U.S. Adults: National Health Interview Survey, 2013." *National Health Statistics Reports* 77 (July 15): 1–10. http://www.cdc.gov/nchs/data/nhsr/ nhsr077.pdf, accessed August 3, 2015.

Wilson, Bianca. 2005. "African American Lesbian Sexual Culture: Exploring Components and Contradictions." PhD diss., University of Illinois at Chicago.

Wilson, Bianca, and Robin Miller. 2002. "Strategies for Managing Heterosexism Used among African American Gay and Bisexual Men." *Journal of Black Psychology* 28 (4): 371–391.

Woody, Imani. 2011. "Lift Every Voice: A Qualitative Exploration of Ageism and Heterosexism as Experienced by Older African American Lesbian Women and Gay Men When Addressing Social Services Needs." PhD diss., Capella University.

———. 2014. "Aging Out: A Qualitative Exploration of Ageism and Heterosexism among African American Lesbians and Gay Men." *Journal of Homosexuality* 61: 145–165.

4

Erectile Dysfunction as Successful Aging in Mexico

EMILY WENTZELL

Introduction: Selling Youthful Sexuality as "Successful Aging"

I found this Viagra ad (fig. 4.1) among the materials a pharmaceutical sales representative gave to a urologist in Mexico. The ad defines "successful aging" as something that requires pharmaceutical assistance. It shows a handsome and fit man, whose back has been scratched by a partner in the throes of sexual ecstasy, sleeping contentedly next to a note that reads, "Thanks, you were incredible! You acted like you were twenty." Viagra is mentioned only in the discreet outline of the now iconic blue pill shape in the lower right corner. Ideals about aging, sexuality, and manliness are embedded in this ad in similarly subtle but powerful ways. It sends the message that youthfulness—having sex like a twenty-year-old—is sexy and masculine, so, conversely, having sex like an older person must be unappealing and emasculating. The ad reassures those who receive this message that a man can maintain his youth, virility, and appeal through drug-assisted sexual penetration.

Viagra came on the scene in both the United States and Mexico in 1998, as one of many "lifestyle drugs" that have emerged in recent decades. Lifestyle drugs are pharmaceutical treatments for bodily changes and conditions that cause social distress rather than physical harm. These treatments—ranging from baldness cures to eyelash lengtheners—can provide real relief from the pain of feeling like one's body is not looking or performing the way it should. However, the marketing and use of these drugs also conceals the fact that the sources of that emotional pain are *social* expectations for how bodies should be. By enabling people to medicate their bodies and behaviors into line with these cultural ideals, lifestyle drugs make those social expectations seem natural. So, rather than questioning or challenging cultural expectations, people

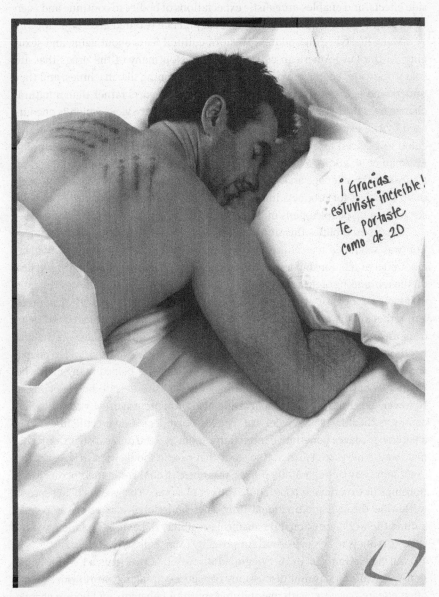

FIGURE 4.1. "Thanks, you were incredible! You acted like you were twenty!" Viagra ad from Mexico.

who cannot meet them increasingly turn to pills that will change their bodies. This situation increases health care costs, exposes people to dangerous drug side effects, and enables unrealistic expectations of bodies to continue and even to be promoted in advertising and medical practice (Conrad and Leiter 2004).

Many lifestyle drugs address Western cultural fears about aging and sexuality. In the Euro-American cultures that develop many of the drugs that are sold worldwide, people often see bodies as functioning like machines, and they understand aging as the breakdown of component parts rather than a natural change over time (Grace et al. 2006). From this point of view, which is encouraged by the expanding market for drug sales to older people, aging itself has come to be seen as a medical problem to be treated (Estes and Binney 1989; Fishman et al. 2008). When this trend meets the longstanding cultural stigma against sex in older age and valorization of youthfulness as a key marker of sexiness, a market for products intended to make older people look, act, and have sex like young people opens up.

Viagra exemplifies this trend. Before Viagra, men's difficulty attaining erection was seen as a typical aspect of aging, or in the cases of younger men, an emotional or relationship issue. The marketing of Viagra and similar drugs relied on the rebranding of these earlier concepts into the biological pathology "erectile dysfunction," or "ED," which cast decreased erectile function as a medical problem rather than a normal change (Tiefer 2006). This medical understanding of decreased erectile function has had a range of social consequences. On the one hand, it has been used to counter the damaging stereotype that older people should not be sexual (Hodson and Skeen 1994) and has helped many men who wanted to have penetrative sex to achieve that desire despite bodily changes. However, ED drugs and their marketing also promote a narrow vision of what counts as "healthy" sex in older age. The idea that decreased erectile function is a pathology makes penetrative intercourse seem like the only satisfying or legitimate way to have sex. Further, it suggests that people should want to have sex the exact same way throughout their lives, regardless of changes in their bodies, relationships or experiences (Gott 2005; Potts et al. 2004). This view is being spread worldwide through multinational drug sales and global marketing, as people around the world are offered the medical possibility of having—and the pressure to use products to achieve—youthful sexuality (Marshall and Katz 2002).

All this is implicit in the Viagra ad discussed above. This ad typifies current medical and cultural discussions of "successful aging" worldwide, which often equate "success" with maintaining youthful behaviors and bodies as long as possible over the life course. However, this emphasis on eternal youth fails to reflect the possibility that people might find meaning and value in bodily and behavioral change over time. Researchers who talk to men and their sexual partners have found that despite these pervasive discussions of the need to medicate away age-related changes in sexuality, many men and their partners do not want to use drugs like Viagra, or do not like them when they try them.

For example, researchers from the United States and New Zealand, where ED drugs are marketed directly to consumers, found that some men reported joy at being able to continue frequent, penetrative sex (frequently with younger extramarital partners). However, other men and many women felt that the drugs precluded a "natural" change toward less energetic but more intimate marital sex, although some felt social pressure to use ED drugs despite this concern (Loe 2004; Potts et al. 2004). Some men also reported not liking the mechanical feel of drug-assisted erections, while some couples felt that men's decreased erectile function led them to be more creative with nonpenetrative sexual activities and increased their pleasure overall (Potts 2005). Worldwide, people also often find meaning and pleasure in the sexual and social changes spurred by decreasing erectile function or other physical aspects of aging. In countries as diverse as India, Ghana, Sweden, and Japan, researchers have found that people often share cultural expectations that sex in relationships will decrease or end with aging and that this is a positive, healthy, and socially productive change (Lamb 2000; Moore 2010; Sandberg 2011; van der Geest 2001).

In this chapter I will discuss this attitude among older, working-class Mexican men. Despite a cultural context where penetrative sex has long been a key marker of masculinity, and the ubiquity of ED drug marketing and the ideas about sexuality it promotes, men in this demographic overwhelmingly reject the idea of using ED drugs. Instead, they see having less sex in older age *as* successful aging. Over the courses of these men's lives, cultural ideals have shifted from expectations that men will be "macho" in their sexual practices, to idealization of men being faithful, caring, and emotionally present for their families. Amid that societal shift, the men I worked with usually came to see decreasing erectile function not as a medical pathology but as a bodily reprieve from macho sexual urges. They believed that this physical change enabled them to become better people by helping them to live out mature, domestically oriented masculinities rather than focusing on penetrative sex after it had become socially and age inappropriate. Their experiences demonstrate the need to investigate what "successful" aging actually means in diverse global contexts and to critique ideas of healthy aging that pathologize bodily changes in ways that increase drug company revenues but limit the range of options older people have for living well.

The Mexican Context

Mexican men make decisions about whether or not to use ED drugs amid heated national debate about who men are and how they should be. For decades, especially in urban areas, people have called for increasing equity between men and women. Divisions of household labor have become more equal as fertility rates have dropped and women have entered the workforce in increasing numbers, and people explicitly see these changes as helping the nation to become modern (Carillo 2007; García and de Oliveira 2004; INEGI 2009). Ideals of love and marriage have also changed. The key reasons people say they want to marry have shifted from economic stability to emotional intimacy (Hirsch 2003).

These changes have all led to widespread public critiques of "machismo," a kind of masculinity associated with womanizing, infidelity, and emotional closure. The belief that machismo is traditional to Mexico is actually relatively new, popularized by poet Octavio Paz in the 1950s ([1961] 1985); many people in Mexico view it as a negative and racist stereotype rather than an accurate portrayal of real men's characters (Gutmann 1996). Nevertheless, in Mexican popular culture it has become understood as something that is innate to Mexican men, and even critiques of machismo tend to frame it as a natural attribute that men should repress, rather than a harmful fiction (Amuchástegui Herrera 2008).

Current ideals of masculinity reflect aspects of machismo, especially the idea that having lots of penetrative sex is a key marker of manliness, but also emphasize responsibility, fidelity, and care for one's partner and family as important ways to be a good man in today's society (Inhorn and Wentzell 2011; Ramirez 2009). Importantly, Mexican men often see bodily changes related to reproductive health, like undergoing vasectomy, as ways to demonstrate this responsibility (Gutmann 2007; Huerta Rojas 2007). Since many Mexican men also see changing over time in socially appropriate ways as a key part of being good men (de Keijzer and Rodriguez 2007; Escobar Latapí 2003), changing the ways they have sex as they age can be a powerful way in which men disassociate themselves from macho masculinities and begin to live out alternative forms of manliness associated with respectable aging (Wentzell 2013).

Yet this trend is in tension with both "traditional" ideas of Mexican masculinity and the marketing messages associated with ED drugs. Viagra and similar drugs have been available in Mexico without a prescription for almost twenty years. ED became a major topic of conversation immediately after the drugs' introduction. Today Viagra jokes figure prominently in TV comedy, and the label "Viagra" is frequently attached to food items thought to have reinvigorating properties. For instance, when I was dining at a seafood restaurant, I received after-dinner mints with "Viagra" printed on the back—the owner explained that it was a joke, since seafood was said to be an aphrodisiac. While direct-to-consumer pharmaceutical ads are not allowed in Mexico, both ED pharmaceuticals and herbal copycats, such as Powersex and Himcaps, are very visible, with colorful signs advertising them on most pharmacy walls. M-force, an herbal supplement said to treat ED, advertises frequently on Mexican network television, and a private clinic specializing in ED treatment runs regular ads in cities' local newspapers. Thus, men experiencing decreasing erectile function in Mexico cannot help but know that their condition could be labeled as the medical pathology ED and treated with drugs.

Whether men can afford ED drugs is another story. ED drug costs are moderate but not cheap, and thus beyond the financial reach of many in a country with marked economic inequality. ED medications have been dispensed free of charge to older men in Mexico City in a government attempt to raise morale among the aged, and an ED pharmaceutical has also been included in the list of drugs that government hospitals must provide cost free to eligible patients (CNN 2008; IMSS 2010). However, at the hospital where I did my research the drugs were actually not offered due to shortages. This is likely also the case at other resource-strapped public health institutions. Thus, working-class Mexican men make treatment decisions regarding decreased erectile function in a context where ED drugs are all around but may be financially difficult to access. Together with social reasons that I will discuss later, these structural barriers contributed to older men's common rejection of the idea of seeking medical treatment for decreased erectile function.

Research Site and Methods

This research was based in the urology department of a government-run hospital in the central Mexican city of Cuernavaca. I chose this setting because it enabled me to meet a large group of men who were experiencing decreased erectile function and was a context in which it was socially appropriate to discuss that issue. The hospital is part of the Mexican Social Security System (Instituto Mexicano del Seguro Social, or IMSS), one of a set of government institutions that offer free health care to Mexican citizens. Since the IMSS provides comprehensive care but sometimes requires long patient waits, IMSS-eligible patients who can afford to often seek private practice care for issues that are not costly to treat. That meant that the urology patients I worked with tended to be working class. This study involved over 250 interviews with male patients, about 50 of which included the wives or family members who accompanied the men to their appointments. The urologists asked patients who they believed might be experiencing decreased erectile function if they would like to participate in a study on health-related changes in sexuality, and most said they would. After I explained my study and the participants signed informed consent forms, we did Spanish-language interviews that ranged from fifteen minutes to over an hour. We talked about their health problems, life histories, sexual function changes, and experiences of medical treatment. Study participants ranged in age from their early twenties to mid-nineties, but most were in their fifties and sixties. Almost 70 percent of participants reported a decrease in their erectile function, although only 11 percent sought medical treatment for this change.

In a context of rushed medical appointments, the vast majority of participants reported that they were happy to talk about their experiences with someone who wanted to listen. Being a woman facilitated these conversations, as men reported that they felt more able to reveal intimate and emotional information to a woman than they would with another man. Being American also helped, since participants often stated that they expected American women to be more sexually knowledgeable than Mexican women, and so they did not feel ashamed to discuss frankly even stigmatized sexual experience.

The Benefits of Decreased Erectile Function

Since I met them in a hospital, it was clear that all the study participants saw medicine as a useful way to deal with unwanted bodily changes. However, they rarely saw decreased erectile function as a medical problem. Instead, they tended to describe it as a normal aspect of aging. Most men explained that their erectile function was simply "not like before," making the matter-of-fact statement that neither men's bodies, desires, nor social lives were the same as when they were younger. For instance, a fifty-five-year-old delivery truck driver reported that he now experienced erections only infrequently, but that this was a normal consequence of age and hard work. He said, "My work is a little rough, heavy. I carry a lot, so I feel a little tiredness. Now, I can't have as much sex as before. This is normal. Now it's not the same—when I was young, more potency. Now with my age, not anymore." Similarly, a retired electrician in his late sixties equated cessation of sex explicitly with the end of youthful occupation, joking, "It's part of being retired—I can't work anymore!"

Rather than believing that men had to have frequent penetrative sex throughout their lives to age successfully, participants overwhelmingly valued respectably age-appropriate forms of manhood. They said that for young men, good masculinity included frequent, often extramarital, penetrative sex, but only in the context of hard work and responsible economic provision for one's family. Although these older men had grown up in a time when it was seen as appropriate for younger men to be highly and extramaritally sexually active—to the point where a man who had always been faithful to his wife apologized that he knew this practice was "not normal"—men saw persistent performance of youthful sexuality as somewhat absurd in older age. In response to a question about whether he continued to engage in sex, a sixty-eight-year-old barber laughed and said, "Here in Mexico we have a saying: 'After old age, chickenpox.' It means that some things become silly when one is older." This absurdity came from the idea that good older masculinity centered on family and home rather than on friends and lovers. Although older men were still expected to provide for their families financially and to work hard, they believed that this work should become domestically oriented. Participants said that as older men they felt duty bound to provide emotional support and family leadership—for instance, in terms of being a "role model" for grandchildren—which they had not seen as important to being good men or husbands in their younger years.

For instance, a fifty-six-year-old planned the following after his retirement from the public health service: "I will dedicate myself to my wife, the house, gardening, caring for the grandchildren—the Mexican classic." Participants frequently described this change of focus as a "second stage" or "other level" of life. They said that erectile function change was a natural element of this stage because it signaled that their youth had ended. They discussed frequent, penetrative sex as a pleasurable practice that had been crucial to their past understandings of themselves as men, but it was no longer an important focus in their lives. For example, a seventy-five-year-old retired factory worker explained, "Erectile dysfunction isn't important. When I was young it would have been, but not now." Similarly, a sixty-four-year-old retired mechanic stated that his "sex life now doesn't exist, doesn't exist. But I'm satisfied, from my youth. I don't miss it." Many participants reported that their onset of erectile difficulty was the catalyst that had prompted them to mature. They also saw maturing over time as a positive process through which they became better men. A sixty-eight-year-old appliance repairman discussed his shift from frequent extramarital sex in his youth to being largely faithful as an older man, explaining, "With age, you start to think more."

ED Drugs as Socially and Physically Harmful

Thoughtfulness about age-related changes extended to the ways men treated their bodies. They often thought that carelessness in their youth had damaged their bodies, for instance attributing current heart disease to a history of anger and violence, or decreased erectile function to the exhaustion caused by decades of grueling physical labor. So, many men who felt that their bodies had become fragile sought to avoid youthfully vigorous sex in order to preserve their health. For instance, a sixty-four-year-old retiree said, "I've had prostate cancer for two years, so [I do] nothing sexual, because I'm taking care of myself. . . . I don't know if it's because of the medications or what, but I haven't felt—for example, I don't even have erections. No desire, I'm calm. I feel good. Very calm, and the only thing that worries me is my health." In general, most participants saw abstinence for health as a responsible move that supported, rather than undermined, good masculinity in older age. For example, a sixty-four-year-old small business owner told

me that he was abstaining after prostate surgery and related complications, but
he noted explicitly that this change did not make him feel like less of a man. He
said, "I don't have much sex because of hygiene, for health, because I'm bleeding,
et cetera. That doesn't mean that I'm no longer a man."

Other participants abstained from sex out of concern for their sexual partners' health. For instance, a seventy-four-year-old who had become faithful to
his wife said that because of her hypertension and recent stroke, "We don't have
sex because my wife is sick . . . but I'm not going to die. It's not necessary, it's not
urgent. In my youth, I enjoyed it enough." Other men did not have romantic partners and so rejected the idea of using ED drugs because it would mean returning
to the casual sex they had had in their youths, which they perceived as risky. For
instance, a single, sixty-eight-year-old retired truck driver told me that he would
not consider using ED drugs "for fear of a [sexually transmitted] illness."

Most men believed that bodily slowing in general and decreased erectile
function in particular were natural consequences of a lifetime of hard work.
Further, they saw this slowing as positive. They often described the reduction
in general and sexual energy that they experienced as part of older age as an aid
for acting in the ways that they thought respectable older men should. Because
of that view, many participants believed that ED drugs would artificially "accelerate" one's body, putting it through socially and physically inappropriate
paces that could hasten aging and potentially cause premature death. Many
men expressed fear of the drugs, making comments like a sixty-eight-year-old
retiree's observation that "Viagra scares me." Elaborating on the cause of this
fear, a seventy-eight-year-old food vendor stated that ED drugs "accelerate you,
to your death. Many friends have told me, they will accelerate you a lot, then
you'll collapse, that stuff will kill you." Participants sometimes worked this idea
into perhaps apocryphal stories of ED drugs harming relatives or neighbors. For
example, a plumber in his late fifties reported that "people are dying of Viagra!
They get excited, have heart attacks. I had an old uncle, he 'got Viagraed.' He
stayed there on top, like a sea turtle—with the girl under him! . . . There are lots
of rumors about Viagra here in Mexico, lots of fear." This idea that the possible
dangers of ED drug treatment outweighed its benefits was rooted in the notion
that youthful levels of sex were simply inappropriate to, and perhaps physically
harmful during, older age. Overall, study participants understood ED drugs to be
physically dangerous *because* they were socially inappropriate.

Accepting Decreased Erectile Function

Given the emphasis that most of these men placed on penetrative sex as a marker
of manliness in their youths, men often appeared to go through a process of
adjustment in which they came to accept that they were older and that the kind

of sex that was desirable for them had changed. Most participants were married, and they reported that their wives were key to the emergence of their desires to mature and cease youthful sexuality. In keeping with changing cultural values for marriage and masculinity, men who had focused on extramarital sex in their youths often saw decreased erectile function as an aid to becoming better, more faithful husbands later in life. For example, a fifty-five-year-old retired laundry worker who said, "I was a womanizer," explained that because of bodily aging, "The truth is, now I don't have the same capacity. I'm fifty-five, I know what I am. I don't want problems with my wife. Like I deserve respect from her, she deserves it from me as well." For him, not being physically able to cheat made it possible to be the kind of husband he thought an older man should be.

Similarly, a sixty-eight-year-old retired power company worker reported that he was not concerned that an upcoming prostate operation might end his erectile function. He said, "I'm satisfied, I passed my best years, I'm happy. We've [my wife and I] enjoyed ourselves." He went on to say that cessation of erectile function would cause a shift in his relationship with his wife, in which he would not only become faithful but strive to support and appreciate her more fully. He explained, "Now I will completely dedicate myself to her. Recognize that she has done everything for me, whatever I did she has always been with me. She cares for me, and I care for her too, and we have to get along well." Men who had already made this shift reported increasing contentment in their relationships. A ninety-year-old retired bodyguard, reporting that he had not had sex with his wife for six years, said, "Life, love, compassion all grow. With time, they are deeper." Rather than feeling like successful men because of their sexual conquests, study participants stated that they now took pride in being loving, emotionally present husbands, fathers, and grandfathers. A sixty-seven-year-old bakery owner summed up this notion, saying, "Married life [meaning marital sexuality] is like a plant that dries up over time, the force ceases. When you get old, you're more tired—spending time together is more important. Spending time together happily."

Despite their acceptance, some of these men were dismayed when they first began to experience erectile difficulty, since it did not fit in with their youthful understandings of themselves as men. Conversations with wives and other family members were crucial for helping them rethink the relationship between sex and masculinity. For example, in a joint interview with a sixty-eight-year-old laborer and his wife, the husband said that he had recently been experiencing less-firm erections and that he was bothered by this change, adding that he believed that his wife "doesn't like it." She corrected him by asserting that the change was natural and acceptable, saying, "It wasn't the same, but it's not serious, it happens with age and health problems."

Most older women interviewed, including those who said that they enjoyed sex, described its cessation as part of the natural life course and reported that helping their husbands feel good about bodily changes was more important to them than continuing to have penetrative sex. Many said that emotional tenderness and physical closeness, without penetration, was satisfying and appropriate for this phase of their marriage. Women who had not enjoyed their marital sex lives more emphatically encouraged their husbands to adopt older age-appropriate masculinities that did not involve sexual contact. For instance, when a retired husband in his sixties somewhat sadly revealed that "the machinery of erection has broken down," his wife interjected, "Now we don't want any more!"

Exemplifying this process of change, a sixty-one-year-old construction worker reported that he initially experienced decreasing sexual function as a threat to his masculinity and marriage. However, he said that interactions with his wife led him to see this shift as socially, mentally, and physically beneficial. When his erectile function began to wane, he said, "I thought, I'll be useless, my wife will cheat on me. But now I've changed. I don't want to wander the streets, I'm dedicated to the home." He reported that his wife convinced him over time that communication and enjoying shared activities were more important to her, and for their marriage, than sex. As the importance of sex to his masculine sense of self lessened and he and his wife grew emotionally closer, he noted that their sex life underwent a "beautiful change." They had sex on the less frequent schedule that she desired, and she now "sets the conditions" for their sexual activity. He said that sex became more pleasurable for them both, rather than an obligation for her. Further, he reported relief at no longer having the "sick mind" that led him to desire sex constantly in his youth, the frequency of which he believes stressed his prostate and caused his current health problems.

Conclusion: Rethinking Successful Aging

Overall, medical and ED drug marketing narratives asserting that "successful" aging requires unceasing penetrative sex throughout older age have not led most of the working-class, Mexican men I interviewed to desire ED treatment. Instead, many of these men believed that decreasing erectile function had social benefits. It helped them to have sex and relationships that they saw as appropriate for respectable older men, which involved changes ranging from cessation of all sexual practice, to newfound fidelity, to less frequent but more tender sex with their wives. These changes were aspects of a broader social shift toward emphasis on the family and home that most study participants believed was appropriate for older men and that also helped men who had grown up with now-outdated ideas of masculinity change with the times. Further, because they came to see decreased erectile function as a natural change that helped them to live out good masculinity in older age, many study participants believed ED drugs to be silly at best, and deadly at worst.

These men's experiences demonstrate the inadequacy of medical models of sexuality and aging that do not account for cultural context, and thus conceal the possibility that people might experience decreasing sexual function as desirable rather than "dysfunctional." By spreading Euro-American ideas of aging as a pathology and defining successful aging as staying young with the help of medicines, ED drugs and their marketing threaten to reduce the diversity of understandings of what positive aging means around the world. Narrowing ideas of how sexuality should be in later life, and of what constitutes healthy masculinity for older men, will increase pharmaceutical company revenues while decreasing the range of options older people have for living well. We can fight against this trend by basing our ideas of successful aging on people's diverse and culturally specific social needs, rather than on the expectation that healthy aging means "staying as young as possible" for everyone, everywhere. Doing that can counter the trend of marketing visions of successful aging that require people to take costly medications that may have significant negative side effects, and that pathologize bodily changes that people might otherwise be inclined not only to accept but to welcome.

ACKNOWLEDGMENTS

I am grateful to all the study participants for sharing the intimate details of their lives with me and for the physicians at the IMSS for making this research possible. I also thank Fulbright IIE, the Wenner-Gren Foundation, and the American Association of University Women for funding this research. This chapter is adapted from my 2013 article "Aging Respectably by Rejecting Medicalization: Mexican Men's Reasons for Not Using Erectile Dysfunction Drugs," published in *Medical Anthropology Quarterly* 27 (1): 3–22.

REFERENCES

Amuchástegui Herrera, Ana. 2008. "La masculinidad como culpa esencial: Subjetivación, género y tecnología de sí en un programa de reeducación para hombres violentos." In *II Congreso Nacional Los Estudios de Género de los Hombres en México: Caminos andados y nuevos retos en investigación y acción*. Mexico City.

Carillo, Héctor. 2007. "Imagining Modernity: Sexuality, Policy, and Social Change in Mexico. Sexuality Research and Social Policy." *Journal of NSRC* 4 (3): 74–91.

CNN. 2008. "Elderly Men to Get Free Viagra in Mexico City." 14 November. http://www.cnn .com/2008/WORLD/americas/11/14/mexico.city.viagra, accessed 8 February 2016.

Conrad, Peter, and Valerie Leiter. 2004. "Medicalization, Markets, and Consumers." *Journal of Health and Social Behavior* 45: 158–176.

de Keijzer, Benno, and Gabriela Rodriguez. 2007. "Hombres rurales: Nueva generación en un mundo cambiante." In *Sucede que me canso de ser hombre: Relatos y reflexiones sobre hombres y masculinidades en México*, edited by A. Amuchastegui and I. Szasz, 241–274. Mexico City: El Colegio de México.

Escobar Latapí, Agustín. 2003. "Men and Their Histories: Restructuring, Gender Inequality, and Life Transitions in Urban Mexico." In *Changing Men and Masculinities in Latin America*, edited by Matthew C. Gutmann, 84–114. Durham, NC: Duke University Press.

Estes, Carroll L., and Elizabeth A. Binney. 1989. "The Biomedicalization of Aging: Dangers and Dilemmas." *Gerontologist* 29 (5): 587–596.

Fishman, Jennifer R., Robert H. Binstock, and Marcie A. Lambrix. 2008. "Anti-aging Science: The Emergence, Maintenance, and Enhancement of a Discipline." *Journal of Aging Studies* 22 (4): 295–303.

García, Brígida, and Orlandina de Oliveira. 2004. "El ejercicio de la paternidad en el México urbano." In *Imágenes de la familia en el cambio de siglo*, edited by M. Ariza and O. D. Oliveira, 283–320. Mexico City: Instituto de Investigaciones Sociales, Universidad Nacional Autónoma de México.

Gott, Merryn. 2005. *Sexuality, Sexual Health, and Ageing*. New York: Open University Press.

Grace, Victoria, Annie Potts, Nicola Gavey, and Tina Vares. 2006. "The Discursive Condition of Viagra." *Sexualities* 9 (3): 295–314.

Gutmann, Matthew C. 1996. *The Meanings of Macho: Being a Man in Mexico City*. Berkeley: University of California Press.

——. 2007. *Fixing Men: Sex, Birth Control, and AIDS in Mexico*. Berkeley: University of California Press.

Hirsch, Jennifer. 2003. *A Courtship after Marriage: Sexuality and Love in Mexican Transnational Families*. Berkeley: University of California Press.

Hodson, D., and P. Skeen. 1994. "Sexuality and Ageing: The Hammerlock of Myths." *Journal of Applied Gerontology* 13 (3): 219–235.

Huerta Rojas, Fernando. 2007. "El cuerpo masculino como escenario de la vasectomía: Una experiencia con un grupo de hombres de las ciudades de México y Puebla." In *Sucede que me canso de ser hombre: Relatos y reflexiones sobre hombres y masculinidades en México*, edited by A. Amuchastegui and I. Szasz, 479–518. Mexico City: El Colegio de México.

IMSS. 2010. Cuadro Basico, Nefrologia y Urologia, vol. 2010: IMSS.

INEGI. 2009. Geográfica, Vol. 2009.

Inhorn, Marcia C., and Emily Wentzell. 2011. "Embodying Emergent Masculinities: Reproductive and Sexual Health Technologies in the Middle East and Mexico." *American Ethnologist* 38 (4): 801–815.

Lamb, Sarah. 2000. *White Saris and Sweet Mangoes: Aging, Gender, and Body in North India*. Berkeley: University of California Press.

Loe, Meika. 2004. *The Rise of Viagra: How the Little Blue Pill Changed Sex in America*. New York: New York University Press.

Marshall, Barbara L., and Stephen Katz. 2002. "Forever Functional: Sexual Fitness and the Ageing Male Body." *Body and Society* 8 (4): 43–70.

Moore, Katrina L. 2010. "Sexuality and Sense of Self in Later Life: Japanese Men's and Women's Reflections on Sex and Aging." *Journal of Cross-cultural Gerontology* 25 (2): 149–163.

Paz, Octavio. (1961) 1985. *The Labyrinth of Solitude and Other Writings*. Translated by L. Kemp. New York: Grove Weidenfeld.

Potts, Annie. 2005. "Cyborg Masculinity in the Viagra Era." *Sexualities, Evolution and Gender* 7 (1): 3–16.

Potts, Annie, V. Grace, N. Gavey, and T. Vares. 2004. "'Viagra Stories': Challenging 'Erectile Dysfunction.'" *Social Science and Medicine* 59 (3): 489–499.

Ramirez, Josué. 2009. *Against Machismo: Young Adult Voices in Mexico City*. New York: Berghahn Books.

Sandberg, Linn. 2011. "Getting Intimate: A Feminist Analysis of Old Age, Masculinity, and Sexuality," vol. 527: Linköping University Electronic Press.

Tiefer, Leonore. 2006. "The Viagra Phenomenon." *Sexualities* 9 (3): 273–294.

van der Geest, Sjaak. 2001. "'No Strength': Sex and Old Age in a Rural Town in Ghana." *Social Science and Medicine* 53: 1383–1396.

Wentzell, Emily A. 2013. *Maturing Masculinities: Aging, Chronic Illness, and Viagra in Mexico.* Durham, NC: Duke University Press.

PART II

Ideals of Independence,
Interdependence, and
Intimate Sociality
in Later Life

5

Beyond Independence

Older Chicagoans Living Valued Lives

ELANA D. BUCH

Eileen Silverman[1] had lived alone ever since her husband died of a sudden heart attack when she was fifty-three. They met as law school classmates and married just before he left to fight in World War II. Mrs. Silverman never practiced law; instead, she ran the family's men's clothing store until after the war and then stayed home raising their children. When Mr. Silverman died, their children were grown and out of the house. Overwhelmed by memories, she sold their home and bought an apartment in a high-rise nearby. She had once had friends in her building and across the neighborhood; they had weekly bridge games and a daily walking group. When we met in 2006 she was in her late seventies and told me that most of her friends were "all gone. Most of them have left me." Some died, some went to warmer climates, others moved to live near children and grandchildren, and still others "wanted to move into buildings where they serve food."

Mrs. Silverman no longer got out that much unless someone could go with her. Severe scoliosis had hunched her back and she walked unsteadily, supported by a cane. Neither of her children could help as much as they would have liked. Her son, a judge, lived several hours away and came up a couple of weekends a month to help her with paperwork, bills, and the like. Her daughter lived only a few blocks away and visited Mrs. Silverman most weeks, but also had her hands full caring for an adult son with significant disabilities. They urged Mrs. Silverman to hire a home care worker, and finally she agreed.

Twice a week, Maria Arellano spent four hours working with Mrs. Silverman, helping her bathe, cleaning the apartment, and doing laundry. The two of them took weekly trips to the grocery store and library, stocking up on the food and books that nourished Mrs. Silverman during the many hours she spent alone. Maria's careful attention to her needs helped Mrs. Silverman sustain her way of life, as her memory and body weakened. As Mrs. Silverman told me, "She does it all and that's a good thing." Despite the differences in their ages and backgrounds—Maria was from Puerto Rico and Mrs. Silverman was Jewish—Maria was able to intuit and anticipate Mrs. Silverman's needs and desires, rarely asking for instructions. On days when Maria missed work, Mrs. Silverman was reluctant to ask the agency for a substitute: so few workers were able to decipher her needs without constant direction. Mrs. Silverman did not like giving her care workers instructions because it felt like she was "bossing them around" or constantly asking for help. As she told me, "My whole family, we aren't leaners, we don't lean on other people. So I don't like asking for help." For Mrs. Silverman to maintain this sense of independence, her care worker had to be attuned to Mrs. Silverman's needs and desires, able to sustain the older woman's way of life without asking for instructions and thereby drawing attention to Mrs. Silverman's growing need for help. For Mrs. Silverman, like millions of other older Americans, home care played a crucial role in her daily life and sustained her sense of independence, making it an important practice for understanding what it might mean to live a valued or successful life in the United States.

Discussions of successful aging in the United States tend to focus on the ways individuals can optimize and expand the amount of time they remain physically vigorous and independent but have comparatively less to say about what might be perceived as "success" for those experiencing age-related debility. Here I focus on the ways that concerns about personhood—and especially the relationship between independence and personhood—shape the aspirations of older adults in the United States who are adjusting to life with increasing impairment.

Across diverse social and cultural contexts, people rely on diverse ideologies and criteria to understand what kinds of beings count as "persons," a designation that has profound consequences for who is included and excluded in social life. Personhood is a fundamentally relational concept describing people's membership, roles, and status in societies; processes of making and unmaking persons are ongoing throughout the life course and inherently social (Mauss [1935] 1979; Strathern 1988). Individual persons in the United States are typically construed as bounded by physical bodies that house a noncorporeal but continuous "self" or "soul" or "will." Normatively, independent persons should exert agency in the world such that they are mentally, financially, and domestically self-determining and self-sufficient (Kaufman 1994; Luborsky 1994). Thus, concerns about personhood become especially salient for older Americans when increasing frailty and social isolation threaten their ability to live in a way deemed "independent."

In the United States, the ability to exercise agency and autonomy over daily life is a key sign of full adult personhood and is seen as intimately connected to control over homes and property (Radin 1982; Stern 2009). Thus, in the United States many young adults aspire to move out of natal homes to gain independence, while older adults fear losing the independence symbolized by living in their own homes. Recognizing these cultural ideals, John Rowe and Robert Kahn included "continuing to live in one's own home, taking care of one's self" as a central part of their seminal definition of successful aging (1998, 42). Yet how do the ideals of successful aging apply to those like Mrs. Silverman who fall somewhere in the middle—continuing to live in their own homes, but unable to care for themselves without significant assistance?

Home care can be seen as a kind of liminal practice introduced at moments when older adults in the United States first acknowledge their need for assistance and the ways this threatens their personhood. Home care workers like Maria are hired to assist older adults who live in private homes and apartments with what gerontologists call "activities of daily living"—the everyday things people need to do to live, such as bathing, toileting, feeding, cooking, cleaning, and grocery shopping. Thus, many older adults value home care for its potential to sustain their sense of independence, in part because it relieves their kin of the "burden" of their care.

By focusing on the experiences of elderly Chicagoans and the home care workers who help them continue living in their own homes, this chapter highlights both the ways that home care relationships help older adults live valued lives and the ways that home care relations can exacerbate inequality. In Chicago home care workers, who are disproportionately poor women of color, often develop forms of embodied empathy to perform the daily tasks listed above in ways that sustain older adults' ways of life and thus their senses of independence. In the process, they navigate complex differences of race, class, generation, and ability. This kind of care enables workers to perform their tasks without calling attention to their labor, sustaining elders' sense of independence by obscuring their reliance on others. Home care practices that obscure workers' labor simultaneously intensify hierarchies of care and empathy such that elders' abilities to live independently take precedence over workers' abilities to sustain their own lives and households.

This chapter also examines alternative ways that disabled older adults in Chicago craft lives they find meaningful. In these cases, the potential for good and meaningful old age arises not from individual actions and choices but rather from the complex, dynamic social relations in which older adults are embedded. In contrast to the emphasis on independence in broader successful aging discourse, many older adults creatively engage in ever-evolving moral communities comprised of neighbors, kin, friends, television personalities, religious institutions, and home care workers. These efforts suggest possibilities for a good old age that emphasize sociality rather than individual actions and abilities.

Home Care in the United States

Over the last century, improved nutrition, sanitation, and medical care have radically lengthened human lifespans. For those who have access, advanced medical treatments transform once fatal injuries and illnesses into chronic conditions. These conditions often leave survivors requiring care of unprecedented intensity and duration. Due to longstanding gendered divisions of labor, in the United States as elsewhere, women historically have provided the bulk of child care and eldercare required by their families. As economic and social pressures push women of all classes into the paid workforce, individuals and families seek paid care services. Government policies have also increased funding to support home-based and community-based services for older adults in an effort to reduce long-term care costs by helping older adults delay entry into nursing homes as long as possible. Home care services for older adults in the United States are funded by either public programs (typically using a combination of federal Medicaid, Older Americans Act, and state dollars) or by private funds (including both personal savings and insurance). Due to these changes, paid home care has become one of the fastest growing occupations in the United States (BLS 2014).

Home care workers are overwhelmingly women and disproportionately from minority and immigrant backgrounds. In exchange for this crucial labor, home care workers earn poverty-level wages and limited benefits—only one third of home care workers receive health care insurance through their jobs, and a majority of home care workers receive some kind of public assistance to support their families (PHI 2015). As a legacy of racially motivated employment laws, home care work in the United States was until 2015 not protected by the Fair Labor Standards Act, which guarantees minimum wage and overtime pay to most workers (Boris and Klein 2012; Glenn 2012).

This chapter draws on ethnographic fieldwork conducted between 2006 and 2008 in Chicago with the employees and elderly clients of one publicly funded home care agency, which I call Plusmore, and one privately funded agency, which I call Belltower. In Chicago, to qualify for publicly funded home care services, older adults had to demonstrate need for assistance and have savings and assets (excluding their homes) totaling less than $17,500. Older adults receiving services from the publicly funded agency were predominately African American, as were their home care workers. Older adults receiving privately funded home care were most likely to be white, and their home care workers were primarily Filipina, African American, Latina, African, and Polish. During fieldwork, I spent two months at each agency's offices, observing supervisors' daily work fielding phone calls, managing workers, staffing cases, and mediating disputes. In the process, I learned about hundreds of older adults beyond those

I was able to observe directly. Afterward, I spent six to eight months visiting a smaller number of older adults on a weekly or biweekly basis while their home care workers were present and conducted formal life-history interviews with these older adults and workers.

Sustaining Independence, Embodying Difference

To sustain elders' preferences and self-determination in the face of threats to their independence, home care workers used their bodies to create continuity between elders' current lives and past experiences. In doing so, home care workers' prioritized the bodily preferences of their elderly clients above their own. For older adults to be recognized and recognize themselves as independent persons, they first needed to feel and be seen as living self-determined lives. When I asked older adults what it meant to take good care of someone like themselves, they repeatedly told me that there was no single measure, attitude, or practice that defined good care. Instead, they suggested that good care would facilitate self-determination and reflect their preferences. For example, Hattie Washington, an eighty-two-year-old African American Plusmore client, told me, "It's according to who you're taking care of and according to what they want." Elders were unwilling to define or label specific practices "good care," because for them good care was care in which they were treated like a person in ways that recognized their continued subjectivity and almost didn't seem like "care" at all. As Maureen Murphy, a seventy-two-year-old Irish-born Belltower client, told me, "If I have my senses at all, I'd like to be treated as though I have some. I'd like to be treated like a person, and not a piece of furniture." Ms. Murphy poignantly argued that being treated like a person required those who care for her to engage her as an active subject.[2]

To sustain elderly clients' personhood, workers shaped their everyday care practices in ways that not only sustained client's biological life but also reflected their clients' preferences and life experiences. As Maria told me, "I always say that your true self comes out when you're old. . . . Everyone is a person of their own. And I always try to find that little thing that person likes. They pretty much tell you what their thing is if you give them half a chance; they tell you what their surrounding was. . . . So you find their thing and you work with that." With one older woman, Maria made sure to take her on regular walks, since "you just ask her out for a walk and it makes her shine. Even if it's just around the block, it makes her shine." With a client who was very religious, Maria made sure to find time to read the Bible and pray together. Another client had spent his career in the navy, so she began taking him to the beach to watch the boats go by.

Workers developed and drew on the embodied, sensory aspects of empathy to shape everyday care practices in ways that not only sustained client's biological life but also reflected their clients' embodied preferences. This was most apparent in the way workers prepared meals for their clients. Losses of smell and taste, so frequently associated with memory and nostalgia, meant that food sometimes lost its power as a direct sensorial link to older adults' earlier lives. While these losses meant that elders struggled to take pleasure in the act of eating itself, they instead felt pleasure when eating foods they remembered enjoying or from the sociality of eating with others. Workers strove to facilitate this through myriad mundane acts of care—they learned just how small to cut meat or how soft to cook vegetables, so that they could preserve a given food's remembered and pleasurable texture while still rendering it chewable for clients who wore dentures. They adjusted the salt in a dish, seeking to make it more healthful for clients with high blood pressure while retaining enough flavor that their client would enjoy it. Workers held at bay their own senses of how a particular dish should be prepared, for example, by learning to cook a clients' favored German-style macaroni and cheese instead of the southern style learned at their mother's apron strings. By constantly attending to food as both physical and social sustenance, workers prepared meals that reflected elders' histories of subjective experience while also protecting the elders' physical well-being.

Grace Washington's efforts to care for Margee Jefferson exemplified the embodied and empathic skill that workers and older adults alike associated with good care. Margee's children hired Belltower to care for their mother after Margee tripped and fell, lying alone on the floor for several hours before her son came home and helped her up. Margee, whose family was of German descent but had lived in Chicago for at least three generations, was a severe hoarder and struggled to manage her diabetes. Margee's home, which she had shared with her in-laws from the time she was married until they died, was filled to the brim with the collected belongings of three generations of continuous habitation. Grace, an African American woman whose family migrated to Chicago in the mid twentieth century, worked tirelessly in these challenging conditions, striving both to make the home safe but still familiar to Margee. Grace's supervisor wanted Grace to impose a strict routine on Margee's day and radically alter the older woman's diet. However, Grace argued that maintaining familiar bodily routines and ways of life was central to maintaining older adults' well-being and personhood. She told me, "They're old. You can't come in here and say, 'Baby, you got to get up at seven AM.' . . . I let them keep with their daily routine. It may be modified a bit, but I'm not trying to modify it too much where it gets kind of confusing."

To find the balance between subtle modification and confusing changes, Grace empathically imagined what it was like to be Margee's embodied self, reaching across differences of age, race, class, and lifetimes of experience to understand what alterations could be made without disrupting Margee's way of life. In this way, the work of sustaining Margee's independence and way of life was deeply embodied—not only requiring physical effort but also requiring

Grace to inhabit her own body differently. Grace used this imaginative, embodied attunement to make minor changes to Margee's home and meals, all the while challenging her supervisor's instructions to completely alter Margee's way of life. In practice, this meant surreptitiously replacing the sugar in Margee's sugar bowl with a no-calorie sugar substitute, but continuing to provide the older woman with her preferred bananas and cereal. Grace explained to me that she could change the sugar without upsetting Margee because the taste and texture of the substitute were so similar, but there was no breakfast other than bananas and cereal that would satisfy the older woman. Similarly, Grace created some daily routine, by encouraging Margee to rise and sit at the sunny dining room table around lunchtime and by enthusiastically listening to Margee's oft-repeated stories. However, she refused to force Margee to wake up at eight in the morning and get dressed as her supervisor had insisted. Grace argued that if Margee wanted to sleep until eleven, that was her business. As Grace told me, "That was her routine. I'm trying to help her, but I'm not trying to change her whole life. I'm trying to make her feel comfortable in her whole surroundings. . . . These are these people's houses. You can't go in there and tell these people, who are paying you their hard-earned money to come here and help them. They are not saying change them. They are saying they need a little bit of help. You cannot go into these people's houses and change these people's lives according to your standard. You cannot change these people's lifestyle." In respecting that Margee had the right to determine what happened in her own house, and to have her preferences respected by those whom she (or more accurately her daughter) was paying, Grace endorsed widespread American ideologies in which self-determination is thought to flow from control over property and capital. By embodying Margee's very different way of life, Grace subordinated her body to Margee's frailer body, enabling Margee to remain at home and sustaining her sense of independence.

Workers were committed to sustaining their elderly clients' bodily well-being and personhood, and thus they generally accepted that they would work in challenging, uncomfortable, and sometimes unhealthy households. This produced notable asymmetry between workers' care for their clients' well-being and their care for their own well-being, intensifying the inequalities already existing between workers and their clients. Care workers frequently told me about the challenges of working in elders' homes, which were often kept unventilated and hot even in summer months, since so many older adults are easily chilled. Recognizing that older adults might get sick from being in cooler spaces, workers managed their discomfort by wearing lightweight clothing and carrying large bottles of ice water with them.

As Grace Washington worked to sustain Margee Jefferson's routine and independence, she did so in Margee's sensorially overwhelming home. As Grace told me, when she first started working there, "The goddamn house wasn't fit for a dog to live in. . . . You got a room literally with garbage damn near filled to the ceiling. . . . Baby, if a dog went in that bathroom, the dog would turn around and walk away. . . . You got mold coming out the sink, whereas it looks like spiders is in infestation." Despite the hundreds of hours Grace and other Belltower workers had since spent clearing the home of debris, it remained a difficult place to work. The downstairs bathroom, which they had cleaned for hours, still did not meet Grace's standards of cleanliness—she told me that she tried her best not to use the toilet when she was there, despite working eleven-hour days. Nevertheless, she told me, "I didn't complain and I didn't have a problem with that because when I go into a senior's house, I take it as if this is my grandmother." Thus, even though Grace felt the house was "a goddamn garbage place. This is no damn house," and was concerned about the effects of spending so much time there on her health, she argued that it was her moral obligation as a carer to stay there and do what she could to protect her client's way of life and improve her well-being.

While care workers labored among and consumed their clients' sensorial worlds, sustaining clients' ways of life and independence also meant that carers worked to prevent the intrusion of their own sensorial worlds into those of their clients. Agencies exhorted workers to bathe every day, never wear unwashed clothes, and carry deodorant so clients would not have to smell body odors that might accumulate. Live-in workers were advised not to cook or bring "ethnic" food that might leave strange odors in clients' homes. For care workers, caring meant subjecting their bodies to their clients' sensory worlds while limiting their clients' exposure to their own worlds and lives.

For example, as Thanksgiving 2006 approached, Grace worried that the restaurant that Margee and her son favored would be closed for the holiday. Wanting to make sure Margee would still be able to celebrate in traditional fashion, Grace brought Margee several plates of the special Thanksgiving delicacies she had cooked in preparation for her own family's feast. Though the dishes were southern-style recipes she had learned to cook from her mother rather than the German-style cooking Margee was accustomed to, they included many foods that she knew Margee liked. She had been cooking for weeks, an expression of the love and care she felt for her family and extended to Margee. A week after the holiday, the plates that Grace brought sat in the refrigerator virtually untouched and Margee suggested that I should eat them, since no one else was going to. Grace looked down, disappointed but not surprised, and shrugged, telling me that someone should enjoy the food. While Grace spent eleven hours a day in Margee's overwhelming home, attuning her body to Margee's embodied tastes and daily rhythms, neither she nor Margee felt that the older woman was morally obliged to similarly partake in Grace's life. The wages Grace was paid for her work—approximately $6.75 an hour—and Margee's vulnerability as an older person in need of care, meant that Grace, like other care workers, used her body to partake in and reproduce her client's sensorial world without ever expecting a similar engagement in return.

Rather than take for granted that this kind of bodily asymmetry is a natural part of relationships between care workers and those for whom they care, it is important to attend to the ways that these asymmetries are connected to ideologies of independence that intensify the social and economic inequalities structuring paid care work. This was particularly apparent in debates over whether to expand the Fair Labor Standards Act to guarantee minimum wage and overtime pay to home care workers. Opponents to this expansion argued that increasing workers' wages would threaten the affordability of home care services and older adults' ability to live independently (NAHC 2013). Such arguments rely on naturalized hierarchies between people in which sustaining elders' independence is seen as more important than workers' abilities to sustain their lives and families. Efforts to promote successful aging that focus on promoting self-determination and independence implicitly prioritize the well-being of vulnerable older adults over the well-being of their also-vulnerable care workers, strengthening existing social hierarchies based on race, class, and gender.

Sustaining Moral Relations

While many older adults valued their independence and hoped that home care would sustain it, elders in Chicago also offered other possibilities for imagining and living a good old age. In particular, many older adults created and participated in both new and old moral communities, often drawing their home care workers into these social worlds. In their classic text, Rowe and Kahn (1997, 433) argue that active engagement with life—by which they refer to both interpersonal relations and productive activities—"represents the concept of successful aging most fully." Many discussions of successful aging imply that older adults need to get out of their homes in order to actively engage life—do things, keep busy, be productive!—yet many older adults in Chicago crafted meaningful engagements with moral and social communities while remaining at home. These engagements with kin, neighbors, and the home care workers themselves gave shape to elders' daily lives, infusing them with vital energy and purpose.

Hattie Meyers, an African American woman in her early eighties, lived alone for decades after the deaths of both her sons and her husband. Over the year I knew her, she had a more and more difficult time navigating the steep stairs up to her second-floor apartment and rarely went out. She had been in and out of the hospital for several years, suffered from increasingly painful kidney stones, and was having difficulty managing her diabetes. During one of the hospital stays, a social worker convinced her to hire a home care worker and helped her fill out the paperwork to qualify for publicly funded services from Plusmore. Despite being increasingly homebound, Mrs. Meyers was anything but isolated. Over the years, she had gathered a rich community around her, and they, along with her African American home care worker Loretta, sustained her. Mrs. Meyers sustained them as well. For example, when a longtime friend in the neighborhood died unexpectedly, Mrs. Meyers spent days organizing the visitation at the neighbor's home, making sure people brought the right foods and came at the right times. Tired and unable to navigate the stairs, Mrs. Meyers did not attend the funeral or visitation, but many neighbors and friends came to see her at home afterward.

Despite the loss of her children, Mrs. Meyers was a matriarch, gathering young people around her, taking them under her wing. For example, her neighbor Mandy had moved into a downstairs apartment with a good view of their building's front courtyard about a decade earlier. The first year she moved in, Mrs. Meyers realized Mandy didn't have anything but sandwiches to feed her young son for Christmas dinner, and so she invited the young family to share hers. They had been close ever since, and Mandy and her son both called Mrs. Meyers "Ma." Mandy took Mrs. Meyers to doctor's appointments and grocery shopping. Together, the two women kept an eye on their building, which was in an increasingly dangerous neighborhood. As Mrs. Meyers told me, "She calls fifty times a day. She tells me what's happening out front and I tell her what's going on out back." Loretta, her home care worker, also called Mrs. Meyers "Ma," and Mrs. Meyers in turn worried about Loretta's seemingly violent boyfriend, offering Loretta maternal advice about romantic relationships, children, and finance.

Most mornings, Mrs. Meyers spent several hours on the phone with her nieces and nephews, offering them wisdom and counsel as they navigated the trials of young motherhood, new jobs, troubled relationships. As soon as she had finished eating breakfast and taken her medication, "the phone rings. My niece called, and then the other one called. I said, 'I'm on the phone with your sister.' Then this other one over here calls. All this is really good because if I was dead they'd be over here." She was glad for the conversation, glad that her kin checked on her and worried about her, but even more, it was important to her that they still valued her advice and experience. She told me, "They are all I have. They just call me all day, all night, whatever. The kids and the grandkids, they make me feel so big."

When Loretta or I were not at her apartment, Mrs. Meyers spent her afternoons watching her favorite game show, her soap opera, and cable news. More often than not, her viewing was interrupted by phone calls. Sometimes she would watch her soap opera while on the phone with another friend who was watching, enjoying sharing their reactions to plot twists. Always current on the news, Mrs. Meyers frequently engaged me in lengthy conversations about the 2008 presidential elections. She spoke with equal parts wonder that a black man might win a national election and fear that he would be assassinated in the process, making sure I understood the shock of his growing success for a black woman who grew up in Jim Crow Alabama and later worked as a county sheriff during the 1968 riots in Chicago. By discussing this with me, Mrs. Meyers invited me into the moral community she constantly forged around her, a community in which she was deeply valued. This community was sustained not only through the pragmatic work of social support but also through the conviviality forged by conversation, debate, celebration, and mourning.

Unlike Mrs. Meyers, George Sampson, an African American man in his late seventies, did not seem to have many friends nearby or spend much time on the phone. He too spent most of his time in his apartment, since his severe asthma made even short trips outdoors risky. Kim Little, an African American Plusmore home care worker, came five afternoons a week, buying his groceries, making sure he had hot, diabetic-friendly meals, and keeping his apartment up to his exacting standards. Mr. Sampson lived in a city-owned senior apartment building on the Chicago's near North Side, and his son visited him for at least an hour or two on the weekends. His daughter lived out of state, but he did not talk about his children much. A quiet, fastidious man, Mr. Sampson was demanding and introverted, nevertheless forging creative engagements with moral communities. Most days when I visited, Mr. Sampson had his radio tuned to the Moody Bible station or another Christian talk station. He told me he liked to listen to the discussions and hear the sermons, and he especially liked the call-in shows. Though he rarely called in himself, Mr. Sampson liked to guess how the host or the interviewee would respond to callers' queries, testing his knowledge of scripture in the process. Mr. Sampson had spent many years studying at the Moody Bible Institute after his wife died, often attending classes in the evenings after working several shifts. He told me, "I wanted to know what the Lord said and what he meant and I wanted to know everything. . . . I wanted to know about Jesus all my life. I have read the Bible about ten times or more and I don't know but I know a little bit." By listening and participating in the radio shows, Mr. Sampson continued to deepen his understanding of Jesus though he could no longer attend Bible study in person. Mr. Sampson thus spent part of each day meaningfully engaged with a moral, religious community he found significant despite his relative isolation.

Mr. Sampson also forged an attenuated moral community with his home care worker, Kim. In the afternoons, after Kim had gone grocery shopping, she would fix Mr. Sampson his lunch and take a short break to eat her own.

Mr. Sampson sat at the edge of his bed, his meal in front of him on a small folding table. Kim perched on a small stool by the window on the far side of the small single bed. As they ate, they watched courtroom television shows, commenting animatedly about the predicaments of the plaintiff and defendant. They argued about what the judge should do, and (usually) acknowledged the judge's wisdom when he or she castigated the defendant for his bad behavior or the plaintiff for allowing himself to be taken advantage of. As they did so, Mr. Sampson's face lit up and became animated, in stark contrast to his normally reserved demeanor. In these exchanges, Mr. Sampson and Kim formed a moral community by debating the norms of correct behavior and punishment. Like many other older Chicagoans, Mr. Sampson and Mrs. Meyers creatively forged social and moral communities, often with the participation of their care workers, which gave meaning to their daily lives and were at least as important to their personhood as their senses of independence.

Beyond Independence

The experiences of older Chicagoans and their home care workers provide a critical perspective on definitions of successful aging that focus only on physical and cognitive ability, independence, and care of oneself. Older Chicagoans who experience debilities that limit their ability to live alone without assistance often seek home care, hoping this will sustain their personhood and independence. For these elders, sustaining a sense of independence means living in their own homes, having their preferences incorporated into daily routines, and being recognized as a person rather than an object. Part of what makes home care valuable to older adults is the way that home care workers subordinate their own bodily needs to those of their elderly clients. Together, these aspects of care promote elders' vision of themselves as still independent persons by obscuring the vital contributions poor women of color made to their daily lives. Workers' contributions are similarly hidden in policy discourses that emphasize the value of maintaining elders' independence while saying little about the ways such efforts contribute to racial and class inequality. Ideologies of independence may thus be intrinsically bound up with social inequality.

The older adults I grew to know in Chicago sustained their personhoods not only through the hidden labor of their care workers but also through the elders' enjoyment of conversation, debate, and watching television with others. In these ways, elders remained engaged and valued members of vibrant moral communities sustained by the varied contributions of elders, family, kin, and care workers. A broad understanding of how to live a good old age might thus look beyond concerns of 'success' and individual action, instead attending to the intertwined fates of elders and those who care for them, and to the ways that social relations and moral communities offer possibilities for even frail, disabled, and home-bound older adults to live valued lives.

NOTES

1. Institutional and personal names have been changed. I preserve the forms of address ("Mrs. Silverman," "Maria," etc.) used by older adults and workers because these forms convey important information about the ways hierarchy operates in these relationships. Notably, Margee Jefferson was the only older adult who asked to be called by her first name, though Grace sometimes still called her Mrs. Jefferson. Workers were typically called by their first names.
2. Material from this section is adapted from Buch 2013.

REFERENCES

BLS (Bureau of Labor Statistics). 2014. "Occupational Outlook Handbook, 2014–2015 Edition." http://www.bls.gov/ooh/fastest-growing.htm, accessed 24 January 2015.

Boris, Eileen, and Jennifer Klein. 2012. *Caring for America.* Oxford: Oxford University Press.

Buch, Elana. 2013. "Senses of Care: Embodying Inequality and Sustaining Personhood in the Care of Older Adults in Chicago." *American Ethnologist* 40 (4): 637–650.

Glenn, Evelyn Nakano. 2012. *Forced to Care: Coercion and Caregiving in America.* Cambridge, MA: Harvard University Press.

Kaufman, Sharon. 1994. "The Social Construction of Frailty: An Anthropological Perspective." *Journal of Aging Studies* 8 (1): 45–58.

Luborsky, Mark R. 1994. "The Cultural Adversity of Physical Disability: Erosion of Full Adult Personhood." *Journal of Aging Studies* 8 (3): 239–253.

Mauss, Marcel. (1935) 1979. "A Category of the Human Mind: The Notion of Person, the Notion of 'Self.'" In *Sociology and Psychology: Essays,* edited by Ben Brewster, 59–94. London: Routledge and Kegan Paul.

NAHC (National Association for Home Care and Hospice). 2013. "The Companionship Exemption Explained." http://www.nahc.org/NAHCReport/nr131001_2, accessed June 15, 2015.

PHI (Paraprofessional Healthcare Institute). 2015. *Paying The Price: How Poverty Wages Undermine Home Care in America.* New York: PHI.

Radin, Margaret. 1982. "Property and Personhood." *Stanford Law Review* 34 (5): 957–1015.

Rowe, John W., and Robert L. Kahn. 1997. "Successful Aging." *Gerontologist* 37 (4): 433–440.

———. 1998. *Successful Aging.* New York: Pantheon Books.

Stern, Stephanie M. 2009. "Residential Protectionism and the Legal Mythology of Home." *Michigan Law Review* 1–7 (7): 1093–1144.

Strathern, Marilyn. 1988. *The Gender of the Gift: Problems with Women and Problems with Society in Melanesia.* Berkeley: University of California Press.

6

Growing Old with God

An Alternative Vision of Successful Aging among Catholic Nuns

ANNA I. CORWIN

At its inception, the notion of "successful aging" offered a welcome paradigmatic shift from previous models that described aging as the slow decline of the body into decrepitude and social isolation (Achenbaum and Bengtson 1994; Butler 1975; Cumming and Henry 1961). Such grim models have been replaced by a vibrant alternative: "successful" or "active" aging, in which elderly individuals enjoy physical and mental health and productivity into their late years. This shift in gerontology and public cultural ideals has been accompanied by a surge of interest in communities in which older individuals are apparently aging exceptionally well (e.g., Buettner 2005; Poulain, Pez, and Solaris, 2011; Reichstadt et al. 2006; Willcox, Willcox, and Ferrucci 2008). Examples abound of individuals living healthy, productive, vigorous lives well into their eighties, nineties, and even one hundreds. Researchers continue to mine such communities to understand why some individuals live longer lives with fewer instances of chronic illness, depression, and other deleterious conditions often associated with old age.

Within this expanding field, some epidemiologists have found that elderly Catholic nuns in particular age exceptionally successfully. As a group, Catholic nuns in the United States have been found to experience increased longevity, be physically healthier in their later years, face fewer instances of Alzheimer's disease, and report higher emotional well-being at the end of life (Butler and Snowdon 1996; Danner, Snowdon, and Friesen 2001; Snowdon 2001). Seeming to embody the standard criteria of successful aging,[1] Catholic nuns are reportedly less impacted by chronic illness and emotional burdens that often accompany late life and dying.

A tremendous amount of research has been conducted to try to understand the nuns' relative success. Epidemiologists have examined convent archives, conducted annual physical and cognitive evaluations, and even examined the structure of the nuns' brains after death (Butler, Ashford, and Snowdon 1996; Butler and Snowdon 1996; Danner, Snowdon, and Friesen 2001; Snowdon 2001, 2003; Riley et al. 2005; Tyas et al. 2007). While contributing factors such as education, nutrition, physical activity, optimistic outlook, and spiritual and social support have been identified through surveys and medical examinations, David Snowdon (2001) notes that the question of how the nuns' daily social and spiritual practices contribute to their experiences of health and well-being cannot be answered using the existing largely quantitative analyses that have been conducted thus far as part of the nun studies.

In June of 2008 I left Los Angeles to fly to a convent in the midwestern United States, where I would spend the next five summers and part of a year living as an anthropologist with 150 elderly Franciscan Catholic nuns.[2] I had begun this journey to try to understand why some people experience greater well-being at the end of life than others. Specifically, I wanted to understand how the lives of religious persons might shape their experiences as they aged.

This chapter draws on ethnographic research spanning over seven years within this community of older Franciscan Catholic nuns, examining how the notion of successful aging is realized among these nuns who have been heralded by researchers to be successful in their aging. While the nuns I lived with indeed struck me as remarkably happy and healthy in their old age, I found that their lives and attitudes provided an interesting counterpoint to the assumptions behind more standard successful aging paradigms. Sarah Lamb's recent work has brought a critical analysis of the successful aging literature, arguing that the model of successful aging as presented both in popular and much of the academic literature promotes a very particular cultural and biopolitical model promoting "individual agency and control; maintaining productive activity; the value of independence and importance of avoiding dependence; and permanent personhood, a vision of the ideal person as not really aging at all in late life, but rather maintaining the self of one's earlier years" (2014, 41; see also introduction this volume). In a *New York Times* interview, actor Frances McDormand commented similarly that nowadays, "There is no desire to become an adult. Adulthood is not a goal. It's not seen as a gift. Something happened culturally; no one is supposed to age past 45—sartorially, cosmetically, attitudinally. Everybody dresses like a teenager. Everybody dyes their hair. Everybody is concerned about a smooth face" (Bruni 2014). Youth is culturally valued to such an extent that as one ages, one is supposed to perform an extension of youthfulness into one's older years. Sociopolitical critiques of successful aging have also drawn attention to the ways in which the values of successful aging are intimately bound to "Western neo-liberal expectations for productivity and independence in a capitalistic society" (Fabbre 2014, 2; see also Calasanti

2004; Dillaway and Byrnes 2009; Liang and Luo 2012). In other words, the expectations associated with successful aging underscore neoliberal ideals in which an individual's value is aligned with his or her independence and earning power.

Through my ethnographic research with the Catholic nuns, I found that their understandings of personhood, temporality, individual agency, and productivity strikingly contrasted such prevailing North American models. This chapter argues, in fact, that the very reasons the nuns "succeed" so profoundly at the end of life may be tied to practices that contradict the premises behind the successful aging paradigm. Specifically, I explore how the nuns' experiences of well-being may be increased precisely because they do *not* uphold the ideals of individual control, independence, productivity, and permanence underlying prevailing successful aging models.

The chapter is organized around the four themes at the heart of contemporary US discourse on successful aging: individual agency and control, independence, maintenance of productive activity, and permanent personhood. I will explore how each of these four ideals emerge in the nuns' everyday practices, arguing that the four ideals promoted in the successful aging paradigm are specifically not upheld, and in most cases devalued, in the nuns' everyday practices. In these ways, the project offers ethnographic insight into the everyday lives of elderly Catholic nuns and the unique ways in which these nuns understand and experience well-being at the end of life.

The Franciscan Sisters of the Sacred Heart Convent

The Franciscan Sisters of the Sacred Heart[3] convent sits cradled between rolling hills in a rural farming community in the Midwest. The majority of the nuns in the convent grew up in large Catholic families. As children, they helped in the house, cared for siblings, and worked with their parents at home or on the farm when they weren't in school. Most of them attended Catholic schools run by nuns. As children, many of the nuns watched as aunts and uncles or older cousins and siblings joined the Church to become nuns or priests. Most of the nuns recounted that their parents expressed pride in having a relative join the Church. In school, many of the nuns were invited to participate in visits to a convent, where they were introduced to monastic life. Most Catholic girls in their community understood that becoming a nun was an available alternative to marriage, and until the 1950s joining a convent was one of the only ways a young Catholic girl could gain an education beyond high school.

However, even though life as a nun offered the option for college or graduate education and work outside the domestic sphere, joining the convent also involved a tremendous sacrifice. When the nuns joined the convent, they had to bid farewell to their families; they were not allowed to visit their families' homes until institutional changes in the Church lifted visiting restrictions in the 1960s. During their training, the novices lived in the novitiate wing of the convent under the strict regulation of a "novice mistress." Having experienced the rigidity of convent life, many young women left the convent after just a few months. Those who stayed were required to abide by a structured schedule of prayer and work for the rest of their lives. At the end of their lives, when the nuns were no longer able to work and live in the main convent, they could retire to the assisted living or infirmary wings of the convent where their peers or (nowadays) convent employees would be available to provide support.

During the time I lived and researched in the convent, there were about 250 nuns there, only 2 or 3 of whom were novices. Like many convents in the United States, the Franciscan Sisters of the Sacred Heart convent has seen few new members in recent decades. The large novitiate wing, built in the 1970s, was designed to house between 100 and 200 new sisters. In the years I was there, it was nearly empty. I spent most of my time in the main convent with retired nuns, who were living in the assisted living and infirmary wings of the convent. Although at first glance these wings resembled the sterile hallways of an assisted living center, I quickly came to realize that aging happens differently in a convent than it does in other North American communities.

Individual Agency and Control

The introduction to this volume makes the argument that one of the central tenets of successful aging is the notion that each individual is responsible for her own health and well-being as she ages and that she should want and desire this responsibility. The concept that each of us is and should be in control of our own body and future is a deeply ingrained North American value. For most people in the United States, this type of individual agency is seen as a fundamental right and its desirability is rarely questioned. Decisions around one's health care, housing, and diet, for example, are all widely viewed as ultimately up to the individual herself. Individuals expect to be the ones in charge of the decisions concerning where they live and what they eat, and physicians often make recommendations that patients are responsible for choosing and enacting.

The values of individual agency and control, however, emerged differently among elderly nuns. As members of a Catholic convent, the sisters took three vows: of poverty, chastity, and obedience. The vow of obedience held two meanings: first, that the nuns be obedient to the divine, and second, that they be obedient to institutional authorities. The nuns believed that the divine held the ultimate authority and power in their lives. Until the 1970s, the image of an eye of God was painted on the convent dining room wall to symbolize the divine watching over the nuns as they ate each meal. When I was there, the image of an eye was still inscribed in stained glass above the chapel door, looking down on the nuns as they prayed. The eye represents divine omnipotence and omnipresence, a constant reminder to the sisters that the divine, the all-powerful, was watching over them.

In addition to this understanding of a divine authority, the nuns were required to be obedient to institutional authorities, from the novice mistress who oversaw them in their first few years in the convent to the convent superiors who, for much of the nuns' lives, have been responsible for day-to-day decisions in the nuns' lives, from the minute to the profound. For example, the novice mistresses dictated minutiae in the nuns' everyday lives such as how much toothpaste can be used on the novices' toothbrushes. Even after they left the novitiate, institutional authorities continued to determine such details of the nuns' lives as what they ate, when they ate, where they lived and worked, who they could socialize with, and when they would retire. Although major institutional changes in the 1960s and 1970s (see Corwin 2012a; Orsi 2005) have changed the meaning of obedience and have given many nuns more freedom to determine the details of their daily lives, elderly nuns have nevertheless lived much of their lives under strict institutional authority.

This authority was designed to strip the nuns of their sense of ego and independence and to deny them individual agency and control in order to "empty them of the self." This practice was theologically devised to strengthen the nuns' sense of divine authority and love (Benson and Wirzba 2005; Clifford 2004; van Riessen 2007). The idea behind this was that if the nuns were stripped of their sense of self they would come to understand that they were not in control of their lives; the divine had ultimate control.

This lack of agency and control seems to have supported the nuns as they aged. From the time they joined the convent, the nuns were encouraged to accept all decisions over their lives with serenity and peace. When they reached old age, they seemed to understand illness and death as inevitable and met these, too, with acceptance, serenity, and a sense of peace rather than with a sense of failure, discouragement, or frustration, as many other Americans and Europeans seem to experience.

For example, when I met Sister Mary Bernard, she was ninety-eight years old, and even in my twenties I could barely keep up with her. Under five feet tall, Sister Mary Bernard rushed down the hallways, greeting everyone in her path. She had a close relationship with God and spoke to me with great enthusiasm and humility about her childhood and loving parents, her decades as a primary school teacher, and her enduring gratitude for what she saw as the many blessings in her life. When she was ninety-nine, Sister Mary Bernard's doctor told her that she needed to have her leg amputated above the knee. When I spoke to her about her impending surgery, she said, "You have to accept what God gives you. I'm still remembering that. The hardest thing is to accept the difficult things, but you know He loves you the most with those, because he's asking you to go through that for Him."

After the surgery, Sister Mary Bernard continued to live an active social life, holding court in the hallways of the convent infirmary from her wheelchair. She confessed that although she had thought she couldn't live without her leg, she ultimately was able to muster her resolve and accept what she saw as God's decision. She told me that her faith carried her though the surgery and continued to buoy her after her recovery.

During the months I was in the convent, I witnessed many sisters encounter difficult medical news, and although coming to terms with illness, pain, or physical decline is never easy for anyone, the majority of the nuns seemed to accept the changes in their physical bodies with remarkable equanimity. It seemed that the nuns' sense that divine and institutional authorities were in control of their lives helped to relieve individuals from the responsibility to control things that they might not be able to change such as illness. In this way, it seemed that the years of practice accepting that they did not have complete individual agency and control over their everyday lives helped prepare the nuns to accept change as they aged.

Independence

A second theme of the successful aging paradigm is the ideal of independence. Most research and popular books on successful aging presume that individuals value independence throughout their lives and would like to maintain it into old age (introduction this volume). Dependence on others is widely seen as not only undesirable but also as a moral failing.

When the nuns joined the convent, however, they made a distinct move away from a life of independence and committed themselves to a lifetime of communal living. The nuns ate, slept, and bathed in shared spaces. They prayed together, worked together, and negotiated all aspects of everyday life with the women in their community. There was little emphasis put on independence and tremendous value put on communal living, sharing, living in harmony, and serving others.

The older nuns in the infirmary continued to spend much of their time serving others and each other. One summer I watched each evening as two sisters who lived in the infirmary would take a walk together, arm in arm, around the grounds of the convent. Sister Noella, who struggled with progressing Alzheimer's disease, was concerned that Sister Agatha, whose arthritis usually confined her to the infirmary, wouldn't get any fresh air without her help, so she helped Sister Agatha physically navigate the hallway, the elevator, and the paths around the convent. But Sister Agatha did not see the interaction in quite the same way. Each evening, Sister Agatha mustered the energy to overcome the limitations of her body to guide and orient Sister Noella so that she would not get lost on her walk around the spacious convent grounds. These two sisters helped each other make it outside for a nightly stroll. The convent ethos of community and service allowed them each to see the walk as a way to serve the other. They did not speak about "dependence," but rather each saw herself as a friend putting herself second in order to serve another sister.

Although the paradigm of successful aging places great value on the ability to live and function independently, epidemiological findings suggest that there are in fact strong correlations between living in a community and "successful aging," defined here as physical and mental health along with the reported sense of well-being (Snowdon 2001). In addition, my own research with the nuns suggests that their strong sense of community, mutuality, and shared life supports them as they age (Corwin 2012b, 2014). This may be informed by the fact that when the nuns transitioned into old age and were no longer able to function independently, they could draw on a lifetime of experience living interdependently and did not necessarily interpret dependence on others as moral failure. Instead, interdependence was seen positively, as a way to serve and to be served.

Active Aging and the Maintenance of Productive Activity

A third theme in the successful aging paradigm is the pursuit of "active aging," the maintenance of productive activity into late life. This includes maintaining physical activity—for example, the ability to walk and exercise. It also includes the ability to remain a "productive" citizen, contributing to one's community into old age.

The nuns' community values informed how they understood the notion of productivity. The vow of poverty required that the nuns turn all of their funds and earnings over to the convent. They were given a stipend to cover monthly expenses such as toiletries, small purchases, and the occasional meal on the road, but all earnings were intended to symbolically and materially serve the community as a whole. The convent community emphasized the value of service through action. The nuns' work was evaluated based on whether it did "good" in the world. While the material contributions the nuns made from their salaries to the convent were valuable as they kept the convent operational, there was little relationship between the nuns' earning power and their sense of productive contribution. The nuns did value each other's material work, and when they retired, some expressed having a hard time giving up positions in which they were able to work and serve others. However, the community viewed "being" good as more important than "doing" good. When the nuns returned home to the convent to retire, they were met with a community of peers who reinforced the notion that being in community and praying was just as important as serving others through physical work. The nuns went to great effort to communicate that the work the retired nuns did in prayer was as important if not more important than the physical work they performed in the world (see Corwin 2012b).

For example, Sister Regina spoke to me about a transition in her life when she began to see being a good person as equal to or more important even than being productive. She explained that she went through a spiritual transformation in which she stopped valuing the things she did and began to value the way she lived her life. In this first quote, she stated that what was previously most important to her was "doing" or accomplishing things in the world, in other words, being productive: "I did, or I say I 'do'd,' from the time I was able to do things, until I was about—I must've been in my early forties. Everything—the biggest thing was doing. That was my biggest prayer."

Sister Regina went on to say that the productive accomplishment of things, even routinized prayer, became less and less meaningful. She said: "And so it got to the point when I was in my forties that that didn't really mean anything to me. I did it because it was part of the protocol. . . . But being is harder than doing. And so I've been being for a long time. For a long time. But the levels of being they have become intensified, you know, I don't hafta—I don't hafta to call God, God is part of who I am." As Sister Regina matured in her spirituality, she became more interested in being, which she described here as a way of being with God. This transformation exemplified the convent's emphasis on valuing who a person is rather than what she accomplishes.

Because the nuns did not associate work with their material livelihood, and because they value "being" good as equal to or above "doing" good, they did not seem to suffer a significant reduction in their sense of self worth as they aged or retired. When retiring or infirm nuns did experience concerns about their ability to serve others or make productive contributions to the community, they were met with enormous support, emphasizing the importance of being rather than doing good. As evidence of this, the nuns who were in the infirmary who could no longer work or serve in other ways were often thanked for their prayers. With these expressions of gratitude, the community signaled the importance they placed on being in relationship with God, something nuns could practice at any stage of life. In this way, productivity in the convent was not necessarily tied to physical activity or material earnings. Instead, the nuns were encouraged to experience themselves as valuable persons both during and after their materially productive years.

Permanent Personhood

A fourth central theme in the successful aging paradigm is that of maintaining agelessness or permanent personhood. Permanent personhood involves "a vision of the ideal person as not really aging at all in later life but rather maintaining the self of one's earlier years, while avoiding or denying processes of decline and conditions of oldness" (introduction this volume; Lamb 2014). This North American vision tends to associate personhood with competent active adulthood. In this model, children are seen as incomplete adults, on their way toward full personhood. Elderly individuals who do not (or cannot) maintain active adulthood can be seen as moving away from full personhood. Those who cannot function productively and competently—namely children, persons who are disabled, as well as older adults—are often segregated from engagement in everyday interaction (Kittay 2010; Rogoff 2003). Children in North America are segregated from engagement in the valued activities of adulthood, such as productive work and often even household chores, only gaining access to these activities when they become adults (Paradise and Rogoff 2009). Research in US nursing homes and continuing care retirement communities has similarly found that when individuals begin to display cognitive or physical decline, they often experience exclusion from existing social networks (e.g., Taylor this volume). These exclusionary patterns run in contrast to many indigenous American communities where all individuals are collaboratively involved in everyday household and production activities (Paradise and Rogoff 2009). Similarly, the Catholic nuns I grew to know collaboratively engaged their elderly peers in everyday activities. In this way, a person was engaged and valued at every stage of the lifespan, and the nuns did not strive for an ageless adulthood.

Catholic nuns also exist in a temporal landscape that provides of a notion of life after death (Robbins 2007). The nuns I lived with did not view death as an end point but rather as a transition from corporeality into another mode of being, a continuation of life in heaven. Death was understood to be a passage or transformation rather than an end, or, as in some Western conceptions, a moral failure. In this way, in the convent, personhood and the values associated with it were not tied to the state of active adulthood. Rather, the nuns located personhood within the soul, which, for Catholics, begins before birth at conception and endures after death, when the soul is understood to live on in an afterlife. The nuns therefore did not limit valued personhood to adulthood; unborn babies as well as those who have died and now reside in heaven were seen to maintain value as persons.

This alternative view of personhood impacted how the nuns treated themselves and each other when they reached old age and infirmity. The notion that they would maintain a mutable personhood and continue relationships with loved ones after death seemed to reduce the nuns' fear of dying. Perhaps even more significant, the notion that they maintain dignified personhood even after physical decline seemed to be evidenced in the ways that they treated each other as they aged.

The nuns in the infirmary, even those experiencing significant physical and mental decline, continued to be meaningfully engaged in everyday activities as dignified, valuable persons. The nuns continued to involve their infirm peers in religious activities, at meals, and in social activities such as card games. For example, when I was in the infirmary, I watched as three older, able-bodied nuns played cards every night with Sister Helen, a peer who was suffering from a degenerative neurological disorder. Sister Helen's face and upper body were contorted and her arms were permanently contracted, held against her body. She had aphasia and could no longer speak. She communicated with extended unintelligible groans and, occasionally, a sparkle in her eyes. Despite the fact that Sister Helen could no longer interact in typical ways, her peers continued to treat her as a person deserving of continued respect, support, and dignified interaction. Each night, two of her peers included her in a card game, often holding the cards for her and helping her move them to the correct location. Even more significantly, the nuns almost never spoke to her in the condescending- or simplistic-register "elderspeak" that Americans often use with older adults, especially those with limited communicative ability. Instead, they spoke to her as a dignified member of their community, engaging her in laughter, conversation, and everyday communication. Even as her body transformed, after she could no longer speak or eat, the other sisters continued to treat Sister Helen as a valuable person. Through this involvement, the nuns showed that they did not link personhood to competent adulthood. They continued to value each other as valuable persons, notwithstanding the inevitable changes encountered over the life course.

Conclusion

Catholic nuns may be heralded as "successes" within the prevailing successful aging paradigm, based on North American ideals of independence, individual agency, productivity, and permanent personhood. However, I hope to have shown in this chapter that many nuns' experiences of physical and mental well-being may be supported by the fact that they themselves do not hold these ideals.

Instead of valuing individual agency and control, the nuns I grew to know located control and agency *outside* of themselves. Over their lifetimes, the nuns learned to accept that divine and institutional authority held ultimate authority in their lives. This understanding that they were not in control of their lives may actually have helped the nuns cope with and accept physical and mental decline as well as death.

Second, because the nuns lived in community, they did not value independence as much as they valued interdependence. From the time they joined the convent, the nuns learned to spend their lives coordinating living space and everyday tasks with others. This lifelong practice of interdependence seems to have supported the nuns as they transitioned into the dependence that often accompanies old age and physical decline. Activities that involved reliance on others at the end of life seemed to be interpreted as ways of serving and being served and were quite easily accepted by the nuns. Dependence therefore was understood not as a failure of individual autonomy, but as a way to be served after a lifetime of serving others.

Further, because the nuns lived as members of a religious community that took vows of poverty, they were not directly engaged in an economy that values production. The nuns did not put as much value on "doing" or being productive as in the wider society. While the nuns worked as nurses, teachers, or church administrators, this work was valued for how it impacted others and whether they had made positive change in the world. Although their service could be valued for its productivity, the nuns received a tremendous amount of socialization into valuing "being good" over "doing good." Through practices and overt socialization, the nuns focused on "being" kind, peaceful, generous, and loving people who have positive relationships with others and with the divine.

Finally, the nuns' sense of personhood was not limited to productive adulthood. The nuns believed that personhood was located in the soul rather than in the embodied person. Personhood extended in time before birth, beginning at conception and beyond death into the afterlife. This sense that individuals were valuable members of the community even when they were not productive adults encouraged them to treat others in the community with respect, dignity, and engagement, even when they displayed significant cognitive or physical decline. To the nuns, the value of a person was not located in a certain stage of the lifespan: they did not strive for ageless adulthood; the value of a person was located in the soul. This perspective allowed the nuns to treat each other with dignity even as their personality, abilities, or physical body changed over time.

Even though Catholic nuns experience many of the pleasures we associate with "successful aging," such as good physical and mental health and an inner sense of well-being, the neoliberal values heralded in the successful aging paradigm seem to be at odds with many of the values held by these nuns. While longevity and physical and mental health are things almost all humans hope for, the values of individual agency and control, independence, continued productivity, and permanent personhood are not universal values. In fact, ethnographic exploration into the lives of elderly Catholic nuns seems to indicate that the nuns hold almost none of these values. The nuns' sense of well-being at the end of life seems to be bolstered by a lifetime of practices

that emphasize relinquishing control over the details of their lives, interdependence, service, and a sense of personhood that extends well before and
beyond adulthood.

NOTES

1. See Baltes and Baltes 1990; Johnson and Mutchler 2013; Rowe and Kahn 1987, 1997;
   and this volume's introduction for more on standard criteria of successful aging.
2. The technical term for the women in this study is *women religious*, a term that
   refers to women who have taken the three vows of poverty, chastity, and obedience
   but continue to work in the world. The sisters in this study are "active" or "apos-
   tolic" sisters, as they work in the world as nurses, teachers, and administrators.
   Technically, the term *nun* refers to women who live contemplative lives. However,
   since the women religious in this study refer to themselves as "nuns," I will use
   the term in this chapter. I conducted fieldwork with the sisters over the summers of
   2008, 2009, 2010, 2012, and 2013, and for a five-month period in 2011.
3. The name of the convent and the names of individuals are pseudonyms.

REFERENCES

Achenbaum, W. Andrew, and Vern Bengtson. 1994. "Re-engaging the Disengagement
    Theory of Aging: On the History and Assessment of Theory Development in Geron-
    tology." *Gerontologist* 34: 756–763.
Baltes, Paul B., and Margret M. Baltes, eds. 1993. *Successful Aging.* Cambridge: Cambridge
    University Press.
Benson, Bruce Ellis, and Norman Wirzba. 2005. *The Phenomenology of Prayer.* New York:
    Fordham University Press.
Bruni, Frank. 2014. "A Star Who Has No Time for Vanity." *New York Times*, 15 October,
    AR1. http://www.nytimes.com/2014/10/19/arts/frances-mcdormand-true-to-herself
    -in-hbos-olive-kitteridge.html?_r=0, last accessed 23 September 2016.
Buettner, Daniel. 2005. "New Wrinkles on Aging: Residents of Okinawa, Sardinia, and
    Loma Linda, California, Live Longer, Healthier Lives Than Just About Anyone Else
    on Earth." *National Geographic* 208 (5): 2.
Butler, Robert N. 1975. *Why Survive? Being Old in America.* Oxford: Harper and Row.
Butler, Steven M., and David A. Snowdon. 1996. "Trends in Mortality in Older Women:
    Findings from the Nun Study." *Journal of Gerontology: Social Sciences* 51B (4):
    S201–S208.
Butler, Steven M., J. Wesson Ashford, and David A. Snowdon. 1996. "Age, Education, and
    Changes in the MiniMental State Exam Scores of Elderly Women: Findings from the
    Nun Study." *Journal of the American Geriatrics Society* 44: 675–681.
Calasanti, Toni. 2004. "Feminist Gerontology and Old Men." *Journals of Gerontology
    Series B: Psychological Sciences and Social Sciences* 59 (6): S305–S314.
Clifford, Catherine E. 2004. "Kenosis and the Path to Communion." *Jurist* 64: 21–34.
Corwin, Anna I. 2012a. "Let Him Hold You: Spiritual and Social Support in a Catholic
    Convent Infirmary." *Anthropology of Aging Quarterly* 33 (4): 120–130.

————. 2012b. "Changing God, Changing Bodies: The Impact of New Prayer Practices on Elderly Catholic Nuns' Embodied Experience." *Ethos* 40 (4): 390–410.

————. 2014. "Lord, Hear Our Prayer: Prayer, Social Support, and Well-Being in a Catholic Convent." *Journal of Linguistic Anthropology* 24 (2): 174–192.

Cumming, Elaine, and William Earl Henry. 1961. *Growing Old: The Process of Disengagement.* New York.

Danner, Deborah D., David A. Snowdon, and Wallace V. Friesen. 2001. "Positive Emotions in Early Life and Longevity: Findings From the Nun Study." *Journal of Personality and Social Psychology* 80 (5): 804–813.

Dillaway, Heather, and Mary Byrnes. 2009. "Reconsidering Successful Aging: A Call for Renewed and Expanded Academic Critiques and Conceptualizations." *Journal of Applied Gerontology* 28 (6): 702–722.

Fabbre, Vanessa D. 2014. "Gender Transitions in Later Life: A Queer Perspective on Successful Aging." *Gerontologist* 55 (1): 144–153.

Johnson, K. J., and Jan E. Mutchler. 2013. "The Emergence of a Positive Gerontology: From Disengagement to Social Involvement." *The Gerontologist* 54 (1): 1–8.

Kittay, Eva Feder. 2010. "At the Margins of Moral Personhood." *Ethics* 116 (1): 100–131.

Lamb, Sarah. 2014. "Permanent Personhood or Meaningful Decline? Toward a Critical Anthropology of Successful Aging." *Journal of Aging Studies* 29: 41–52.

Liang, Jiayin, and Baozhen Luo. 2012. "Toward a Discourse Shift in Social Gerontology: From Successful Aging to Harmonious Aging." *Journal of Aging Studies* 26 (3): 327–334.

Orsi, Robert A. 2005. *Between Heaven and Earth: the Religious Worlds People Make and the Scholars Who Study Them.* Princeton, NJ: Princeton University Press.

Paradise, Ruth, and Barbara Rogoff. 2009. "Side by Side: Learning by Observing and Pitching In." *Ethos* 37 (1): 102–138.

Poulain, Michel, Gianni Pes, and Luisa Salaris. 2011. "A Population Where Men Live as Long as Women: Villagrande Strisaili, Sardinia." *Journal of Aging Research* 1: 1–10.

Reichstadt, Jennifer, Colin Depp, Lawrence Palinkas, David Folsom, and Dililp Jeste. 2006. "Building Blocks of Successful Aging: A Focus Group Study of Older Adults' Perceived Contributors to Successful Aging." *American Journal of Geriatric Psychiatry* 15 (3): 194–201.

Riley, Kathryn P., David A. Snowdon, Mark F. Desrosiers, and William R. Markesbery. 2005. "Early Life Linguistic Ability, Late Life Cognitive Function, and Neuropathology: Findings from the Nun Study." *Neurobiology of Aging* 26 (3): 341347.

Robbins, Joel. 2007. "Continuity Thinking and the Problem of Christian Culture: Belief, Time, and the Anthropology of Christianity." *Current Anthropology* 48 (1): 5–38.

Rogoff, Barbara. 2003. *The Cultural Nature of Human Development.* Oxford: Oxford University Press.

Rowe, John, and Robert Kahn. 1987. "Human Aging: Usual and Successful." *Science* 237 (4811): 143–149.

————. 1997. "Successful Aging." *The Gerontologist* 37 (4): 433–440.

Snowdon, David. 2001. *Aging with Grace.* New York: Bantam Books.

————. 2003. "Healthy Aging and Dementia: Findings from the Nun Study." *Annals of Internal Medicine* 139: 450–454.

Tyas, Suzanne L., David A. Snowdon, Mark F. Desrosiers, Kathryn P. Riley, and William R. Markesbery. 2007. "Healthy Ageing in the Nun Study: Definition and Neuropathologic Correlates." *Age and Ageing* 36 (6): 650–655.

van Riessen, Renée. 2007. *Man as a Place of God: Levinas' Hermeneutics of Kenosis.* Dordrecht: Springer.

Willcox, Bradley J., D. Craig Willcox, and Luigi Ferrucci. 2008. "Secrets of Healthy Aging and Longevity from Exceptional Survivors around the Globe: Lessons from Octogenarians to Supercentenarians." *Journals of Gerontology Series A: Biological Sciences and Medical Sciences* 63 (11): 1181–1185.

7

Aspiring to Activity

Universities of the Third Age, Gardening, and Other Forms of Living in Postsocialist Poland

JESSICA ROBBINS-RUSZKOWSKI

One afternoon over sweet wine, pastries, and tea, Pani Anna and Pani Honorata, two Polish women retirees, discussed the pleasure they both took in participating in a University of the Third Age (UTA) in Wrocław, the city in southwestern Poland where they lived.[1] The UTA is a type of educational and social institution for older people popular both within Poland and world-wide. Anna loved learning English and thereby being able to communicate with her grandchildren growing up in England, while Honorata loved improving her poetry-writing skills and participating in a cabaret group. I had met these women through the UTA, where I was conducting ethnographic fieldwork about aging in Poland and also teaching a conversational English-language class. Anna was a participant in the English class I was teaching, and Honorata was a member of the leadership of the UTA.

This gathering took place at Anna's home in Biskupin, a neighborhood that was not destroyed by bombing at the end of World War II (unlike many others in Wrocław). The neighborhood is leafy, full of small narrow streets lined with nineteenth- and early twentieth-century villas, strikingly different from the large mid-twentieth-century apartment buildings common elsewhere in the city. At Anna's three-story house, where she lived by herself after the death of her husband, we sat in the formal living room while she served wine in cut-glass goblets, pastries on floral-patterned china, and tea in delicate teacups with a matching pattern.

In addition to the social and intellectual pleasures of the UTA, that after-noon Anna and Honorata spoke proudly of the successes of their kin who lived abroad in England and Germany—and disparagingly of their age-mates who did not participate in UTAs and instead joined neighborhood senior clubs or parish clubs. Even worse, Honorata said, were those who sat at home and watched TV. These activities, she asserted, were not as valuable as those at the UTAs, for they consisted of gossip or laziness. Honorata went so far as to link watching TV with illness in later life, suggesting that these people would end up sick and dependent on others, possibly even living in a medical care institution, such as one of my other fieldwork sites that we had been discussing.

In this harsh judgment of her peers, Honorata was commenting not only on the merits of poetry writing as opposed to TV watching but also on the proper way to grow old. And it is not just Honorata who holds such beliefs about how to age. In fact, UTAs have become tremendously popular in contemporary Poland as exemplars of what gerontologists and policymakers have called *active aging* (see the introduction to this volume). UTAs and other organizations that promote active aging can transform old age from a negative to a positive experience for those who attend them. However, I wish to explore how older people in Poland engage in other forms of meaningful sociality that do not easily fit into the category of active aging, some of which are subject to others' negative evaluations. Indeed, even experiences of illness and residing in institutional care, which Honorata described as opposite to her participation in the UTA, can provide opportunities for meaningful social relations in later life.

Honorata's comment, the rise of the UTAs in Poland, and the opposition of active aging to illness and dependence are not natural facts but instead demand explanations as to how certain forms of sociality—and life itself—become valued and others devalued. In this chapter I seek to understand the moral dimensions of a range of practices of aging by examining them within their particular cultural historical contexts. I compare the UTA with other forms of social life for older people in Poland, namely, allotment gardening and residing in a rehabilitation hospital run by Catholic nuns. By juxtaposing this range of experiences of aging, I aim both to shed light on contemporary forms of exclusion in old age and to offer inclusive visions of aging that go beyond binary constructions of activity and passivity, success and failure, productivity and unproductivity, and health and illness.

This chapter draws on twenty-two months of ethnographic research in a range of contexts for older adults in Poland. I conducted fieldwork between 2006 and 2014, with the longest period of research occurring between 2008 and 2010, in Wrocław and Poznań, two cities in western Poland that have around 600,000 residents. In addition to UTAs, other fieldwork sites included a rehabilitation hospital run by Catholic nuns, a state-run home for the chronically physically disabled, a day center for people with early stages of Alzheimer's disease, and other social groups for older people (such as a neighborhood senior club, parish club, retired technical workers association, and allotment gardeners association). I also conducted interviews with older people who do not take part in any formal social group.

Histories and Politics of "Active Aging" in Poland

In contemporary Poland, UTAs are the most visible example of active aging. "Active," "successful," "healthy," and "productive" aging together constitute a response to earlier visions of aging as a time primarily marked by decline (e.g., Cumming and Henry 1961). These newer models frame aging as a time of life characterized by continued growth, development, and positivity. Many studies have shown that what counts as a positive old age can vary cross-culturally (e.g., Lewis 2010); that is, people across the world differently imagine what "successful" or "active" aging means and engage in varying practices to achieve these ideals. There is no universal model.

In Europe, active aging is an increasingly important cultural norm that is supported by local, national, and transnational governments. In 2012 the European Union sponsored a year of programming under the name "European Year for Active Ageing and Solidarity between Generations"; in Poland there is a governmental initiative running from 2014 to 2020 called Government Program for the Benefit of Social Activity/Active-ness of Older People (Rządowy Program na rzecz Aktywności Społecznej Osób Starszych). In the Polish program, UTAs receive special attention as especially popular institutions worthy of support. Through UTAs and other organizations, the government supports a range of social and educational programs for older people (meaning over the age of sixty), many of which focus implicitly or explicitly on maintaining health.

UTAs are a global phenomenon that vary in terms of institutional content and form. Founded in France in 1973, UTAs can now be found in many parts of the world.[2] All UTAs share a commitment to education in old age as a means to make old age a positive time in the life course and tend to be experienced as overwhelmingly positive for people who participate in them (Swindell and Thompson 1995). However, underpinning this notion of the UTAs' transformative power is the assumption that without intervention, old age is somehow a less valuable time in the life course. This fundamentally negative view of old age is also evident in the term "third age" itself, which is imagined to be a life stage in which one has retired from formal employment, does not have care obligations, and is still healthy. The "third age" is opposed to the "fourth age," which is supposedly characterized by "dependence and decrepitude" (Laslett 1996, 192; see the discussion of "real" old age in the introductory chapter in this volume). Thus, like the concepts of "successful," "active," "healthy," and "productive" aging, there is an undercurrent of negativity running through such seemingly positive phenomena as UTAs, as demonstrated in the opening vignette.

Having more than doubled in number in Poland from less than two hundred to over four hundred in the years between 2004 and 2012, UTAs are a visible part of the postsocialist Polish social and cultural landscape. In Polish UTAs the cultural specificity of active aging—or, to use the Polish term, *aktywność* ("active-ness," "activity")—is associated with living, and aging, in a particular historical moment. Specifically, active aging at Polish UTAs consists of practices and ideals that signify the country's transition from state socialism to market democracy, a process marked by democratic elections in 1989 and membership in the European Union in 2004. These changes brought about not only political and economic reforms but also transformations in society and culture (Verdery 1996).

One transformation has been that older people now often experience discrimination partially because of their association with this past world order (Robbins-Ruszkowski 2013, 2014b). This discrimination can take the form of both experience and representation, in which older people are negatively presented in the media. At the group level, these negative representations often depict a demographic fear of waves of dependent elders draining state coffers. Older people were also more likely to have been disadvantaged by the structural changes in Polish society after 1989. Taken together, these factors can create a hostile experience for some older people in Poland. In this context, participating in UTAs becomes a way for older people to counteract the negativity associated with oldness—one that is often understood in terms of the national imagination.

In the UTAs where I conducted fieldwork, shifts in world view were evident in the activities in which older people engaged and in their understanding of the meaning of such activities. For instance, the UTA in Wrocław offered a range of classes, activities, and workshops, on topics ranging from academic (e.g., physics, philosophy, and foreign language classes) to artistic (e.g., choirs, poetry lessons, handicraft groups) and athletic (e.g., sailing, swimming, Nordic walking). Especially popular were classes in English-language instruction and computer skills. One reason for this popularity is the number of Poles living abroad in English-speaking countries, spurring older people like Anna (described in this chapter's opening) to want to learn English and to learn Skype to communicate with relatives abroad.

More than just communicative tools, speaking English and knowing how to use a computer are symbols of the global capitalist economy in which Poland now participates. Growing up during state socialism, older Poles learned Russian, not English. Having retired before or soon after the political economic changes of 1989, older people have largely been left out of the "computerization" of Polish society, in the words of a Polish NGO leader. By learning English and computer skills, then, older people are not only learning skills that can help them connect to family abroad, but also demonstrating their belonging in the contemporary world order.

Institutional leaders and participants alike emphasize that such educational activities transform old age from a time in the life course characterized by social stigma, isolation, and withdrawal from the broader social world to a time characterized by personal growth, new social roles, and education. Indeed, one former director of the UTA spoke of creating "Euroseniorzy," or "Euroseniors," through educational activities that create "openness" in the older generation, who had learned to be "closed" during state socialism. To this former director, participating in UTA activities has transformative potential not only for individuals but for entire generations that came of age and lived decades of adult life during state socialism. Active aging is thus not only a personal project but also a political one.

Yet transformations since 1989 have not been uniformly positive for Polish society. Inequality has increased since socialist times, and certain segments of the population, including older people, are experiencing poverty, decreasing access to health care, and other structural hardships (e.g., Watson 2011). Thus, in the next section I consider how UTAs may reproduce forms of inequality in Polish society, both in the ways they implement a certain concept of active aging and appeal largely to the middle and upper classes.

The Limits of Universities of the Third Age: Gender, Class, and Health

In Wrocław there are currently ten UTAs. Many, but not all, are affiliated with higher education institutions. During interviews with institutional leaders, I learned that these ten institutions are oversubscribed, as older people in Wrocław wish to attend UTAs at higher rates than there are available spaces. Found not only in major cities but also in small towns, UTAs are a well-known phenomenon across Poland. However, despite this popularity, UTAs have some exclusionary characteristics that raise questions about their suitability for the aging Polish population as a whole and as a normative model for aging. Specifically, UTAs appeal more to women than men, to people of higher socioeconomic status, and to those who are in good health. I raise these limitations not to detract from the value they hold for the many who participate in them but rather to question how such seemingly positive forms of social life like UTAs and those related to active aging more broadly may also contain within them histories and practices of inequality.

Many who attend UTAs describe the experience as transformative because the UTA provides an opportunity "to do something for oneself" for the first time in one's life.[3] Notably, all participants who framed the UTA as an opportunity to "do something for oneself" were women, who comprise over 80 percent of participants nationwide (Robbins-Ruszkowski 2013). Although it is true that women do live longer than men in Poland (GUS 2014),[4] this difference in longevity is not enough to explain the dramatic difference in participation rates in UTAs. Throughout the history of the UTA in Wrocław, a majority of its women members have been either widowed or unmarried (Robbins-Ruszkowski in press). This held true during my fieldwork, in which over half the women participants I met were widowed. With many having kin living abroad, as discussed above, older women who attend UTAs tend to lack a geographically proximate kin network that constitutes the cultural norm for older women, leading them to seek out other forms of social connection.

Additionally, gendered cultural ideals of sociality over the life course shape participation in UTAs in Poland (Robbins-Ruszkowski 2013, 158, 163n.3). Both women and men explained to me that women are connected to the world of people and social relations, while men are connected to the world of things and nature. This holds true across the life course, as girls and women become socialized into taking responsibility for maintaining social ties (both kin and non-kin) and managing the domestic sphere (through household work and care for kin)—in addition to labor outside the home—while boys and men primarily become socialized into the sphere of work outside the home. In old age, and particularly after retirement, older women and men thus have different forms of sociality available to them. This was borne out in conversations with UTA participants. When I asked women UTA participants how older men occupied themselves if not at UTAs, common answers were "Oh, my husband prefers to stay at home, watching soccer and drinking beer," or "He hangs out at his allotment garden." These answers were presented as common knowledge, as if I was asking something so obvious it did not need to be articulated. The few men with whom I spoke at the UTAs told me that they attended because they were interested in particular course offerings or sought to remedy loneliness, or in the case of one older man, because his wife had suggested they attend together. However, their differing comportment in classes (e.g., his reticence and cynicism, her gregariousness and eagerness) gave the distinct impression that he was tagging along.

Importantly, no one critiqued the UTAs for this greater appeal to women than men. However, gender segregation at the UTA connects to broader discourses of gender and aging in Poland. Indeed, many suggested to me that Poles understand older men to be weaker than older women. For instance, a doctor at the rehabilitation center explained that there were many more women than men at the center because rehabilitation was hard work, and men did not have the strength for such work in old age. Men either die of heart attacks, she said, or have a stroke and do not have the strength to recover. In the words of a woman UTA participant, "[Men] are not suited for old age." These comments about men did not convey a harsh judgment or moral failing, but rather a sort of matter-of-fact description about what they saw as a sad reality. This "old-men-are-weak, old-women-are-strong" narrative of aging highlighted in UTA-gendered participation rates may then be reproducing forms of gender inequality in Polish society.[5]

Additionally, there are socioeconomic class limitations in the appeal of UTAs. Most of the participants I met had retired from certain kinds of careers, as teachers, accountants, engineers, and medical workers. Although their professions had not all been particularly high paying, they were jobs that required and valued some form of higher education, meaning that participants would tend to feel that something called a university would appeal to them. Very few of my research participants from UTAs had worked in manual labor, service industries, or technical professions. This class distinction is common to UTAs in other parts of the world (Formosa 2006), but there is a particularly Polish dimension of these class dynamics that has to do with longstanding divisions in Polish society dating back to at least the eighteenth century (Jakubowska 2012).

Indeed, the ethnographic scene that opened the chapter only becomes understandable in light of historical class distinctions. The physical location of Anna's home, along with its decorative style, represented her family's relative wealth. Although I never learned the occupation of her husband, it was clear from some of his belongings, such as hunting gear that was passed down from his father, and from the age of some of the furniture, which Anna described as belonging to her family, that her family had been one of considerable means for multiple generations. This home was a stark contrast to the furnishing of other homes I visited, which were filled with items dating primarily to the mid-twentieth century, and were notably less elaborate in their style. The bourgeois and antique style of Anna's belongings symbolizes a connection to the Polish nobility and intelligentsia. The content of their conversation was similarly classed, as Anna and Honorata spoke of pursuing knowledge of foreign languages, poetry, and theater and denigrated other forms of sociality like TV watching or gossiping. This distinction between nobility and peasant or working class has proven remarkably durable from the presocialist time of the eighteenth and nineteenth centuries through the present, despite almost sixty years of state socialism (Jakubowska 2012). In both the form and the content of this social interaction, Anna and Honorata were establishing themselves as older Polish women of a particular type—and setting themselves apart from other types of older Poles (Bourdieu [1979] 1984). UTAs are thus sites in which forms of social inequality can become reinforced and maintained.

Finally, Anna and Honorata's conversation implicitly devalued those with poor bodily health, resonating with broader active, successful aging discourses prevailing in the UTAs and wider society. Despite attending events at UTAs in two cities over a period of four years, I never saw anyone in a wheelchair. Very few people used a cane. All meetings were held in university spaces across the cities, to which most people arrived by bus or tram. In other words, people with physical disabilities were almost entirely absent from UTAs. Additionally, the topic of illness was notably absent from programming at the UTA. Although health was a frequent topic, evident in lectures on cooking and shopping nutritiously, as well as numerous physical activity groups, discussions of illness itself did not form a part of the UTA curriculum. Given the common stereotype of older Polish people as overly preoccupied with illness and disease, this absence is striking. Indeed, given the probability of illness at some point in old age, and somewhat poorer health of older people in Poland compared to other European countries, this absence is all the more remarkable. However, within the "third age" model, explicitly imagined as a time in the life course in which one is healthy, there is no discursive possibility for conceptualizing illness, for to do so would move the institution out of the third age and into the fourth age. The concept of the third age thus makes illness unthinkable.

Taken together, the gendered, classed, and bodily nature of both the form and content of activities at the UTA render these institutions exclusionary for some older Poles. In writing this, I do not mean to suggest that UTAs themselves are not worthy institutions, or that all participants come from elite backgrounds or are models of perfect health. Rather, I aim to draw attention to the fact that the vision of active aging they promote has implicit gendered, classed, and bodily biases that make it inaccessible to some segments of the population. Inasmuch as UTAs promote an increasingly valued cultural model of aging, it is necessary to highlight the hidden ways that they can reproduce existing inequalities. In the next section I will draw connections between UTAs and two other forms of sociality—gardening and living in institutional care—to suggest other possibilities for creating inclusive models of aging.

Gardening and Other Forms of Living

Another meaningful site of sociality and opportunity for aktywność, or "activeness," for older people in Poland is the allotment garden, a site in many ways different from the UTAs. For instance, allotments are popular among both men and women, and among people from a range of class backgrounds. Moreover, they are not iconic of a postsocialist active aging paradigm because of their clear association with the socialist past. Grouped together on large plots of land in urban centers, many allotments were established by state enterprise during socialist times, although in some parts of Poland the gardens date back to the nineteenth century (Bellows 2004). Currently, allotments are managed by the Polish Union of Allotment Gardeners, although the state is taking an increasing interest in controlling allotments because of their high property value and desirable locations. Although some younger people acquire allotment gardens to use primarily for recreation (e.g., barbecues, lawn games), allotment gardens are understood in the popular imagination to be largely a pastime of older people. Indeed, when I would tell Polish friends in their twenties and thirties that I was studying allotments, they would let out a kind of knowing chuckle, followed by a description of stereotypical allotment gardeners: an older man standing shirtless in his allotment, drinking beer and chatting with a friend at the neighboring garden; an older woman meticulously tending her flowers and growing vegetables and fruits for canning, pickling, and making jam. As opposed to younger families who have allotment gardens, older people tend to spend more time there; some visit the plot every day year-round. As two older women gardeners gave me a tour of their block of gardens, they pointed to the overgrown gardens as evidence that younger people maintained those.

Although the UTAs and gardens are quite distinct, they both promote aktywność. Indeed, one man explained the reason for so meticulously maintaining his flower and vegetable gardens thus: "It's necessary to be active." Like participating in classes at UTAs, the ability to grow vegetables, fruits, and flowers gives people a sense of purpose and provides opportunities to maintain and create social relations. Several people told me that their gardens help to keep them alive and healthy. Lech, a man in his eighties who worked as a treasurer of his allotment garden organization, told me that "I am alive, thanks to my garden," as he described his struggles with cancer and other health issues. He contrasted the healthy, flavorful food he grows at his allotment, including fresh cucumbers and peppers, with the less healthy, tasteless food available at large supermarkets such as Tesco. (Much to his chagrin, his middle-aged son preferred the taste of supermarket cucumbers.) However, it was clear from how he spoke that it was not only the food he grew but also the acts of tending the garden and managing the organization's finances and social relations that Lech found restorative.

Another man, Zbyszek, made explicit the value he saw in engaging in allotment gardening. When we first met via a common acquaintance and he learned that I was studying gardens, he immediately said that allotment gardens are popular in Poland because Poles have a need for their *own* plot of land, their *own* property, contrasting Poles with "czarists" to the east. By framing gardening in terms of property rights, connection to the land, and an opposition between Poles and Russians (whom he called "czarists"), Zbyszek was placing himself within a presocialist history, in which part of what is now Poland was ruled by the Russian Empire. This historical framing both differs from and resonates with forms of activity at the UTA: It is older than the contrasts with the state socialist past made in the UTA's classes but similar in historical depth to the class distinctions evident in Honorata and Anna's conversations. However, Zbyszek drew on a national rather than a classed form of difference, suggesting that the aktywność of the garden includes more Poles than that of the UTAs (but, notably, is still based on a form of opposition).

In seeming contrast to both allotment gardens and UTAs would be places dominated by illness. Indeed, during my research in two long-term care institutions and a day center for people with Alzheimer's disease, the language of aktywność or active-ness was notably absent. However, I did find a similar sense of satisfaction, meaningfulness, and even self-transformation in old age among some people in these contexts. Most notable were two women living at a rehabilitation center run by Catholic nuns in Wrocław, who understood their lives to have been positively transformed by their experience in the center. Most Poles view long-term care institutions as places of last resort, given the cultural ideal of caring for older relatives at home, and thus often experience these institutions as places of abandonment. However, some in elder-care institutions create meaningful lives for themselves, despite the barriers to doing so. In telling these women's stories, I aim to point out similarities to the satisfaction that older Poles in other contexts express, using the language of aktywność, as part of my broader project of searching for understandings of aging that hew close to local meanings and values.

Marta was a farmer from a village outside Wrocław until her multiple sclerosis became so debilitating that she could no longer live at home.[6] She moved to the rehabilitation center, where she was to live in one of the beds set aside for permanent residents (most patients are supposed to stay for only a few months, although in practice many stay for longer as their condition fails to improve). Marta's room on the third floor was a center of social life, as family, friends, and other patients stopped by to visit, although some staff interpreted her chattiness as too gossipy. Seasonally appropriate trinkets (gifts from family and friends) decorated the small table in her room. Marta always insisted on making visitors a cup of instant coffee, a show of hospitality that was not possible for most people in the center, either because of limited physical capacity or because they did not have such homelike goods in their rooms. The few times I had to decline her offer because of time, I was scolded for my rudeness. When she was well enough, Marta returned to her home for Christmas and Easter, but she was always relieved to return to the center, where she felt she was getting appropriate care, where it was calm, and where she could attend chapel daily. Although she longed for home, Marta came to prefer the physical care of medical staff to that of her family, the calmer social interactions in a medical room to those with rambunctious grandchildren at home, and the spiritual possibilities of attending chapel in the same building daily rather than struggling to attend weekly in a more remote location. Indeed, Marta became so

content with life at the center that she described feeling *u siebie* ("at home")
there.

Only one other person I knew at this Catholic rehabilitation center similarly described feeling this way there. Like Marta, she was one of the permanent
residents at the center. After a lifetime of working various jobs (as a merchant
and a groundskeeper), Dorota moved to the center when her arthritis became
too debilitating for her to manage on her own and her only living relative, her
grandson, was not able to care for her. A devout Catholic, Dorota took great
satisfaction in attending chapel daily. She helped to wheel her roommate down
the fourth-floor hallway to the chapel; they sang devotional songs together each
morning. Frequently visited by staff and volunteers because of her good humor
and storytelling ability, Dorota commented on the quality of care in the institution by remarking that the staff would even bring her tea if she was thirsty. This
contrasted with the earlier life that she evoked in her stories, in which she cited
struggles to find food during the war and efforts in various jobs to support her
family. In this context, having someone to bring her a cup of tea was a sign of
good care. For Dorota, the rehabilitation center provided physical, spiritual, and
social comforts that fit her ideals.

Although the cases of Marta and Dorota seem to present contrasting
examples of experiences of old age to those of the allotment gardeners and
UTA participants, I see in these lives a similar kind of contentment, satisfaction, and purpose. On a daily level, each person has access to forms of sociality
that provide meaning, whether this be weeding and pruning a garden maintained for decades amid neighbors, learning English and writing poetry among
women of the same social class, or serving coffee and singing hymns with core-
ligionists. Although it may seem trite to highlight seemingly mundane activities, it is exactly through such everyday practices that persons, social relations,
and worlds are maintained and transformed. Paying attention to such practices can help to serve as a counterpoint to the dominant macro-narratives of
active aging promoted by the European Union and governmental initiatives
that threaten to blind us to the complexities of life as it is lived.

Paying Attention to Practice for an Inclusive Future

Despite a national and international context in which the "third age" of health,
activity, and independence is contrasted to the "fourth age" of illness, passivity,
and dependence, research focusing on the sociality of daily life in Poland shows
that such a binary framework cannot explain the meaning and satisfaction that
people experience in old age. What if funding was directed not toward programs
focusing on active aging as such but toward ensuring that people have the ability to support whatever kinds of social activity they find meaningful? Could such

financial support work against dominant cultural ideals that value some kinds of social life—and, by extension, some groups of persons—to the exclusion of others?

In raising such questions, I aim to move toward an understanding of aging that is less polarizing, less exclusionary, and less subject to moralizing judgments. In fact, it is my hope that the examples presented here show that people in Poland already *do* find diverse methods for achieving an old age that feels worthy and valuable. The challenge, then, is how to create cultural models and visions of old age that reflect the diversity of meaningful practices that already exist. Paying close attention to daily practice and sharing stories that emerge from these observations—in short, ethnography—suggests one way forward. Given the demographic realities of global aging, ethnographic research thus becomes crucial to creating a world that is more accepting of the diversity and complexity of human experiences of aging—and, indeed, of living.

ACKNOWLEDGMENTS

My greatest thanks are to the people and institutions in Poland who welcomed me into their lives during my research. I am also grateful to Sarah Lamb, Elana Buch, and Kristin Yarris for their insightful suggestions on earlier drafts of this chapter. Research and writing were supported by grants from the National Science Foundation (DDIG #0819259), the Wenner-Gren Foundation (Dissertation Fieldwork Grant #7736), Elderhostel/Road Scholar, IREX Individual Advanced Research Opportunity award (with support from the US Department of State Title VIII), and several units at the University of Michigan (Center for Russian, East European, and Eurasian Studies; Department of Anthropology; Institute for Research on Women and Gender; and Rackham Graduate School), and Wayne State University. None of these organizations is responsible for the views expressed herein.

NOTES

1. *Pani* is the formal term of address for women in the Polish language. All names are pseudonyms. For ease of reading in English, I have omitted "pani" throughout this text; however, it was the standard term of address throughout my fieldwork and served as a form of respect.
2. The first UTA was founded by the French scholar Pierre Vellas at the University of Toulouse in 1973. Within a few years, UTAs were created in other parts of Europe and Canada, and they flourished in Britain in the 1980s. Marvin Formosa (2012, 2–7) reports that by 2012 UTAs could be found in sixty countries around the world.
3. See Robbins-Ruszkowski 2013 for more detailed discussions of this phrase ("*robić coś dla siebie*").
4. In 2013 the average life expectancy for men was 73.1 years and for women 81.1 years (GUS 2014, 15).
5. However, it should also be noted that this idea of men as weak and women as strong is inversely correlated with other forms of power in society; for instance, men still

control government, corporations, expectations of women at home. See, for example, Graff 2009 and Pine 2002 for more on gendered domains of life in Poland.

6. This ethnographic example and the one that follows have previously appeared in Robbins 2013 and Robbins-Ruszkowski 2014a.

REFERENCES

Bellows, Anne C. 2004. "One Hundred Years of Allotment Gardens in Poland." *Food and Foodways* 12 (4): 247–276.

Bourdieu, Pierre. 1984. *Distinction: A Social Critique of the Judgment of Taste,* translated by Richard Nice. Cambridge, MA: Harvard University Press.

Cumming, Elaine, and William E. Henry. 1961. *Growing Old, The Process of Disengagement.* New York: Basic Books.

Formosa, Marvin. 2006. "A Bourdieusian Interpretation of the University of the Third Age in Malta." *Journal of Maltese Education Research* 4 (2): 1–16.

———. 2012. "Four Decades of Universities of the Third Age: Past, Present, Future." *Ageing and Society* 34 (1): 1–25.

Graff, Agnieszka. 2009. "Gender, Sexuality, and Nation—Here and Now: Reflections on the Gendered and Sexualized Aspects of Contemporary Polish Nationalism." In *Intimate Citizenships: Gender, Sexualities, Politics,* edited by Elżbieta Oleksy, 133–146. New York: Routledge.

Jakubowska, Longina. 2012. *Patrons of History: Nobility, Capital, and Political Transitions in Poland.* Burlington, VT: Ashgate Publishing Company.

Laslett, Peter. 1996. *A Fresh Map of Life: The Emergence of the Third Age.* London: Macmillan Press.

Lewis, Jordan P. 2010. "Successful Aging through the Eyes of Alaska Natives: Exploring Generational Differences among Alaska Natives." *Journal of Cross-Cultural Gerontology* 25 (4): 385–396.

GUS (Główny Urząd Statystyczny). 2014. Trwanie życia w 2013 r. [Life expectancy tables of Poland 2013]. Edited by Departament badań demograficznych i rynku pracy. Warsaw: Zakład Wydawnictw Statystycznych.

Pine, Frances. 2002. "Retreat to the Household? Gendered Domains in Postsocialist Poland." In *Postsocialism: Ideals, Ideologies, and Practices in Eurasia,* edited by C. M. Hann, 95–113. London: Routledge.

Robbins, Jessica. 2013. "Shifting Moral Ideals of Aging in Poland: Suffering, Self-Actualization, and the Nation." In *Transitions and Transformations: Cultural Perspectives on the Life Course,* edited by Caitrin Lynch and Jason Danely, 79–91. New York: Berghahn Books.

Robbins-Ruszkowski, Jessica C. 2013. "Challenging Marginalization at the Universities of the Third Age in Poland." *Anthropology and Aging Quarterly* 34 (2): 157–169.

———. 2014a. "National Dimensions of Personhood among Older People in Poland." *Etnografia Polska* 58 (1–2): 159–174.

———. 2014b. "Thinking with 'Postsocialism' in an Ethnographic Study of Old Age in Poland." *Cargo: Journal for Social/Cultural Anthropology* 12 (1–2): 35–50.

———. In press. "Responsibilities of the Third Age and the Intimate Politics of Sociality in Poland." In *Competing Responsibilities: The Ethics and Politics of Responsibility in Contemporary Life,* edited by Susanna Trnka and Catherine Trundle. Durham, NC: Duke University Press.

Swindell, Richard, and Jean Thompson. 1995. "An International Perspective on the University of the Third Age." *Educational Gerontology* 21 (5): 429–447.

Verdery, Katherine. 1996. *What Was Socialism, and What Comes Next?* Princeton, NJ: Princeton University Press.

Watson, Peggy. 2011. "Fighting for Life: Health Care and Democracy in Capitalist Poland." *Critical Social Policy* 31 (1): 53–76.

8

Should Old Acquaintance Be Forgot?

Friendship in the Face of Dementia

JANELLE S. TAYLOR

"Successful aging" represents a vision of how to age well that has proven compelling for many in North America and beyond, shaping how people think and act in regard to their own aging. At the heart of this vision, as found in John Rowe and Robert Kahn's influential formulation, are three main components: (1) low probability of disease and disease-related disability; (2) high cognitive and physical functional capacity; and (3) active engagement with life (Rowe and Kahn 1997, 433). Aging successfully is, in this vision, not just a matter of living longer but of living in good physical and cognitive health, and in the company of others.

It is worth noting, however, a certain ambiguity in the role assigned to social relations and friends within this discourse. On the one hand, having friends is one of the ends of successful aging, in that it exemplifies "active engagement with life." On the other hand, friends also appear as a means to achieve successful aging, insofar as they are understood to promote the maintenance of the physical and cognitive health of the individual. Rowe and Kahn write: "Being part of a social network is a significant determinant of longevity. . . . Social support . . . can have positive health-relevant effects" (1997, 437–438).

Much subsequent research has followed up on the latter point, with particular attention to asking whether "engagement in . . . social interaction . . . has a protective effect on cognition" (Beland et al. 2005, 320) among the elderly, slowing or delaying the onset of dementia or reducing its incidence. For example, researchers inform us that "greater social resources, as defined by social networks and social engagement, are associated with reduced cognitive decline in old age" (Barnes et al. 2004, 2322), and "larger social networks have a protective influence on cognitive function among elderly women" (Crooks et al. 2013, 1221).

Although it might seem to have to do only with how one person will age, the idea of successful aging thus also presupposes an entire social world. Implicitly, it is envisioned as a social world in which other people are not also aging in complicated ways alongside one. If friends are to fulfill the dual functions assigned to them in successful aging discourse, they too must remain active and healthy and free of dementia. Whether as means or as ends, friends appear as important props supporting the pursuit of successful aging as a fundamentally individual project. Having friends, it seems, is good and important because it keeps you active and engaged and because it can reduce your risk of developing dementia. As Sarah Lamb astutely points out, however: "The only certainty in the human life course is that we each will die. And few are able to live life in perfect health until suddenly dropping dead at age 100. Rather, most experience some degree of decline for months or years leading up to death, and/or profoundly experience a spouse's, partner's or close friends' decline and dying" (2014, 437). In what follows, I will focus on this last point: many people as they age do experience the decline of a close friend.

One of the most dreaded forms of decline is also one of the most common. Dementia, as a clinical syndrome involving progressive decline in cognitive abilities and capacity for independent living (Prince et al. 2014), affects approximately 7 percent of people over age sixty, its prevalence approximately doubling for every five years of additional age—rising from about 2 percent at age sixty-five, to about 50 percent at age ninety (Prince et al. 2013, 68). It is worth noting that recent and projected increases in the numbers of elderly people living with dementia are in fact an ironic consequence of the same advances that have set the stage for contemporary reimaginings of old age as at least potentially a period of continued vibrancy in the successful aging discourse. As the anthropologist Sharon Kaufman notes: "We can see the problematic ramifications of medicine's life-extending capabilities all around us: in the 'epidemics' of Alzheimer's disease and heart failure that exist because medical interventions have enabled people to live long enough to suffer those consequences of old age" (2015, 110). Even those rare individuals who might reach age ninety in good physical shape and cognitively intact would likely find that a very high proportion of their peers and friends, if they are still alive, will be living with dementia.

What is it like for people to experience the onset of dementia in a friend, and how do they respond? How and why do friends so often fall away after dementia sets in—and how and why do some individuals nonetheless remain engaged? I was led to such questions by my own observations as the daughter of a mother living with very advanced dementia. On the one hand, I was painfully struck by how quickly most of my mother's friends faded away as her dementia progressed, particularly following the death of my father; on the other hand, I was (and remain) deeply grateful and moved by the loving loyalty of one old friend who has continued to visit her even as memory, mobility, and language have abandoned her (Taylor 2008, 319). As the psychologist Susan McFadden and the chaplain John McFadden note, "Most empirical research on the social relationships of persons who have dementia is directed toward families and paid caregivers. . . . However, . . . it is time to consider the challenges dementia poses to friendships and community connections that have often been nurtured over the course of many decades" (2011, 4). Hoping to contribute to this effort, I am currently engaged in an ongoing research project that seeks to document the perspectives and experiences of people who have found themselves facing the onset of dementia in a close friend. This research project, which has been supported in its initial stages by a grant from the Fetzer Institute, is focused primarily on finding and interviewing people who self-identify as friends of someone with dementia who are (in whatever way) trying to keep up the friendship. Borrowing the language of "exemplars" employed by the Fetzer Institute, I refer to such individuals as "exemplary friends." As of this writing, interviews have been conducted with thirteen "exemplary friends," seven family members, and three health professionals who work with people with dementia (most in the United States, one in the United Kingdom, and one in the Netherlands). Some of these interviews were conducted in person and some by phone or Skype; with permission from the individuals interviewed (and following research protocols approved by the University of Washington's Human Subjects Division), all have been recorded and transcribed. Drawing on preliminary findings from this research, I offer here some critical reflections on successful aging discourse, inspired by considering the perspectives and experiences of people who have found themselves facing dementia as it affects a friend.

Friendship and Dementia as Moral Laboratory

The onset of dementia symptoms, and/or receipt of a formal diagnosis, are generally acknowledged to be devastating, for spouses and other family members as well as for the person affected. Interviews with people who speak from the position of close friends suggest that the onset of dementia can also be very difficult for them.

The voluminous literature on successful aging is mostly silent concerning this situation. What place do friends suffering incurable progressive ailments have, in the life of a successfully aging elderly person? The narrowly individualistic framing of much successful aging discourse might seem to suggest that one should step back from such friendships when cognitive impairments set in and seek instead to maintain relations with others who, being healthier, may be more stimulating company, and thus better suited to contribute to one's own (individual) pursuit of successful aging.

My interviews suggest, however, that for at least some elderly people, the onset of dementia in a close friend calls into play a quite different understanding of the self, as realized in and through relations with others. As the philosopher Charles Taylor puts it, "One cannot be a self on one's own" (1989, 34, quoted in Mattingly 2014, 22). As the anthropologist Cheryl Mattingly has argued, devastating and unforeseen events present people with moral challenges. Mattingly calls such situations "moral laboratories," to highlight the way that people striving to do the right thing, in circumstances where it often is unclear, become "researchers and experimenters of their own lives," experimenting with different ways to sustain the moral values, selves, and relationships that they hold most dear. In the process, bad luck can open paths toward developing or revealing unsuspected dimensions of familiar people and relationships: "New projects of becoming may be set in motion through the accidents of fortune. So, a chain of events . . . conspire to provide radically altered circumstances and set a new story in motion. Such events . . . demand virtues not needed before. Accidents create new situations that demand new or more well-developed virtues in order to even perceive a 'best good' in uncharted waters" (Mattingly 2014, 82). This resonates strongly with how "exemplary friends" with whom I have spoken describe how they have experienced the onset of dementia in a close friend.

For some, an impulse to "do the right thing" in response to news of dementia prompts an immediate commitment to stick with a friend as they move forward into uncharted waters. Helen, a very slim and well-groomed professional in her early sixties, sat with me in her office overlooking a fabulous water view and described to me her relationship with Naomi, who has early-onset Alzheimer's disease that is by now very advanced. She and Naomi had been very close at one point, but they had then had a falling out and had "broken up" for some years. Soon after they eventually reconnected, Naomi told Helen about her diagnosis. Helen relayed: "And then *soon* after that walk she told me. And one of my first responses was just to say: 'I'm in it till the end.' And I have held that quite seriously. And I think some of that was about my guilt about this ruffle that we had, but also just because it felt like the right thing to do. It came out of the moment. I don't think I would have thought it out. Yeah." When asked whether she had any previous experience with dementia, to have a sense of what might lay ahead, Helen replied, "No. Clueless!"—and she laughed. We shall return to Helen's story a bit later, to discuss some of the unforeseen forms of growth that later emerged from this spontaneous commitment.

Esther, who at age eighty-three has several close friends who have developed dementia, described her ongoing commitment to them, especially to her dearest friend Maura, as the natural continuation of their longstanding friendship: "We were out for dinner, and it was very clear she forgot what the last sentence was. And I would say that was at least ten years [ago]. . . . It's a relationship that goes back maybe sixty years. And she was an unbelievable woman. . . . And we watched our children grow up to a certain age, and I loved her; so it never occurred to me that I didn't want to see her again." The progress of dementia eventually rendered impossible some of the shared activities, such as talking about politics, around which Esther's friendships had always been organized. But for her, as for others I have interviewed, the commitment to keeping up these relationships was a fundamentally moral commitment—not only to the friend but to a sense of oneself as realized in and through these relationships. Esther reflected: "In a sense Maura really disappeared. She who was so fabulous—she's definitely not fabulous anymore. . . . [But] I want to see them as long as I can. . . . I do it for me. I do it for them too, but I really—it's really important to *me*. Friendship has always been such an important part of my life."

As dementia progresses over time, waning capacities and new needs spur new forms of interaction, and friendship as a "moral laboratory" becomes a site for experimentation, creating conditions for the emergence of new virtues. This is clear in the comments of Liv and Bert, a couple in their sixties, who spoke to me about their experiences with their friend Peter as he developed dementia and eventually died, about three years previously. Turning to Bert, Liv said: "I will say that at the end you were fantastic with Peter." Then, to me: "I will say that Bert is not always the most understanding, sympathetic person [laughs]. But with Peter [turning again to Bert], the last few days when he was sort of almost unconscious, you were the one who was holding his hand and talking to him, and even [Peter's wife] was absolutely flabbergasted that she saw that side of you that we've never seen under any other circumstances."

For Thea, her husband Arne's interactions with his friend Joe on a boat trip similarly brought to light previously unrealized virtues. Sailing had been a passion of Arne's for many years, but the progress of his dementia, as well as his Parkinson's disease, had rendered this favorite activity newly perilous. Speaking an English lightly inflected by her native Dutch, Thea said:

> I am so surprised, it is a new experience for me to see how men, their friendships—now I realize that they are so caring, and tender to each other. Joe, the man on the boat, he was so caring for Arne all the time. I could observe him observing Arne. So he was not, like I sometimes am, overbearing about caring for him—like I will say, "Oh, don't stand on the staircase!" Joe didn't do that, but he would *observe* him: "Is it safe, or not?"—and to not have to *talk* about these painful things, he *did* something to prevent that something bad would happen. So he was in his mind all the time caring for Arne on the boat. So that was really touching.

In such ways, friends report that their continued engagement following the onset of dementia can serve as a moral laboratory, providing the opportunity for realization of the moral self, as well as the development and expression of moral virtues.

Gossip and the (Re)making of Moral Communities

When I began interviewing people about their experience with the onset of dementia in a friend, one detail that caught me by surprise was how prominently these stories feature talk among friends about other friends who are not present—gossip, if you will.

Talk among friends often figures as part of the process by which the reality of dementia is first acknowledged. Debbie first noticed during a camping trip that her friend Ellen was repeating herself in conversation and having difficulty playing familiar card games and completing some quite basic tasks. Immediately upon returning home, she reached out to another mutual friend: "I talked to my dear friend Teresa who lives in Colorado. . . . She saw [Ellen and her husband] last winter, but very briefly; and she said she didn't notice anything. I said, 'Teresa, I got to talk with you about something. I didn't want to e-mail you, because I just wanted to get your reaction.' And I just told her what I told you about the visit with them."

Once the presence of dementia is established as a shared understanding, talk among friends centers on establishing a shared understanding of how the condition is progressing. Lorraine, speaking of her friend Harry, describes talking about him regularly with other mutual friends in their social circle: "We take care of him. . . . Oh, yes, we're all aware of it. Yes. We all talk—oh, we talk about it. . . . Everybody sort of compares notes on how Harry's doing, what he's doing." Note that in Lorraine's framing, talk about the mutual friend with dementia is explicitly linked to collective efforts to care for him.

This has come up in other interviews as well. For example, Cora, a very sharp-minded eighty-three-year-old woman, described how she and others talk about and care for a friend with dementia who has been part of a monthly bridge group. Bridge is a very complicated game, of course, that requires considerable cognitive abilities; finding ways to continue to include this friend as her dementia progresses has therefore required adapting some of the ways that they play together:

> So she's there, but not active. And she loves to go around and sit and what have you. And she has a friend that lives there that's also in our bridge group that helps her get the dessert ready or what have you, because she still wants to have her friends over, which I think is healthy and really good. This last month when we played bridge, she opened the cards and looked puzzled, and somebody said, "Just separate them by suits," and told her that. And then she said—so she had presence of mind enough to say,

"You know, I haven't played this for a long time. Maybe I should take some lessons." And we all just sort of chuckled.

Cora told me that she often speaks by phone with other members of the bridge group, sharing observations about their mutual friend and arranging plans for who will pick her up and bring her to the next meeting. Talking about her was integrally part of their process of collectively devising ways to continue to include her in the group's shared activities. Cora explained: "Because we don't want to exclude her, we *won't* exclude her, because as I say it could happen to anybody." Cora went on to tell me that they had noticed that their mutual friend had lately forgotten many details of her children's and grandchildren's lives; the bridge group members were talking about making up a list of their names and activities to give to her, a sort of "cheat sheet" that they hoped might help her continue to engage in an important form of social talk.

Gossip is, as the anthropologist Niko Besnier notes, "a form of inter-action that in most societies variously provokes scorn, derision, and contempt," but it is also an activity that many people find intensely interesting and pleasurable, and it can have significant social and political consequences. "Confined to the intimacy of domestic contexts," he writes, "gossip can nevertheless have a long reach, affect important events, and determine biographies. Through gossip, people make sense of what surrounds them, interpreting events, people, and the dynamics of history" (2009, 3). I would like to suggest that one of the other things people sometimes can do through gossip is engage in what the philosopher Hilde Lindemann calls "holding the individual in personhood," in other words, "the social practice of personal identities" (2014, 3). Cultural anthropology has in many contexts demonstrated how, as Lynn Morgan succinctly phrases it, "people are made by people" (2009, 22); when it comes to dementia, gossip and talk can be critical to the making or unmaking of relational personhood.

I like best the term used by Lorraine (whom we heard from above), to describe how she and her friends compare notes about their mutual friend Harry, who has dementia, as a means of taking care of him. Lorraine described one of these conversations: "As one of the friends in Michigan said, 'When Harry's in the cocoon that we create'—this particular group creates the cocoon. We've been traveling together for years . . . and that's the group that Harry feels comfortable in." Through talk, the onset of dementia in an elderly individual can be made into a collective experience, and a collective response mounted. In the process, a group can make and remake itself as a moral community and offer itself to vulnerable members as a "cocoon"—in other words, a safe place within which to undergo a transformation.

Tragedy, Transformation, and the Growth of Love

Not only can the onset of dementia, as moral laboratory, spur new ways to sustain existing relationships—it can also serve as the catalyst for the creation of social bonds that are new.

This possibility emerges clearly in the comments of an elderly professor I will call Carol, who is still working and very active at age eighty-three. She spoke to me about her experience with dementia in a dear friend and former colleague, about eleven years younger than herself, who years ago developed early-onset Alzheimer's disease that is by now quite advanced. Carol now lives in California, but she travels a couple of times each year to the city where her friend still lives:

> Every time I go East I go with Alan [the friend's husband] and visit her. And I've learned that almost no one—including the colleagues of hers—makes the forty-minute drive or whatever to go visit her. Everybody has kind of almost written her out. So even though I'm in some ways her furthest-away friend, aside from her husband who actually goes *every* single day to feed her lunch, I think I'm almost the only person that goes to visit. And I sit with her; she no longer talks. She mostly just sits there and sometimes babbles sounds. . . . Mostly what I do when I'm with her, and it feels like a connection, is to hold her hand or have her head rest on my shoulder, look in to her eyes, say sweet things. . . . And I go because I love her, and I still feel that in some ways I'm with her, although I have to say that I kind of alternate between thinking that her soul is still somehow locked up there inside her and other times that it's blown away. . . . And I go, I must say, in some ways because I've come to love *him* and his devotion. And so I would say partly because I continue to love her or my memories, but also because I feel such deep, *deep*, deep love and connection with him and his loyalty. I mean my partner, Rebecca, and I just say it over and over again: he has become to us a real *model* of devotion. Spousal devotion. I think that the main thing has been the unintentional way in which this challenge to him has transformed him. Yeah. And being able to live with that.

What interests me about this story, which resonates with other accounts I have heard, is how love for and ongoing commitment to the friend with dementia is tangled up with love and admiration for the caregiver. In this case, this was a new development following the onset of dementia and not merely the preservation of an existing relationship. Carol explained to me that Alan was her friend's second husband, and she had never really gotten to know him nor wanted to; she hadn't liked him much. But after her friend developed dementia, as she witnessed Alan's care and devotion, Carol grew to love and admire him, and indeed to regard him as a model.

As Carol describes it, her experience of witnessing the onset of dementia in her friend contained some of the features of the classical genre of tragedy. Indeed, "if tragedy holds any lesson at all for its viewers, it is not how to *avoid* tragic outcomes but how to *endure* them, as we observe the nobility with which the protagonist faces his demise, and learn what it means to exhibit virtue in the face of a tragic reversal of fortune" (Taylor 2003, 163).

In her critique of successful aging, Sarah Lamb (2014) identifies, as one of the problematic assumption in this discourse, the idea of "permanent person-hood": the assumption that one's personhood is already fully formed earlier in life, and that the task in old age is to preserve and maintain it. Carol's story reveals a very different vision: a whole series of interlocking transformations of people happening in late life amid new difficulties and challenges. The disease transforms the friend, the challenge of caring for her transforms the husband, and the experience of witnessing his devotion transforms Carol and her relationship to both of them. There is important life work happening in this moral laboratory, real learning and personal growth and the formation and deepening of friendship bonds—not only despite dementia but in some ways because of it.

Such Different Things Back

Finally, I would like to share a few examples of what friends describe as new pleasures, new forms of shared activities, and new dimensions of friendship opening up as a direct result of the changes brought on by dementia.

Celia, a sixty-year-old woman, spoke to me about her friendship with Maude, age eighty-five. As Celia recounts, going for walks together was always something the two of them had enjoyed; these days, however, Maude is much frailer and more easily tired, so they walk only very short distances. After one such short walk, they sat together on a bench looking out over Puget Sound at the islands and mountains in the distance, and the boats coming and going. Celia describes with amused pleasure Maude's newly childlike responses:

> And so we were sitting there and watching the ferries and watching the trains and—she's very girl-like now. Like we're sitting on the bench and watching, there's a train coming and there's the ferry coming, and it's also kind of cold and it's kind of at the edge of a little cliff and there's a bunch of blackberry vines and stuff there, and she says, "Oh, I just feel like rolling down that hill, just like Jack and Jill." [laughs] "I'm just going to *tumble* right down there." . . . I don't think she would, she wasn't really going to do it. [laughs] But my inclination was to say, "There's a lot of blackberries there."

Similarly, Liv (whom we heard from above, in conversation with her husband, Bert), spoke of dementia as having revealed hitherto hidden, and very lovable, sides of her friend Peter's personality: "I learned to appreciate Peter *more* as he got sicker for some reason; we all have strengths and weaknesses and goods and bads about us. . . . He did soften, and you *saw* that what was the real Peter was really this wonderful, caring, considerate guy. And that really was the power about him that shone through toward the end. I became fonder of him as he got ill and the rigidity wore off."

When dementia has progressed much further, to the point where many shared activities are no longer feasible and even language may be beyond reach, some friends do continue to find new forms of connection and enjoyment in their ongoing interactions with the person with dementia. Helen (whom we heard from earlier on, as well) told me that she is, at present, the only person who still visits her friend Naomi; even Naomi's daughters no longer come to see her. She said:

> I stay a half hour, maybe forty-five minutes, an hour. Not long. Invariably, when I leave, I'm glad I went. And one of the things [laughs] is I'm really physical with Naomi. So she's in a chair like this and I literally pull her up, give her a big hug, and then she sometimes sort of halfway hugs me back, . . . and then we'll walk around. I've even walked her in the streets of Capitol Hill, and I *love* that part with her. There's something tactile that I get back from that that's nice. We'll walk around, which requires me sort of holding her; and as she gets more comfortable walking, then sometimes I'll just hold her hand. That's enough for her. Sometimes we'll sit on the steps of the stairs in the house and we'll *sing*. She actually loved music, and she hums a lot. And I just . . . even though I don't know very many songs and I'm a horrible singer, we sing. [laughs] And then sometimes I'll just sit with her. I just think you get—I want to say so little back, and that's true, but you also just get such different things back. . . . The thing I [am] talking about is really the physicality of being with Naomi that I really enjoy, and I get something from that. That's not something I sought out of our friendship ten years ago.

Conclusion

It seems fair to say that dementia epitomizes the opposite of "successful aging." It progressively erodes the capacities for memory, language, and cognition that we tend to regard as the necessary foundation of individual identity and personhood. In the process, dementia also strikes a major blow to friendship relations: the friend with dementia may lose the capacity to engage in the activities that have been enjoyed in common, may lose the memory of shared histories, and may no longer be able to produce the expected signs of recognition. Time spent with a friend who has dementia does not readily fit the image of the kind of social engagement envisioned as part of "successful aging," nor is this is the kind of social interaction considered likely to reduce one's own chances of developing cognitive impairment. The predicament of the successfully aging individual whose friend develops dementia makes visible the tension between two unrecognized assumptions inherent within the discourse of successful aging: successful aging both *requires* friendships and *denies* them—or at least it offers no clear vision of the value of friendships, once a friend becomes impaired.

To the extent that active social engagement with others figures as an end of successful aging, it arguably might seem to require that such engagements be robust enough to survive some of the losses and difficulties common to the experience of aging. There may be alternative possibilities dormant within the discourse of successful aging, which could provide openings for developing this vision in directions that could render it less narrowly individualistic and more humane. It is at least conceivable, for example, that "active social engagement" could include volunteer work—or indeed friendships—that might draw a relatively healthy and cognitively intact elderly person into various forms of engagement with other elderly people who are more impaired than they.

At stake in how people take up or resist the discourse of successful aging is nothing less than the social making and unmaking of persons and relationships. If persons are socially constructed, then it becomes vital to understand how this happens in contexts where the outcome is very uncertain. Will friends step up and reach out in the ways needed to "hold someone in personhood" when cognitive losses render claims to personhood fragile—or will they not? Will they retreat, withdraw, and thus contribute to the erosion of personhood in situations of dementia? If the discourse of successful aging contributes to nudging people toward disconnecting from friends when they begin to show signs of dementia, then it may do very real harm to real people living among us.

The individuals I have interviewed share with me perspectives that "speak back" to the discourse of successful aging in ways that I think are instructive. These individuals describe the onset of dementia in a friend, in terms that resonate with Cheryl Mattingly's idea of a moral laboratory: faced with a terrible turn of fortune, they strive to respond in ways that uphold their sense of a moral self, a self that exists in and through relations to others, and they develop new virtues and forge new realities in the process. Their accounts of friendship in the face of dementia offer important resources for critically reexamining the assumptions upon which so much of the discourse of successful aging is premised. These exemplary friends describe *collective* rather than only individual responses to age-related decline; they describe friendship after dementia as a relationship that is capable of *changing*, rather than simply enduring; and they describe dementia as an impetus for personal and interpersonal *transformations* that can involve learning, growth, and unexpected gifts, in addition to very real experiences of sadness and loss.

ACKNOWLEDGMENTS

The Fetzer Institute is a private philanthropic foundation whose mission is "to investigate, activate, and celebrate the power of love and forgiveness as a practical force for good in today's world" (http://fetzer.org/about-us; accessed July 23, 2015). I acknowledge with gratitude their generous support, and thank as well the many colleagues and friends who have provided indispensible help and encouragement for this project, especially: Marigrace Becker, Catherine Besteman, Bettina Shell Duncan, Ilana Gershon, Iben Mundbjerg Gjødsbøl, Sharon Kaufman, Mary Jane Knecht, Sarah Lamb, Ann O'Hare, Uta Poiger, Jeannette Pols, Lillian Prueher, Priti Ramamurthy, Lorna Rhodes, Michael Rosenthal, Aaron Seaman, Lesley Sharp, Mette Nordahl Svendsen, Lynn Thomas, Marieke van Eijk, Lisa Vig, and Kathleen Woodward.

REFERENCES

Barnes, L. L., C. F. Mendes de Leon, R. S. Wilson, and D. A. Evans. 2004. "Social Resources and Cognitive Decline in a Population of Older African Americans and Whites." *Neurology* 63: 2322–2326.

Beland, F., M.-V. Zunzunegui, B. Alvarado, A. Otero, and T. del Ser. 2005. "Trajectories of Cognitive Decline and Social Relations." *Journal of Gerontology: Psychological Sciences* 60B (6): 320–330.

Besnier, Niko. 2009. *Gossip and the Everyday Production of Politics*. Honolulu: University of Hawaii Press.

Crooks, V. C., J. Lubben, D. B. Pettiti, D. Little, and V. Chiu. 2013. "Social Network, Cognitive Function, and Dementia Incidence among Elderly Women." *American Journal of Public Health* 98 (7): 1221–1227.

Kaufman, Sharon R. 2015. *Ordinary Medicine: Extraordinary Treatments, Longer Lives, and Where to Draw the Line*. Durham, NC: Duke University Press.

Lamb, Sarah. 2014. "Permanent Personhood or Meaningful Decline? Toward a Critical Anthropology of Successful Aging." *Journal of Aging Studies* 29: 41–52.

Lindemann, Hilde. 2014. *Holding and Letting Go: The Social Practice of Personal Identities*. Oxford: Oxford University Press.

Mattingly, Cheryl. 2014. *Moral Experiments: Family Peril and the Struggle for a Good Life*. Berkeley: University of California Press.

McFadden, Susan H., and John T. McFadden. 2011. *Aging Together: Dementia, Friendship, and Flourishing Communities*. Baltimore: Johns Hopkins University Press.

Morgan, Lynn M. 2009. *Icons of Life: A Cultural History of Human Embryos*. Berkeley: University of California Press.

Prince, M., E. Albanese, M. Guerchet, and M. Prina. 2014. "World Alzheimer's Report 2014: Dementia and Risk Reduction, An Analysis of Protective and Modifiable Factors." London: Alzheimer's Disease International.

Prince, M., R. Bryce, E. Albanese, A. Wimo, W. Ribeiro, and C. P. Ferri. 2013. "The Global Prevalence of Dementia: A Systematic Review and Metaanalysis." *Alzheimer's and Dementia* 9: 63–75.

Rowe, John W., and Robert L. Kahn. 1997. "Successful Aging." *Gerontologist* 37 (4): 433–440.

Taylor, Charles. 1989. *Sources of the Self.* Cambridge, MA: Harvard University Press.

Taylor, Janelle S. 2003. "The Story Catches You and You Fall Down: Tragedy, Ethnography, and 'Cultural Competence.'" *Medical Anthropology Quarterly* 17 (2): 159–181.

———. 2008. "On Recognition, Caring, and Dementia." *Medical Anthropology Quarterly* 22 (4): 313–335.

PART III

National Policies and Everyday Practices

Individual and Collective Projects of Aging Well

9

Getting Old and Keeping Going

The Motivation Technologies of Active Aging in Denmark

ASKE JUUL LASSEN AND ASTRID PERNILLE JESPERSEN

During a game of billiards at a Danish activity center for older people, Kåre raises his glass of schnapps and says jokingly: "Cheers! This is active aging." At the time of fieldwork, he was eighty years of age and one of the daily players of billiards at the activity center the Cordial Club. Placed in the suburbs of Copenhagen, the Cordial Club is a self-organized activity center housed in municipal dwellings with approximately one hundred members, who use the club to play billiards, cards, darts, bingo, and dice, as well as to socialize. A group of thirty to forty core members run the club and attend three to four times a week. Many mainly play billiards, often six hours daily four days a week. To become a member one must be a retiree, and most members are over seventy, with some members well into their nineties playing billiards for as long as the center is open. Both genders attend the center, with a small majority of men, but most activities are divided between the genders, so men mostly play billiards and women mostly play cards. Aske Juul Lassen conducted ethnographic fieldwork at the club as part of a broader study of how life in old age is organized and lived in Denmark.

Since the end of the 1990s, active aging has been a key agenda for policies regarding older people in Europe (Lassen and Moreira 2014; Walker 2009). Taking an active life in old age as the means to increase quality of life and postpone decline and dependency, active aging policies facilitate different types of social, physical, mental, and productive activities for older people. Although the interlocutors in this study did not use the term "active aging" until Aske told them about his research project, they all saw themselves as active individuals who wanted to keep going and engage in life. However, at the same time interlocutors like Kåre distanced themselves from any exterior pressure to conduct life in a certain way. Kåre made sure to continuously point out that he swam eight hundred meters every morning and, as such, acknowledged that he felt the need to stay physically active. In the next moment, however, Kåre would ward off any idea of a healthy old age as the ideal, as he felt that he had labored hard his entire life and had now earned the right to relax and live as he pleased. So when Aske told about active aging policies in the European Union, these were seen as both an unwelcome intrusion into the members' life conduct, as well as an object of ridicule.

In many ways, Kåre lives out the ideal of active aging. His daily swimming and his engagement in the local community through the Cordial Club tells a tale about an old man who has the zest to live an active life physically and socially. He has a wife twelve years younger than he, and this helps to keep him young, he says. They travel a lot, attend concerts, and go on long bicycle trips. But Kåre also lives what could be perceived as an unhealthy lifestyle in many ways. He suffers from type 2 diabetes and cardiovascular diseases, but these do not impede him from drinking a lot, and he does not wish to be bothered by any advice on diet or exercise from his general practitioner. He talks about the contemporary Danish focus on lifestyle and health as a "health regime," and he says: "I don't want to be put under administration just because I have a couple of diseases. I really wish they [the doctors] would just leave me alone." While doing gardening work some years ago, he suffered a thrombosis. He engaged in a rehabilitation program but constantly argued with the doctors at the clinic, saying that they were intruding into his private affairs: "I have worked hard and always contributed. I wish they would just let me enjoy retirement without all the hassle."

Kåre regards his diseases as part and parcel of growing old and does not see them as a reason to be concerned, nor as a reason to slow down in any way. He feels a wish to "keep going" but sees this as his own wish that has nothing to do with active aging policies or any type of intervention into the way old age is lived. For him, "keeping going" is about taking an interest in life; it is about swimming, playing billiards, listening to jazz, traveling, socializing, and drinking—it is not about health, exercise, diet, or activity for the sake of activity itself. In this way, Kåre partially bends the premises of active aging and partially integrates them in his everyday life.

The Danish Welfare State and the Emergence of Active Aging

As a senior citizen in Denmark, Kåre's everyday life as well as his ongoing negotiations with the ideal of active aging is taking place in a particular social context. The Danish welfare state is often referred to as the Nordic Model, grouping the Scandinavian countries (Denmark, Norway, Sweden, and Finland) together in a specific societal regime sharing similar characteristics, such as tax-financed public provision of a large number of social services: child care, basic and advanced education, hospital care and health services, and care for the elderly. Access to these basic social services is independent of income and employment status.

For the elderly population in particular, the Nordic Model is characterized by a universal system combining national old age and occupational labor market pensions. Together with publicly provided and subsidized social services for the elderly—including activity centers, home care, nursing homes, and reduced prices on public transport—the pension schemes essentially ensure an acceptable income and life for the elderly population. Local authorities deliver the social services and forms of eldercare under a common legislative framework, ensuring universal support while allowing for local differences. Historically, the welfare state expanded in the twentieth century when there were "many to support few," in the sense that the working age population was increasing relative to the number of children and old. With the current demographic changes of population aging, the Nordic Model is seriously challenged, and a number of reforms and initiatives have been launched, spanning from a gradual increase in the age of retirement from sixty-five today to sixty-seven in 2022, to the focus on staying physically and mentally active—that is, the ideal of active aging.

As active aging paradigms focus on physical and mental activity, they challenge stereotypical categorizations of the old as passive and declining. The European welfare states reinforced these categorizations through the twentieth century, as old age was increasingly concurrent with public welfare services: "[The] association between older people and the welfare state produced both positive and negative outcomes for this group: . . . On the one hand, it raised [older people's] living standards substantially in most Western European countries, but on the other hand, it contributed to their social construction as dependent in economic terms and encouraged popular ageist stereotypes of old age as a period of both poverty and frailty" (Walker 2009, 77).

However, since the late 1990s the concept of active aging has been at the heart of European and World Health Organization policy programs related to aging. Active aging can be regarded as a new ideal for old age, focusing on older people's possibilities for participation in socially and physically active pursuits. Active aging is based on a wide range of scientific results and aging theories, which, generally speaking, show the rejuvenating effects of various types of activity. This is a departure from the version of old age that was formed throughout the twentieth century, which equated old age with being dependent on the community and the welfare state. The new ideal for old age supports a reorganization of the social institutions associated with old age, such as old-age pensions and nursing homes. Furthermore, it requires a fundamental transformation in the expectations persons have regarding their old age. It is no longer a matter of reaping what one has sown. Instead, continuing to "sow" and participate actively is a precondition for living a good life, throughout a person's entire lifetime. British gerontologist Peter Townsend describes how elderly people's social dependency is in important part structural, socially constructed, and dependent on the ways in which work and the life course are organized, such as the proliferation of a compulsory retirement age and universal pension schemes (1981). The hypothesis behind the active aging agenda seems to be that if the structural framework is changed, the dependency that accompanies old age can also be fundamentally changed.

As a supranational institution, the European Union only indirectly organizes the way old age is lived in Denmark, as active aging is translated differently across European countries and in different Danish municipalities. But as an overall referential point, active aging steers the various old age policies toward more participation and independence among elders, and away from providing to elders as passive recipients. Furthermore, in line with the ideal of participation in active aging, older people in Denmark increasingly participate in policy building and local administration, through organizations like DaneAge and Senior Citizens Councils and through collaborations between municipalities and local organizations for the old.

In the following sections we show how active aging plays out in Denmark through concrete initiatives and current debates about rehabilitation, prevention, and loneliness, exploring how policies and everyday lives are entangled and how active aging ideals shape late life in new ways.

Fieldwork

The insights we present in this article are based on parts of Aske Juul Lassen's PhD dissertation (Lassen 2014a). The fieldwork consisted of participant observation at two activity centers for the elderly in the Copenhagen area—the Cordial Club and Wiedergården—as well as semistructured interviews with a total of seventeen users at the centers. The two centers have very different user profiles. In the Cordial Club, the members mainly come from working-class backgrounds, whereas those who frequent Wiedergården have more mixed backgrounds, while most have completed medium-length or longer higher education. The two centers have mixed gender profiles, with a small majority of men at the Cordial Club and a small majority of women at Wiedergården. Most activities are predominantly used by one of the genders, although activities such as Ping Pong, darts, and language clubs attract both genders equally. The interlocutors were aged between fifty-eight and ninety-two, with an average age of seventy-six.

Both of the activity centers are housed in municipal dwellings but organized by the attendees themselves. Thus, the older people themselves take the initiative to organize the various activities and manage the daily running of the centers. The municipality calls the people who lead the activities volunteers, but the volunteers distance themselves from this label, since the line between organizers and users at the centers is blurred. Some people are responsible for activities, others prepare lunch, others fetch newspapers, others organize parties, and the frailest are allowed to simply participate in the activities. Wiedergården has a manager and canteen staff employed by the municipality, but otherwise the older people themselves are responsible for running the centers. Although they represent a broad socioeconomic spectrum, the members of both centers are all older people for whom an activity center is a central part of their social life, and who all, to a certain extent, engage in their communities through these centers and who believe that it is important to remain active in later life. In spite of their different approaches to active aging, it seems that part of the ideal of the new European good old age—the imperative to stay active—has gained a foothold across the board.

The Motivation Technologies of Active Aging

Active aging policy suggests activity as the solution to problems associated with old age such as dependence and decline, implying that the problems of old age stem from the inactive lifestyles and everyday life behaviors of old people: if older people would only become more active, the problems of old age could be solved for both the individual and society. This premise leads to different types of interventions into the lifestyle of old people, including both rehabilitation (regaining ability after decline or disease) and prevention (proactive action to postpone decline or disease) programs and legislation. Although both rehabilitation and prevention programs predated active aging as health promotion methods in Denmark, in recent years these programs have been incorporated into the active aging agenda to transform old age. The ways rehabilitation and prevention aim at promoting health through activity and individual responsibility for the aging process seem, in fact, a perfect fit for active aging. Active aging, rehabilitation, and prevention all emphasize the importance of individual motivation for the aging process and healthy life conduct.

Rehabilitation and prevention can be seen as motivation technologies (Otto 2013). They attempt to change everyday life behavior by stimulating inner motivation, with focal points such as continuance of functional capacity and recommencement of activities of daily living after periods of functional decline. This stimulation is, for example, created through the nationwide evidence-based "motivational conversations," which "aim to help a person to become clarified regarding his/her values and lifestyle, in order to create an inner motivation to change a specific behavior or lifestyle" (National Board of Social Services 2013, 20–21, author's translation). Moreover, Danish health authorities attempt to support and engender this motivation through health promotion, home health care visits, and patient schools, which place the responsibility for health on the individual and position the inner motivation to stay healthy and active as key for behavioral change. As we will describe in the following sections, this motivation is not always easily found, nor is it necessarily inner. Older people both adapt to and resist the expectations associated with active aging; they express the individual and societal importance of leading a healthy life as well as refuse any interference with their well-earned golden years. As such, they relate in paradoxical ways to active aging and the inner motivation it both engenders and relies on.

Rehabilitation Programs and Dependence

One of the ideals of active aging is elderly people's independence, understood within Danish policy as being independent as far as possible both of welfare institutions and of assistance from others. Dependency might mean receiving home care, being completely immobile, or relying on the help of one's spouse to get out of bed or clean the house, but active aging policies aim to minimize or eradicate such forms of dependency—which had been closely associated with old age in Europe throughout the twentieth century—thereby problematizing the everyday lives of individuals who are dependent on other people's help.

In January 2015, for instance, the new Danish Law on Social Service was instituted, requiring citizens with rehabilitation potential to complete a rehabilitation program before home health care can be provided. This amendment (§83 para. 3) states that "prior to the assessment of the need for help [home care and/ or assistive technology] . . . the local council must assess whether a tender regarding §83a would improve the person's functional capacity and thus reduce the need for help" (Folketinget 2014, 1, author's translation). Rehabilitation is usually used as a term for a program that a person undergoes after an accident or a drop in functional capacity. Rehabilitation programs focus not only on physical activity but more holistically on the citizen's everyday life, social relations, and mental state, encouraging the citizen to participate in establishing goals for rehabilitation. The aim is usually to regain the skills to handle activities of daily living, and sometimes this can be obtained through the use of aids—such as devices that enable the older person to put on support stockings in the morning and take them off at night by him- or herself—thereby freeing the citizen from waiting for home care personnel to arrive and saving public resources.

When the national parliament debated the amendment in 2014, one of the central points was whether it should be permitted for an elderly individual to refuse rehabilitation and still retain the right to home care. Eventually it was added to the law that the older person cannot be refused help by the municipality solely based on the recipient's inability to complete the rehabilitation process, but the biggest national organization for older people, DaneAge, has questioned whether this addition is sufficiently clear. Through rehabilitation, elderly individuals are expected to find their own internal motivation to be rehabilitated. Professionals should aim to "elicit the citizen's motivation" (National Board of Social Services 2014, 7), but it is a difficult space to navigate when they encounter those who are unable to find the motivation, and in whom it cannot be elicited. As such, the legitimacy of the dependence of old people is

problematized and turned into a question of motivation. In this regard, rehabilitation is a motivation technology that aims to internalize the need for activity
and healthy behavior, thereby postponing or avoiding dependence.

In general, participants in the activity centers were afraid of being dependent on someone else's help, and in this way the ideal of independence and
autonomy permeated their everyday lives. Several of the interlocutors had
noticed how they were expected to fight for their independence as part of the
rehabilitation process. They described how much their independence means
to them, but also that they do not want to be "disempowered" or "placed under
administration" just because they suffer from a few illnesses. When their everyday lives were problematized, and their motivation to fight for their mobility
brought into question, many reacted with defiance and a resistance against
what several called the "health regime."

Kåre displayed this kind of resistance when he, following a blood clot, was
referred to a rehabilitation program. He felt that the staff interfered too much,
and he refused to take his blood-thinning medication, because he believed that it
gave him too many bruises and because he felt just fine. When the doctor tried to
get him to take his medicine, he became angry. As we described in our introduction, he did not want to be put "under administration" because of some diseases.

During his rehabilitation program, Kåre often argued with his nurses,
because they wanted him to drink cordial instead of beer and would not let him
ride his stationary bike with as much resistance as he himself would like: "If
they had just asked, they would have discovered that I was quickly up and swimming a thousand meters again after the operation. Although I was two minutes
slower than before the operation. But they only focused on the cycling. When a
doctor finally asked me, it turned out to be bloody unnecessary for me to go all
the way over to Bispebjerg [the hospital]. The way they treat an old man is completely hopeless, of course. I have always worked hard and contributed. I wish
they could just let me enjoy my retirement years without all the hassle." Kåre felt
that the doctors questioned his motivation to regain his heart function, and that
his beer drinking was problematized. More than just a potential dependency
was problematized—at that stage, Kåre had not yet received home care—his beer
drinking and even his preferred exercise habits were also questioned. The goal
was a particular form of independence: independence from care, but not an
independent or autonomous approach to the rehabilitation process.

This ambivalent goal of independence is also evident in Daisy's story. She
cared for her ill husband for a period of five years until his death twenty-five
years ago. The constant heavy lifting of her husband and her work as a cleaning lady meant that Daisy suffers from joint pain, and she cites hard work as the
cause of her osteoarthritis. Furthermore, she has type 2 diabetes and high blood
pressure, and she was given an artificial wrist after a fall two years ago (see also

Lassen 2015). Of her many diseases, her wrist and her arthritis worry her the most, because she fears that they may jeopardize her independence. She considers her elevated blood pressure and blood glucose levels to be primarily her doctor's problem. They are too difficult for her to deal with and do not seem to have any obvious impact on her independence, although the doctor often points out that it is dangerous to ignore these diseases. She evaluates the severity of her various diseases based on the immediate threat they represent with regards to her independence. Her fear of being dependent on home help leads to a unilateral concern about, and motivation to take care of, individual diseases, while she neglects other diseases, which have less noticeable (yet potentially lethal) consequences.

Thus, both Daisy and Kåre are motivated to stay independent, but they adapt this expectation to their everyday practices and desires. Kåre drinks beer, swims, and would like to be left alone by his doctors; Daisy takes care of her arthritis but not her diabetes. Both express motivation toward maintaining independence, but their stories show how motivation and independence are formed differently in everyday lives. It is not something innate, nor is it something determined by the authorities. Rather, it is formed through their life stories, habits, and social relations.

Prevention Programs and Decline

In addition to striving to eradicate dependence, Danish active aging paradigms also aspire to reshape other problems previously associated with old age, such as the physical decline experienced by many elderly people and the passive lifestyles many seem to initiate once they have retired. In this regard, decline and passivity are being fashioned as problems that can be solved through correct activities and proper lifestyle choices. Central to this solution are prevention programs, which intervene in the lifestyle of healthy people, that is, before they suffer from eventual conditions. The premise is that risk factors such as smoking, alcohol consumption, unhealthy diet, and lack of exercise lead to poor health and quality of life. Instead of spending huge amounts on health care for people suffering from lifestyle diseases, government prevention initiatives set in beforehand, trusted to benefit both national expenditure and individual quality of life. Such initiatives emphasize inner motivation: changing health behavior prior to the onset of diseases requires motivated citizens who are able to understand the long-term consequences of their behavior and act accordingly. Initiatives include patient schools, motivational conversations with public employees, health campaigns focused on lifestyle, and preventive home visits.

The Danish preventive home visits (PHVs) have previously been analyzed by Lene Otto as one form of implementing the active aging scheme (2013). Since 1998 Danish law mandates that municipalities offer a PHV to all citizens aged seventy-five or older. The PHVs take place in the home of the citizen, as a dialogue between the citizen and a health professional, aiming to improve self-care and detect physical, functional, and mental problems in the early stages. As Otto states, the PHV's main objective when introduced in the 1990s was to prevent functional decline, but today the PHV seems to have taken on a broader perspective, placing physical activity, diet, and social participation as focal points of discussion. The goal is to empower the citizen to look for the potential to self-care. The PHV provides the citizen with a language and an understanding of their aging bodies, enabling a space where their functional capacity can be negotiated. Although this might help to improve quality of life, it also increases the individual responsibility for self-care (Otto 2013). Where rehabilitation programs set in after decline and dependence, prevention programs intervene prior to decline and dependence and do not accept these as a consequence of old age.

However, many center members subscribe to a different understanding of the correlation between old age and decline, and they point out that decline inevitably accompanies old age. For example, seventy-three-year-old Kisser says, "Of course, it is part of getting old." Several of the interlocutors have a number of chronic diseases that require treatment, as is the norm for their age group. Thus, there seems to be a significant discrepancy between elderly people's perception of decline as something inevitable and the way decline is articulated in active aging policies. In Danish active aging policy, decline becomes a problem rooted in an unhealthy lifestyle and the individuals' lack of motivation. Yet in the interlocutors' everyday lives, decline is ever present, as they notice that they are capable of doing fewer and fewer activities with age despite their often very active lives. The interlocutors Valter and Kisser had stopped cycling together, and Kisser had been forced to give up her part-time job selling sandwiches and sodas to the local choir, because she experienced breathing difficulties. She explained that "I almost couldn't drag myself home anymore, and I needed to just stop right away, but what will be next?" She feared her decline would become a self-perpetuating problem, as she could participate in fewer and fewer activities.

The imperative to stay active in order to avoid an intensification of their physical decline seems to be an integral part of the interlocutors' perception of the aging process. However, at the same time they experience decline as an inevitable aspect of growing older, not something they welcome but, at the same time, not something they strive to avoid (or believe they may avoid) altogether.

Like dependence and decline, active aging discourse also envisions passivity as a problem of lack of inner motivation. However, interlocutors like Kisser dread the way decline and passivity often enhance each other as inscribed into the aging process.

The activity centers in Denmark must be seen in the light of this widely perceived entanglement between passivity, decline, and dependence. Activity centers are often a part of nursing homes in Denmark, where older people from the municipality, usually those with mild impairments, can attend a range of activities during the day for free, in order to keep going despite beginning dependence. In the last decades more and more private initiatives—usually supported by the local municipality—attract older persons with other activity requirements who do not wish to frequent the premises of nursing homes. The Cordial Club and Wiedergården are examples of such initiatives that run almost solely on volunteer work. Most center members are active in their communities outside of the centers and engage in, for example, volunteer work, crafts, and sports, and since Aske met the interlocutors at an activity center they were all active to some extent. But the activities that the interlocutors engaged in—such as billiards, bingo, and darts—often differed from the ones promoted through active aging programs, which tend to emphasize physical exercise and social work and volunteering for the community. All of the interlocutors stressed the importance of getting on with their day and generally disapproved of their inactive acquaintances, but they also stressed that rest and relaxation are important parts of their everyday lives. They both adhere to the ideal of an active old age, as well as resist the idea that activities like running or doing volunteer work fit better with a good old age than billiards or darts. In fact, many interlocutors stressed billiards as an ideal old-age activity, due to the way the game allows for activity and passivity to intertwine when waiting between turns and chit-chatting between games (Lassen 2014b). The smooth rhythm of the game enables them to play for many hours daily, and thus, even though they think of billiards primarily as a social activity, they are physically active during the entire day. But it is a kind of physical activity that is made possible by the passivity that also pervades the game.

So, What about Loneliness?

As we have shown throughout the chapter, the Danish welfare state intervenes heavily in the lifestyle of aging citizens under the rubric of active aging. But in recent years, the focus on the lifestyle of citizens has broadened from the parameters of diet, physical activity, smoking, and drinking to also include the mental health of its aging citizens. This is evident in the campaigns against loneliness launched by DaneAge, the Senior Citizens Councils, and many Danish municipalities, all in 2015, wherein initiatives such as volunteering, visiting friends, cafés for the "lonely old" at community centers, and discussion groups for newly retired males (regarded as especially at risk for becoming lonely) all aim at reducing loneliness in what has been labeled the People's Movement Against Loneliness. This coincides with numerous epidemiological studies that point to poor social relations as an important risk factor for the onset of disability (e.g., Lund, Nilsson, and Avlund 2010).

In the realm of the Danish welfare state, loneliness in old age has been rein-forced, one might argue, by the institutionalization and professionalization of care, which has removed care for the old from the family and community. Although lone-liness is a significant problem for the elderly people who experience it, loneliness is not an automatic consequence of growing old. A recent study shows that in the older group, 7 percent of men and 10 percent of women are lonely (Danish Health and Medicine Authority 2014, 110–111). The loss of one's spouse or friends, one's chil-dren living in a different city, or limited mobility may bring about loneliness, but it is important that aloneness (voluntary) is not mistaken for loneliness (involuntary).

Many of the interlocutors in this study experienced some degree of loneli-ness. Many had lost contact with their old friends, and only a few lived close to their family. For example, Daisy felt that the weekends were a difficult time, because the activity center was closed and most of her social contact took place there. During the weekends, she sometimes went for walks alone in an amusement park, but she no longer went to the cinema or the theater in the evening due to changed bus routes and her fear of being out after dark. Her friend's husband had fallen ill, and her friend spent all of her time looking after him, so they no longer saw each other during the weekends. She had a brother who lived close by, and he was her only sporadic weekend social con-tact. Other interlocutors had no friends left outside of the activity center, and the activity centers were often used to find a partner or a date. As such, the activity centers were a large part of many people's social life, and due to sick or deceased spouses and limited contact with friends and ex-colleagues, the centers were often the elderly people's opportunity to spend time with others.

At the same time, the active, social, and engaged communities that active aging engenders do not seem to be the good old age for all. The good old age can also be experienced alone, or momentarily alone. Some interlocutors explained how they sometimes need to take a break from all the togetherness they experience at the center and in their community. Kåre feels just fine spending his day listening to jazz records and staring out the window from his library in solitude. Sometimes Valter needs his solitude at nights after a long day of chores in the center, where he is the daily manager. He loves to see family and his ex-wife during weekends, but finds nights during the week to be "his own," where he cooks, reads, plays on the computer, and watches television. In the same way, Iris would not do without her nights alone where she surfs the net and finally gets some time to herself after a day of working in her company and taking care of her demented husband. And Lisbeth constantly tries to keep her schedule as open as possible so she will not be overwhelmed by social company and have time to do impulsive activities.

As such, many interlocutors buy into the ideals of active aging, but life is not only social activity, exercise, and engagement. The interlocutors also want to be left alone, and perceive time alone as quality time. Togetherness and activity are not constants. Activity and passivity constitute each other, and so do loneliness and togetherness. Aloneness can be momentary, and aloneness can be wanted. Constant engagements with other people may be an ideal for many younger people continually online connecting with peers and sharing narratives. But for many older persons, the constant engagement in active aging is experienced as youth-centric and as a disruption from their life stories. They want to participate and be active, but not necessarily in the ways expected by the local authorities.

This is not opposite to active aging but something that policies of active aging must not forget in their eagerness to create the active old age. Loneliness complicates the message from active aging. By focusing on the active community, active aging risks creating a feeling of loneliness in people who were previously fine in their own company, and it risks giving all passive or solitary situations a negative spin. More-over, the focus on independence, which we have shown is central in active aging, also risks creating loneliness. Where old people in Denmark previously to a larger degree were dependent on home care and health care, rehabilitation and prevention programs risk engendering motivated, lonely citizens who are able to take care of themselves in their own homes. Loneliness nuances the debate of active aging and questions how much the good old age can be designed by the Danish welfare state.

Conclusion: Active Aging in the Welfare State

The shifts in the discourse on old age and population composition challenge how old age was previously organized in Denmark. Through the twentieth century a range of public institutions, such as home care, nursing homes, and public pensions, formed old age into a period of provision and care. At the turn of the millennium this was increasingly seen as a strategy that pacified older people, which was bad for both quality of life and public funds. Under the international policy framework of active aging, the Danish aging policies began to focus on independence and active participation in one's own health and community. This has fostered a very specific form of growing old, wherein the institutions of old age have gradually been reformed. In the realm of the Danish welfare state, active aging policies target every aspect of the lifestyle of old people, and they are not just about physical activity or diet but also about social activity and mental health.

In addition to fostering independence, active aging aims at eliminating passivity and loneliness. While this is a remarkable ambition, in its eagerness to stimulate constant engagements, relations, and participation, active aging risks changing the perception of aloneness into something inherently negative. While some interlocutors experience loneliness, aloneness is often seen as valu-able. Older Danes both buy into many of the ideas behind active aging, but they also bend it and change it as they go.

This ambivalent attitude toward active aging is recurrent in our data. The old people it targets see many benefits from aging in active ways but find Danish active aging policies to be too meticulous and far reaching, as they aim to intervene in every aspect of the elders' daily lives. In current Danish politics it is very evident that the schism between care and independence is urgent. Older people form a crucial group of voters, and care and provision reforms challenge the way many Danes perceive old age in the welfare state. When the national budget for 2014 was negotiated, the central-left coalition fell apart due to one of the parties' insistence on elderly people's right to two weekly baths. This insistence coins the active aging dilemma in Denmark: What are the basic rights to care and provision in a welfare state, and how much self-care and self-provision can be expected from the increasingly larger group of people approaching retirement? While active aging provides the answer that independence and activity are good for all, it does not answer what happens to those who cannot live up to the expectations of an active and healthy old age, and who might envision other ways of aging well.

REFERENCES

Danish Health and Medicine Authority (Sundhedsstyrelsen). 2014: *Danskernes sundhed—Den nationale sundhedsprofil 2013*. Copenhagen: Sundhedsstyrelsen.

Folketinget. 2014. "Lov om ændring af lov om social service (Rehabiliteringsforløb og hjemmehjælp m.v.)." http://www.ft.dk/RIpdf/samling/20141/lovforslag/L25/20141_L25_som _vedtaget.pdf, accessed 25 August 2015.

Lassen, Aske Juul. 2014a. "Active Ageing and the Unmaking of Old Age." PhD diss., University of Copenhagen.

———. 2014b. "Billiards, Rhythms, Collectives—Billiards at a Danish Activity Centre as a Culturally Specific Form of Active Ageing." *Ethnologia Europaea* 44: 57–74.

———. 2015. "Keeping Disease at Arm's Length: How Older Danish People Distance Disease through Active Ageing." *Ageing & Society* 35: 1364–1383.

Lassen, Aske Juul, and Tiago Moreira. 2014. "Unmaking Old Age: Political and Cognitive Formats of Active Ageing." *Journal of Aging Studies* 30: 33–46.

Lund, Rikke, Charlotte J. Nilsson, and Kirsten Avlund. 2010. "Can the Higher Risk of Disability Onset among Older People Who Live Alone Be Alleviated by Strong Social Relations? A Longitudinal Study of Non-disabled Men and Women." *Age and Ageing* 39: 319–326.

Otto, Lene. 2013. "Negotiating a Healthy Body in Old Age: Preventive Home Visits and Biopolitics." *International Journal of Aging and Later Life* 8: 111–135.

National Board of Social Services (Socialstyrelsen). 2013. *Brug af redskaber i rehabilitering til hverdagens aktiviteter på ældreområdet*. Odense: Socialstyrelsen.

———2014. *Rehabilitering på ældreområdet—inspiration til kommunal praksis*. Odense: Socialstyrelsen.

Townsend, Peter. 1981. "The Structured Dependency of the Elderly: A Creation of Social Policy in the Twentieth Century." *Ageing and Society* 1: 5–28.

Walker, Alan. 2009. "Commentary: The Emergence and Application of Active Aging in Europe." *Journal of Aging and Social Policy* 21: 75–93.

10

Foolish Vitality

Humor, Risk, and Success in Japan

JASON DANELY

Furukawa-san sat in the gently filtered sunlight at the front table of her daughter's café, slowly, carefully prying the meat from the bones of her fish with a pair of chopsticks. She had been coming to the café for lunch about three times a week since moving from the far north of Japan, where she had lived alone since her husband passed away several years ago. Her health had deteriorated at an alarming pace during a recent hospitalization, and her daughter had been so worried that within three months she had arranged for Furukawa-san to move to an older person's apartment (*kōreisha jūtaku*) in Kyoto, maintaining her independence but staying close to her daughter's home.

Furukawa-san was in a good mood when I arrived, taking a seat next to her and showing her the front page of the day's newspaper. The headline running down the side of the front page in bold, angular print read, "520,000 Wait for a Care Home."

"Can you believe that?" she said to me. "There are so many older people now in Japan! I heard that at most places you have to wait in a queue of about a hundred people [before you can get a bed]! The country doesn't want to spend money, that's why. In a few years it will be a couple million." She sighed, then carefully lifted a bowl of miso soup to her lips.

"Well, everyone gets old," she continued. "The things that you used to do, just going shopping, doing the cooking—I stopped being able to do those things. Now I live in a place where a helper comes along every few days—in my case, she comes in the afternoon—and she'll ask me, 'Have you washed your face? Have you changed your underwear? Have you brushed your teeth?'" Furukawa-san mimicked the slow sing-song of a young carer's voice. "It's not bad," she explained. "She just sort of cleans up a little. It's a different person every time."

Unsure of whether I should delve further into this delicate topic, I asked, "What do you think about when you consider how you'll spend your later years [rōgo no seikatsu]?" Furukawa-san replied, "Well, we all just want to live well. How you do that is another matter, you know. We want to have a nice end, but humans don't really get to choose that. I'm eighty-three. Right when I turned eighty my body just started failing me. I was going to the clinic for this and that all the time. [It happened] all of a sudden! I would forget to eat, or I would forget about what I ate, and with my diabetes, it would really cause trouble!"

As she talked about her failing body and mind, she was giggling. Perhaps this was just the reflexive embarrassment that permeates the Japanese culture of propriety, or maybe it was because we were talking about hospital food and failing bodies while still nibbling our lunch. I couldn't quite tell. She giggled even more as she continued: "I went to the doctor and he said I had some sort of condition, I don't recall the name of it now, but I said to him, 'Well, I don't mind so much if [I die] this year, but it would be nice to make it to the next!' He had a laugh at that! 'I don't know how long you'll live, but it may still be quite a few years!' he said, and I had to just agree [laughing]! But my life has been all right [māmā] so far, I guess, you know?"

After catching her breath and taking a sip of tea, it was Furukawa-san's turn to ask me a question: "How's your life been? Wouldn't you say it was all right?" Normally I would have tried to be more reserved, but the sun, the conversation, and even the food was making me feel so giddy, and without really thinking about it, I blurted out, "I'm happy [shiawase]!"

"Oh, that's unusual that someone would say that! Not just all right, but really happy!" Furukawa-san replied after a surprised pause. Then she started giggling again. "You know, after you said that, I thought to myself, there's nothing strange about saying you're happy! I am happy! I'm going tell people I'm happy, too!"

There we were, both laughing, basking in the pleasure of a moment of spontaneous connection, playing with that funny world of words, despite or perhaps because we were talking about old age, illness, and death. In a sense, we were both laughing at "successful aging," that ongoing process of self-betterment that in Japan also includes a sense of seriousness, modesty, restraint, and endurance. For Furukawa-san, exclaiming that she was happy with her life felt exciting, like she was breaking the rules, and I was happy to act as her accomplice.

Conversations between older people in Japan often include these moments of levity, and as average life expectancies edge into the late eighties,[1] there is ample source material for humor. This doesn't mean, however, that Japanese people have been immune to the ideology of successful aging (see introduction, this volume); on the contrary, it pervades much of the current elder welfare system and gerontological research. In this chapter, I want to consider whether the uptake of successful aging in Japan has contributed to the ability of people like Furukawa-san to let down their guard and exclaim that they are happy. Does it encourage or inhibit the development of an attitude and feeling toward aging that provides the opportunity for foolishness and laughter despite hardships accompanying what is for many today a long, slow decline stretching out into one's nineties and beyond?

"Old Age Ain't No Place for Sissies"

"Successful aging" is not funny. Of course, when you slip the phrase into a conversation with someone who is unfamiliar with all of the scientific literature on the subject, you might find that they react with a low chuckle, as if to say, "Nothing's 'successful' about getting old!" But to the geriatricians and gerontologists who have studied and embraced the idea, successful aging is serious business. After all, the implied alternative is some kind of less-than-successful, or even failed, process of aging—the kind of aging, perhaps, that is indicated in the well-worn phrase attributed to Bette Davis: "Old age ain't no place for sissies." As an academic, I've learned to take old age seriously as well. Guided by the work of developmental social scientists, like Erik H. Erikson, I learned to pay attention to the ways old age constituted a psychosocial crisis between *ego-integrity* and *despair.* To me, this meant rolling up one's sleeves and digging into matters of responsibility and the defense of dignity—what Erikson called the "patrimony of [the] soul" ([1950] 1993, 268). I viewed old age as a time to grapple with weighty existential issues, the steady drumbeat of mortality, and maybe even the terror and despair of losing (or having already irrevocably lost) a sense of importance, belonging, and understanding of the world.

So during my first extensive fieldwork in Japan in the early 2000s, I decided to look at spiritual practices and subjectivities of mourning and resilience (Danely 2014). Again, hardly funny stuff. When I would try to casually mention my research topic to older people I met, it would invariably shift the mood of the conversation toward the serious. But gradually I grew more and more conscious of my own assumption that tearful confessions and wringing hands were somehow better indications of what was important to older people than the smiles and laughter. It is hard to keep such assumptions from affecting the ethnographic narrative, especially in a place like Japan, where a high value is placed on enduring suffering and accepting the unhappy ending (Benedict [1946]1976, 254; da Rosa et al. 2014; Levy 1999). Even when Japanese older people do find life satisfying and meaningful, they are usually modest in admitting this about themselves and tend to emphasize the "negative" aspects of aging (cf. Grossmann et al. 2014; Levy 1999).

But stoicism and modesty are not the only ways of embodying old age in Japan. In his classic ethnography of a Japanese village, *Suye Mura* (1939), John F. Embree observed that "the old people may do and say what they like without fear of criticism. . . . Both men and women tend to be more individualistic and free as they get older" ([1939] 1964, 214). We might also consider the beloved Zen hermit Ryōkan, who was also known as the "great fool" (*taigu*) for his fondness of playing with children and writing humorous poetry. One of his poems reads:

> While I bounce the ball, they sing the song
> Then I sing the song and they bounce the ball
> Caught up in the excitement of the game
> We forget completely about the time
> Passersby turn and question me:
> "Why are you carrying on like this?"
> I just shake my head without answering
> Even if I were able to say something how could I explain?
> Do you really want to know the meaning of it all?
> This is it! This is it!
>
> (Abe and Haskel 1996, 132)

Reflecting on these representations of aging made me wonder if I too had been lured by a monolithic view of successful aging as the fruit of hard work rather than of humor and play.

Humor opens up a gateway into understanding well-being and quality of life in old age, and in Japan, this appears most pronounced among the oldest old[2]—those who are most engaged in the process of what Sarah Lamb (2014) has called "meaningful decline" (48). Rather than a somber, serious standoff with death, Japanese men and women who have reached advanced old age (in their eighties and older) often speak to me about the importance of keeping things light, an attitude I call "foolish vitality." Foolish vitality is the playful, unashamed, acceptance of old age, wrinkles and all. It brings together the joy, creativity, and liberation found when one no longer resists the signs of aging, and even comes to embrace them in ways that are silly and saucy but not self-deprecatory or ageist.

A recent example of this kind of foolish vitality in Japan is the pop group KBG84 (derived from the first letters of Kohama Bāchan Gasshōdan (Granny Chorus of Kohama), and the average age of the thirty-three members: eighty-four) (Agence France Press 2015). In 2015 the group made international headlines with their energetic and spirited Okinawan songs and dances.[3] Their name and performance style pokes fun at the youthful pop-idol industry epitomized by the group AKB48 (average age of the forty-eight girls that comprised the group in

2015: 13.8), but KBG84's message is not a social critique of youth-centered media, nor is it simply meant to exemplify successful aging. They inspire because they are willing to risk the vulnerability—exposure to both fame and ridicule—that comes with foolish vitality. In their upbeat music video "Come on and Dance Kohamajima," the grannies dressed in bright summer kimono and red head-bands appear to lead the ordinary townspeople of their island (students, shop-keepers, farmers, etc.) in a series of simple rhythmic dance moves, encouraging everyone to join in their silly fun.

Foolish vitality subverts the power of stereotypes by airing them openly, showing off wrinkles and yellowed teeth with a hearty laugh. This is a risk, a way of being vulnerable that also confers empowerment,[4] as in the phrase frequently overheard in groups of older Japanese people, "At my age, I can say what I like!" Humor itself seems to hinge on this sense of risking vulnerability, tickling us by scuttling along the edge of our comfort zone.

Successful aging, too, deals with risk, but in a different way. In political terms, the successful aging paradigm appears to legitimate neoliberal patterns of withdrawal of the state from the provision of welfare assistance (Dillaway and Byrnes 2009; Rubinstein and Medeiros 2014). Rather than take on the risk of an aging society on a societal level, successful aging supposes that individuals can and should assume the risk themselves as self-reliant agents (Rubinstein and Medeiros 2014, 3; Stowe and Cooney 2015, 45). Conspicuous exuberance and humor turns this around, laughing in the face of risk, playing with it in the way a comedian raises the tension in their audience just before delivering a zippy punchline.

Serious Play in Senior Centers

The use of humor as a therapeutic intervention or strategy for interacting with older people has roots in our understanding of humor as a form of "coping" (Freud [1916] 1993).[5] Professor of Nursing Roland Berk (2001) found no less than fifteen clear psychophysiological benefits of humor and laughter for older adults. While Berk is careful to note the evidence of some risk for those with existing medical conditions, he concludes that the risks are low enough that "it is highly unlikely that a warning label will appear on the prescription for laughter anytime soon" (2001, 333). Successful aging theories have themselves at times included the notion of humor (e.g., Baltes and Baltes 1990, 346; Vaillant and Mukamal 2001, 841), though rarely is humor at the center of research stud-ies, but more often only one of dozens of factors presumed to lead to well-being in later life, including spirituality, education, and mental health.

In the process of importing the successful aging perspective to Japan, those designing senior activities likewise also tend to overlook humor in favor of physical programs emphasizing active aging and exercise (*taisō*), the movement of the body above all else, in order to promote an ethic of self-care (Ricart 2015). In my observations of several light exercise groups for seniors, for example, instructors would stress the way each movement was linked to some capacity to remain independent, or at least to avoid looking like an older person. While doing leg lifts, an exercise instructor at one adult day care facility would say things like, "If you let these muscles get weaker, you'll be shuffling along looking like one of those *old* people! And what will happen? Pretty soon you'll trip and fall over!" He didn't have to elaborate. Everyone knew what happened after a fall, and they would redouble their efforts with faces locked in stern resolve.

The seriousness of successful aging could be seen in senior welfare centers as well. These centers are managed by municipal wards (*ku*) and provide spaces for club activities that had typically been organized by community volunteers of the Old Person's Association. Urbanization, welfare reforms, and longer lifespans have led many retirees to distance themselves from the title of "old person" and age-grade associations,[6] and these welfare centers have come to fill the gap, promoting educational, social, and exercise programs to attract the "third-agers"[7] who feel there is still time and energy to prevent physical and mental decline later in life. Popular center activities included ballroom dance, table tennis, and karaoke. There was a "busy body" (Katz 2000) atmosphere at work here, a drive to not only look and feel vital (*genki*) now, but to prepare for and prevent, if possible, prolonged decline in the future. This was what John Traphagan (2006) called "being a good *rōjin* [old person]," or embodying an ethics of self-care that performs and produces an autonomous self in order to remain enmeshed in appropriately interdependent relationships. In seeking to preserve this version of successful personhood, spaces for older people sanction against displays of foolish vitality, erecting institutional barriers between the more active young-old and those of more advanced age, many of whom, like the man I describe next, possessed a sense of humor that would have made Ryōkan proud.

The Doctor Dancing in Diapers

When I returned to Kyoto after finishing my degree and starting a new research project, most of the cohort I had met at senior centers had stopped attending for various reasons. Sometimes they stopped when their friends had left, but in other cases deteriorating health—mostly regarding eyesight, hearing, or mobility-related issues like having arthritis—just made it harder to get to the centers and more difficult to participate fully. What happens, then, to the aspirations of successful aging, nurtured for years in places like the community center, when the body and mind begin to fail? When walking requires being steadied by a cane, when one begins to move or talk or look like an "old person"? Furukawa-san had stated sagely that we humans can't decide how or when we are to become old or die. And yet this kind of uncertainty does not mean giving up on the hopeful project of well-being, belonging, meaningfulness. Instead, the ethics of well-being become an experiment in self-making where uncertainty, suspense, and tension become the fertile grounds for laughter.

I owe much of this insight on foolish vitality to Dr. Hayakawa, a ninety-year-old physician who held regular "study groups" at his home to discuss issues around life and death, health, welfare, and various other topics. Hayakawa-sensei[8] was articulate and charismatic, and agreed to help me understand this transition to what gerontologists have termed the "fourth age."[9]

H: When I go to talk to people about getting old, I always tell them, "Hey, I'm wearing adult diapers!" You should see everyone's faces! They all laugh! That's fine, right [*ee yan ka*]? I didn't have problems with incontinence until I was about ninety years old, and I was shocked when it happened. I'd feel as if I had to go and rush to the toilet, and then it would feel like only half was able to come out! The muscles relax, sort of sag and get loose, but that's what happens when you age. So that's why I have adult diapers.

D: But you haven't had to use them until you were ninety!

H: You're right [laughing]! But now when I say it, people think, "Oh, we're the same as sensei [teacher]!" And their faces change immediately. All that holding back of real feelings falls away. "Ee yan ka!" everything fine, it doesn't matter! Right? Have you ever been to Tokushima in Shikoku? They have a dance there that they do every August; [they say], "If we're all fools, we might as well all dance!"[10] The whole town dances for a week. If you're a dancing fool or you're just sitting there watching the dancing fools, you must be a fool as well, and if everyone is a fool, then it's all the same, so why not dance together? You see, if there is no difference, isn't it better to dance? Ee yan ka? That's a kind of liberation: What's wrong with dying? What's wrong with getting sick? We all get sick! What's wrong with becoming senile [*boke*]? Isn't it fine forgetting things? What's wrong with any of it? It doesn't mean giving up.

D: Not the same thing as giving up, right? It's more like acceptance?

Hayakawa-sensei was nearly jumping off the ground at this point, his eyes pinched as he burst into a wide, open-mouthed smile.

H: Yes! That's it! [You have] incredible Japanese! Giving up [*akirameru*] is just saying, "I can't do anything about it." *This* is about becoming *clear* [*akiraka ni suru*].

He clapped his hands, both in praise and to close our thoughts there. We'd come to the point that he had been trying to convey: the ordinary acceptance found in late life, dancing fools and diapered elders.

Hayakawa-sensei's version of well-being was the spirit of "*ee yan ka*." His eyes twinkled as he said the phrase, drawing out the first syllable from deep in his throat. "Eeeee" (pronounced "AAY") as if slowly dragging the word through wet gravel. Taken literally, the phrase simply means something like, "Fine, don't you think," and might be either a declaration that things are good, or a question, "Aren't things fine, after all?" And yet, like Ryle's playful discussion of the meanings of a "wink" (Geertz 1973, 6–7), even this double meaning did not exhaust the thickness of Hayakawa-sensei's ordinary phrase. No wonder he used the phrase so often each time we met, always in the casual, familiar form of the local Kansai dialect, locating it squarely in the quotidian realm of a conversation on the street, the dialect most commonly employed in Japanese stand-up comedy (*manzai*).

Like a haiku, consolidating the sensory richness of a moment into seventeen short syllables, Hayakawa-sensei's phrase was able to draw in all of the sweetness and light of his own personality. On another occasion he elaborated on the clarity this gave him:

> If I'm a little slow, or forget things, that's just old age. It's natural, and so we can just say, "Who cares?" Aging is when you no longer have

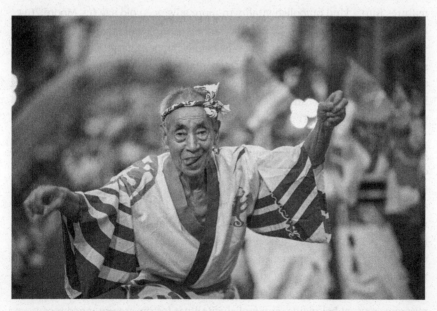

FIGURE 10.1. A deaf man dances the *awaodori* ("fools' dance") at the Koenji Awaodori festival in Tokyo. (Photo by Jason Arney)

regrets [kui]. That's what aging is. The difference between the satisfaction of being able to say that you've lived a life, and the feeling that you
have been given a life by others who will remain afterward, diminishes.
Life and death [he clasps his hands together]. It's as if you are sleeping,
uncertain if you are living or dead. "To die as if asleep" [nemuru ga gotoku
daiōjō]. That's why they say that there is only one wall between life and
death. So the real "good death" is to live and to be given life. Between
life and death is the Buddha, between life and death there is liberation
[nehan]. That's what they say [laughing]!

Dancing in diapers was a way of affirming one's place in an ongoing cycle of life
and death by embodying loss without shame or regret. At first glance, the liberating foolishness that Hayakawa-sensei described seems to contrast with the serious play happening at places like the senior centers, where the emphasis is on the
prevention of physical and mental decline that may lead to frailty and death. But
it would be unfair to draw this contrast too sharply. While the ideology of the centers was squarely founded on the principles of successful aging, the leisure activities happening there were considered (sometimes grudgingly) by participants as
"playful," and they also provided opportunities to experience leisure in ways that
were unavailable in earlier adulthood due to family and/or work responsibilities.
For some, the attitude of discipline and perseverance that center activities engen-
dered could set the stage for the development of a spiritual self-formation that
matures into a kind of foolish vitality in more advanced old age (cf. Moore 2014;
Rohlen 1978). But it should be emphasized that individual creative exploration,
spiritual tuition, or foolish merrymaking largely happens despite the formal mission of successful aging promoted in the contained spaces of community centers
and similar groups. Someone like Hayakawa-sensei would find it difficult to fit
in at the senior center, and "fitting in" is key to participation in the active aging
programs of places like the senior centers.

Perhaps there is a turning point in the life course between the serious play of
the third age and the foolish vitality of the fourth that a successful aging ideology
does not fully acknowledge but that is nevertheless on everyone's mind. What
that turning point is between the pursuit of lifelong active betterment and the
acceptance of old age and death without regrets, with a full and foolish abandon,
is difficult to say. Hayakawa-sensei may be somewhat exceptional in his achievement of such vitality, but for a physician to take a step back from the medical
world and explain his experience as a lively Japanese festival or Buddhist sermon
was inspiring. Maybe dancing in diapers won't be the next great policy achievement of the Ministry of Health, Labor, and Welfare, but the kind of living in the
moment, mutual belonging, and foolish vitality it fosters are untapped resources
that get lost in the shuffle of paper and pain for many at the end of life in Japan.

Successful Aging, Time, and Risk

Successful aging—as it is envisioned by gerontologists both in Japan and elsewhere—is predicated on a system of optimal adjustment to aging such that the active and independent life is long and the time spent in the final age of life is short. In policy, this temporal framework and the values that inform it guide programs focused on prevention. In everyday conversations with older adults and caregivers during my fieldwork, everything was marked as a potential method of prevention, from how to eat one's food (using chopsticks protects against neural degeneration), to the kind of foods that should be eaten (foods high in collagen were popular), to the minutiae of how to exercise, socialize, and enjoy leisure time.

Why such an emphasis on prevention? In some cases, older Japanese people, many of whom had to care for older family members themselves, feel apprehensive toward accepting care and resist the transition to old age. But Hayakawa-sensei's almost mystical description of the good death (diaōjō) as the quintessence of good living suggests an alternative: a narrative not of prevention but of preparation (kokoro gamae) and, eventually, liberation. Prevention and preparation are similar, in that they are both ways to manage risk. But while preparation sets up the conditions of suspense ripe for a punchline, prevention seeks to avoid the joke altogether. Aging then becomes a matter of timing one's dying process: raging against the dying of the light rather than seeing the ways one's light continues to burn in different ways or in different people. The logic of formal service provision and the active aging programs proliferating in its wake envisions aging as a time of active prevention or rehabilitation rather than preparation and liberation, but it does not always account for the risks or anxieties this logic creates.

Successful aging does not eliminate risk but displaces it from social communities or state institutions onto individual. Japan's universal mandatory Long-Term Care Insurance (LTCI) system, put into place in 2001, is a classic case of a modern bureaucracy's ability to normalize categories and displace anxieties related to risk from the social to the personal.[11] For example, I noted numerous instances where the LTCI vocabulary of a seven-degree numeric progression of care needs and levels of risk (yōshien 1–2, or "needing support" and yōkaigo, "needing care," 1–5, with the higher number representing the more advanced need)[12] was used by older adults in everyday conversations to discuss the health of friends and neighbors and even oneself. For example, my eighty-four-year-old neighbor told me, "I never thought about going to day service [adult day care], but when I moved up to yōshien 2, the care manager said that I could go once a week, so I thought, it is better than just being home by myself." Here, the decision to engage in preventative care by going to the day service was made on the basis of the LTCI categories. The choice to avoid the day service meant deviating from the prescribed mode of aging: it was too risky. Older adults, especially those at the level of (where there is already significant difficulty walking, bathing, and using the toilet by oneself), constantly appraised themselves and others according to these administrative categories, sometimes contesting them (to receive coverage for services) or complaining about their inability to account for day-to-day fluctuations of need. Some chose to opt out of the system entirely (cf. Tsukada and Saito 2006), refusing to fill out diagnostic checklists—a last resort, perhaps, to retain a sense of autonomy in the aging process.

Institutional factors guided by the ideology of successful aging and prevention heighten the risk of failure by narrowing the scope of possible aging trajectories, attitudes, and narratives. Alternative perspectives, such as those articulated by Hayakawa-sensei, are typically not available in care settings, where no one can simply say "Ee yan ka" at all of life's little embarrassments.

Conclusion

To say that humor, and especially the ability to laugh at oneself, is a key factor in quality of later life has been observed time and again by anthropologists and cultural gerontologists working in various places around the world. Even in Japan, I would sometimes recall the wry humor of the Jewish community described in Barbara Myerhoff's *Number Our Days* (1980) to supply a vivid reminder that laughing at age is a vital cultural glue, even when differences of faith or background become sources of friction. Older comedians like Betty White are popular across the age spectrum not because they simply joke about aging, but because they are able to reveal the foolishness of our own insecurities about aging and teach us to (successfully) laugh at ourselves. This kind of humor is different from the self-deprecatory, ageist stereotypes found in mainstream culture (think of the way birthday cards for anyone over forty are all about the pitiful, sexual, and mental inadequacies of old age!) and instead embodies something of the foolish vitality described by Hayakawa-sensei: "Ee yan ka?"

There is an important difference between making fun of older people and making fun of the stereotypes about older people. The ability to shrug off the embarrassing qualities of old age and say "Ee yan ka!" with confidence and gusto seems to have a remarkable ability to restore dignity and ground acceptance of old age. Insofar as the "successful aging" model encourages psychosocial well-being and resilience, there is plenty of room for foolish vitality.

But have the policies, practices, and social forms of life that have emerged around neoliberal interpretations and implementations of successful aging programs actually supported the development of foolish vitality? Here I would argue that despite the popular images of seemingly positive "successful aging" and its appealing promise of continued quality of life, its translation into attitudes and behaviors has done more to heighten anxiety, shame, and isolation rather than diminish them. Active aging groups at senior welfare centers and community groups emphasize the dangers of a deteriorating body and mind, the insecurity of family-provisioned care in an aging society, and the need to take aging seriously. But longer lives have not resulted in compression of morbidity (or reducing the time at the end of life when a person is sick or disabled), and there is increasingly less room not only in care homes but also in the popular imagination for those who find themselves "failing" at old age.[13] These are not realities that are easy to laugh off.

From my time in Japan, I've learned that when living past ninety is no longer unusual, aging is no place for sissies. Nor is it a spectator event that one can safely watch from the sidelines, even if sometimes that means boisterously joining the rest of the old fools (and at least this anthropologist) and dancing with abandon.

NOTES

1. As of 2013, Japanese life expectancy at age sixty was twenty-nine more years for women and twenty-three more for men, and Healthy Life Expectancy (HALE) at birth was age seventy-eight for females and seventy-two for males (http://apps.who.int/gho/data/node.main.688, accessed 5 October 2015). In other words, people who reach the age of sixty are expected to live between two or three decades but experience about twelve of those years in poor health.

2. "Oldest old" is used in gerontology to refer to persons over eighty-five. Those age sixty to seventy-five are generally considered "young old," while those about seventy-five to eighty-five are the "old-old." These categories refer only to chronological age and not to a person's health or lifestyle.

3. Okinawa is considered a "blue zone" where supercentenarians have been able to flourish in good health (Davinelli et al. 2012; Wilcox et al. 2007). Okinawans are also known for their unique folk culture and easy-going manner that contrasts with the conservative north.

4. Though not addressing aging in particular, Judith Butler (2006) writes extensively on the ways vulnerability of those in positions of precarity mobilizes resistance to dominant representations even as it exposes one to more public vulnerability.

5. For more on humor as coping, see the special issue of *Social Work in Mental Health* (2015) 13 (1). See also the Woody Allen corpus and graphic novels like Roz Chast's *Can't We Talk about Something More Pleasant?*

6. See Traphagan 2000, 85–107, for a detailed discussion of structuring and contestation of age-grading practices in Japan.

7. The period of relatively active, healthy, and independent late adulthood is distinguished from a more dependent, frail, and declining late adulthood with the categories "third age" and "fourth age."

8. "Sensei" is a form of address usually reserved for teachers of any sort as well as medical doctors, whether women or men. Its literal meaning is "one who has come before."

9. For more on the category of the fourth age, see note 30, introduction to this volume.

10. Held during the Obon season in mid-August, the "Fool's Dance" festival's origins date back four hundred years. The nickname comes from the lyrics to a common dance song, which translates: "Fools dance and fools watch; if both are fools, you might as well dance!"

11. This is not limited to LTCI; see Callaghan 2012 for an excellent discussion of the ways life insurance shaped Japanese experiences of vitality, life-course, and risk. LTCI does for late life what life insurance did for midlife in the early twentieth century.

12. In 2014 a revision of LTCI began a two-year implementation of reforms to this classification system so that those at the levels of yōshien 1 and 2 would no longer receive many of the service benefits directly but would work with local self-governing associations and community groups instead. While the Ministry of Health, Labor, and Welfare has insisted that this would not decrease the level of services to about 1.5 million people receiving such services, it has been criticized by those who feel unqualified volunteers will be inadequate (see http://www.mhlw.go.jp/topics/kaigo/topics/0603/dl/data.pdf).

13. Anne Allison (2013) examines this using the idea of *ibasho*, or a place where one belongs. This lack of a place for older people is not only physical (as in the long waiting list for care homes, or being abandoned by family) but also symbolic (the formal categories of care need, e.g.), and is heightened by the high rates of poverty and isolation.

REFERENCES

Abe Ryūichi and Peter Haskel, trans. 1996. *Great Fool: Zen Master Ryōkan: Poems, Letters, and Other Writings.* Honolulu: University of Hawai'i Press.

Agence France Presse. 2015. "Japan's New 'Girl Band,' Average Age 84." *The Guardian*, July 10, 2015. http:// www.theguardian.com/world/2015/jul/10/japans-new-girl-band-average-age-84, accessed 24 September 2015.

Allison, Anne. 2013. *Precarious Japan.* Durham, NC: Duke University Press.

Baltes, Paul B., and Margret M. Baltes. 1993. *Successful Aging: Perspectives from the Behavioral Sciences.* Cambridge: Cambridge University Press.

Benedict, Ruth. (1946) 1976. *The Chrysanthemum and the Sword.* New York: Meridian Books.

Berk, Roland. 2001. "The Active Ingredients in Humor: Psychophysiological Benefits and Risks for Older Adults." *Educational Gerontology* 27: 323–339.

Butler, Judith. 2004. *Precarious Life: The Power of Mourning and Violence.* New York: Verso.

Callaghan, Sean Koji. 2012. "A Disagreement of Being: A Critique of Life and Vitality in the Meiji Era." PhD diss., University of Toronto.

Danely, Jason. 2014. *Aging and Loss: Mourning and Maturity in Contemporary Japan.* New Brunswick, NJ: Rutgers University Press.

da Rosa, Grace, Peter Martin, Yasuyuki Gondo, Nobuyoshi Hirose, Yoshiko Ishioka, and Leonard W. Poon. 2014. "Examination of Important Life Experiences of the Oldest-Old: Cross-Cultural Comparisons of U.S. and Japanese Centenarians." *Journal of Cross-Cultural Gerontology* 29 (2): 109–130.

Davinelli, Sergio, D. Craig Willcox, and Giovanni Scapagnini. 2012. "Extending Healthy Ageing: Nutrient Sensitive Pathway and Centenarian Population." *Immunity and Ageing* 9: 9.

Dillaway, Heather, and Mary Byrnes. 2009. "Reconsidering Successful Aging: A Call for Renewed and Expanded Academic Critiques and Conceptualizations." *Journal of Applied Gerontology* 28 (6): 702–722.

Embree, John F. 1939. *Suye Mura: A Japanese Village.* Chicago: University of Chicago Press.

Erikson, Erik H. (1950) 1993. *Childhood and Society.* New York: W. W. Norton.

Geertz, Clifford. 1973. *Interpretation of Cultures*. New York: Basic Books.

Grossmann, Igor, Mayumi Karasawa, Chiemi Kan, and Shinobu Kitayama. 2014. "A Cultural Perspective on Emotional Experiences across the Life Span." *Emotion* 14 (4): 679–692.

Katz, Stephen. 2000. "Busy Bodies: Activity, Aging, and the Management of Everyday Life." *Journal of Aging Studies* 14 (2): 135–152.

Lamb, Sarah. 2014. "Permanent Personhood or Meaningful Decline? Toward a Critical Anthropology of Successful Aging." *Journal of Aging Studies* 29: 41–52.

Levy, Becca R. 1999. "The Inner Self of the Japanese Elderly: A Defense against Negative Stereotypes of Aging." *International Journal of Aging and Human Development* 48 (2): 131–144.

Martinson, Marty, and Clara Berridge. 2014. "Successful Aging and Its Discontents: A Systematic Review of the Social Gerontology Literature." *Gerontologist* 55 (1): 58–69.

Moore, Katrina L. 2014. *The Joy of Noh*. Albany: State University of New York Press.

Myerhoff, Barbara G. 1980. *Number Our Days*. New York: Simon and Schuster.

Ricart, Shana Noelle. 2015. "Japan's Aging Society: The Crisis of Care and the Hope of Prevention." Ph.D. diss., University of Chicago.

Rohlen, Thomas P. 1978. "The Promise of Adulthood in Japanese Spiritualism." In *Adulthood*, edited by Erik H. Erikson, 129–147. New York: W. W. Norton.

Rubinstein, Robert L., and Kate de Medeiros. 2014. "'Successful Aging,' Gerontological Theory and Neoliberalism: A Qualitative Critique." *Gerontologist* 55 (1): 34–42.

Stowe, James D., and Teresa M. Cooney. 2015. "Examining Rowe and Kahn's Concept of Successful Aging: Importance of Taking a Life Course Perspective." *Gerontologist* 55 (1): 43–50.

Traphagan, John W. 2006. "How to be a Good Rōjin: Senility, Power, and Self-Actualization in Japan." In *Thinking about Dementia: Culture, Loss, and the Anthropology of Senility*, edited by Annette Leibing and Lawrence Cohen, 269–287. New Brunswick, NJ: Rutgers University Press.

Tsukada Noriko and Yasuhiko Saito. 2006. "Factors that Affect Older Japanese People's Reluctance to Use Home Help Care and Adult Day Services." *Journal of Cross-Cultural Gerontology* 21 (3): 121–137.

Vaillant, George E., and Kenneth Mukamal. 2001. "Successful Aging." *American Journal of Psychiatry* 158 (6): 839–847.

Wilcox, D. Craig, Bradley J. Willcox, Sanae Shimajiri, Sayuri Kurechi, and Makoto Suzuki. 2007. "Aging Gracefully: A Retrospective Analysis of Functional Status in Okinawan Centenarians." *American Journal of Geriatric Psychiatry* 15 (3): 252–256.

11

Nurturing Life in Contemporary Beijing

JUDITH FARQUHAR AND QICHENG ZHANG

Yangsheng is an ancient term that can be translated as "nurturing life." The phrase appears in the philosophical and medical literature of ancient China, dating from the last centuries before the Common Era, most famously appearing as the main subject of the third inner chapter of the Daoist classic the *Zhuangzi* (ca. 3rd century B.C.E.). After many and various appearances in China's vast medical literature, yangsheng saw a popular revival in the 1990s. These days it names a category of activity that includes practices of self-cultivation, wellness, illness prevention, and enjoyment that are widely adopted, especially by retired people, in Chinese cities.

The following chapter incorporates extracts from our book *Ten Thousand Things* (Farquhar and Zhang 2012), in which we investigate yangsheng in practice, hoping with ethnography to better understand the everyday lives and forms of embodiment of ordinary city dwellers in Beijing in the early 2000s. More specifically, we hoped to better discern the historicity and specificity of values, fears, hopes, enjoyments, and tactics of people who had lived through very rapid social change over several dramatic decades of transition—from Maoist communism to a neoliberal "socialism with Chinese characteristics" (He 2001). The book was structured as a series of approaches to and conversations about life. Our topic was not exactly life itself, or the life histories of persons, or the bodily life that is preserved through medical intervention; perhaps, rather, we wanted to engage the notable vitality, always somehow in excess, of the Beijingers we found all around us. We wanted to ask, what is local (Chinese? East Asian? cultural? historical?) about these overflowing vital spirits?

We did not set out to study an aging population, though most of the people we encountered who were interested in yangsheng were fifty years old or over and retired. Though for a while we regretted that few life-nurturing young people were available to talk with us—working lives in Beijing are usually more than full-time and often involve long commutes—we came to especially appreciate the middle-aged and older Beijingers who were so happy to share their lives with us. The great virtue of this population, for an anthropological study of the arts of life, is that these aging individuals, like us, have lived through very marked social changes in their capital city. They reflect on, and can be articulate about, the sorts of things we were interested in ourselves: urban life (chapter 1), how to live (chapter 2), everyday life (chapter 3), and even the meaning of life (chapter 4). In other words, we saw our informants in the parks and back alleys of Beijing's West City District as experts in life, from whom we could learn. Thus, we do not think of our study as providing specific insight on aging alone; we would resist treating "the aging" as a discrete demographic cohort with a culture. Rather, we think yangsheng practitioners are addressing a persistent question that interests many kinds of people at all ages: how can I live well, under my particular circumstances?

We still may wish to consider, however, why practices of nurturing life seem to be especially cultivated by older, retired Chinese. And readers will no doubt want to consider how our study of yangsheng in Beijing might speak to—resonate with or diverge from—the broader "successful aging" movement interrogated in this volume's introduction. One reason older Beijingers seem to be ardent practitioners of yangsheng may have to do with the relatively early mandated retirement ages typical of Beijing work units. Retirees in their fifties and above have time to "look for fun" (zhao le) by exercising, dancing, singing, and swimming with their age-mate friends, and many of them feel that, after lives of hard work and much deprivation, they are entitled to cultivate the quality of their own lives. This is not to say that they have abandoned all responsibilities to their family. On the contrary, we found in Beijing a widespread sense, not always explicitly articulated, that self-care and self-health—the nurturance of life—are the clearest expressions of a sense of responsibility to family and community. Although Chinese and others often think of China as a culture embracing "filial piety" (and indeed a new law was passed in 2012 mandating that adult children visit their elder parents "frequently" and attend to their financial and spiritual needs), over the past several decades the Chinese state has increasingly fostered ideals of elder self-reliance.[1] In the 1980s and 1990s climate of withdrawal of the state from public health care, for instance, and as the parents of the one-child generation have grown older, retired individuals are increasingly providing their own preventive self-care. Everyone hopes that life-nurturing habits will keep extended hospital stays and prolonged illnesses at bay for China's senior generation.

But we would also like to suggest that aging with yangsheng in Beijing is not a project that can succeed or fail; the self-care and self-cultivation sought by life nurturers is not usually thought of as an instrumental health care modality. After all, almost everyone we talked with told us that they nurtured their lives "for fun." Sometimes those we talked to spoke of achieving "a long and fortunate life," voicing China's old cultural ideal of longevity, or *changshou*. We cannot claim to understand changshou in depth, and we remain curious about what people mean by this word. We could only conclude, as we wrote the book, that the ten thousand ways of growing old and having fun in Beijing would have to stand as the only proper answer to this question. We hope the extracts below may indicate some China-specific approaches to successful aging.[2]

Introduction to the Project

In the late twentieth and early twenty-first centuries, a culture of nurturing life has become a widely recognized feature of Chinese public life and "local color." Parks are full of exercisers and hobbyists who speak of their activities as life nurturance, and media outlets provide much advice on how most effectively and enjoyably to nurture life. Yangsheng discourses and practices are forms of modern self-help (or self-health), but the term itself is ancient. The nurturance of life is locally spoken of and globally recognized as peculiarly Chinese and particularly traditional. A recent study by François Jullien (2007) has reminded us that the third chapter of the influential Daoist writings attributed to Zhuangzi is all about the nurturance of life, and a globalizing traditional Chinese medicine claims the term *yangsheng* as rubric for its classical orientation toward preventive medicine, or "treating the not yet ill." Some in the Chinese intellectual movement known as National Studies would place a great deal of the national heritage under the heading of yangsheng as well. This impression of Chinese traditionalism in a popular health movement holds even though the techniques drawn on in the literature of modern yangsheng are often indebted to global science, medicine, and psychology and are propagated through a modern state's public health apparatus.

The prototypical life-nurturing citizen, in the highly mediated images that circulate especially through photojournalism, is an elderly person who practices *taiji quan* (t'ai chi) or *qigong* among friends in a public park. But there are many other activities that fall under the heading of yangsheng, including exercises such as calisthenics, jogging, swimming, and walking backward; hobbies such as water calligraphy (performed outdoors with large sponge brushes on

pavement), dancing, singing, and keeping birds (which must be exercised outdoors in their cages); forms of connoisseurship such as the appreciation of tea,
wine, and medicinal cuisine; and many forms of self-cultivation ranging from
meditation to learning a foreign language.

A popular ditty explains what sort of culture yangsheng is:

> The Way [*dao*] of yangsheng is eating and sleeping, talking and singing,
> playing ball and taking pictures, writing and painting,
> writing poetry line by line, playing chess to banish the blues,
> chatting of heaven, speaking of earth.

This bit of lore suggests considerable variety within the category of life nurturance. The proverb mentions the most necessary and obvious elements of
everyday life, "eating and sleeping," alongside physical exercises such as playing
ball and cosmopolitan hobbies such as taking pictures. This Way is pleasant,
good for "banishing the blues." Some things are even philosophical: "chatting of
heaven, speaking of earth." This list of activities, short as it is, belies any resort
to oversimplification that the term "nurturing life" might suggest. Instead, we
glimpse a manifold culture of the everyday, one that is global and local, embodied and discursive, even ecological and cosmic.

We have elsewhere discussed the political and social contradictions experienced by Beijingers before the present reform era truly got underway, and we
have considered the influence these lived histories might have had on the emergence of a yangsheng movement. It could be argued that nowadays the state and
its Communist Party politics is more benign and that its violent sovereignty has
become the generative and cajoling voice of a classically Foucauldian power/
knowledge apparatus.[3] Power most often appears as the voice of the state-
supported expert, pushing good nutrition or "quality births," explaining why
a cancellation of state social supports amounts to a greater freedom to thrive.

Indeed, most important for the topic of yangsheng is the withdrawal of the
state from the provision of health care. In the 1980s, a great deal of national
government support was withdrawn from hospitals, medical schools, and clinics, and there was a rapid shift to fee-for-service models of payment. In the
1990s there was a massive growth in health insurance schemes, bringing with
it many of the same problems we see in North America. Health insurance is too
expensive for many, the premiums and copay amounts are too high, and the
costs of medical care are rising fast. In this anxious climate, an aging population
is bombarded with state-sponsored public health information and free disease-
screening programs, even while they complain ever more vociferously that it is
almost impossible to "find a doctor," much less pay for medical services. Where
their health is concerned, most people realize that they are on their own.

In the 1980s, references to "Chinese backwardness" were everywhere in the urban popular media in China. The very generation we speak of here, the midlifers and those later in life who have enthusiastically claimed one of the world's most modern cities as their own, and who fill public spaces with the mundane purposes of their own lives, not so long ago thought of themselves as suffering from a chronic backwardness as the world developed all around them. This identification with lack was, of course, the predictable other side of that pervasive emphasis on modernization characteristic of the reform era. Backwardness was the explanation given for everything from failed public services and daily discomforts to corrupt back-door dealings and inegalitarian gender relations. But the language and the stigma of lagging behind is no longer plausible for many Beijingers. Witness the well-pressed and brightly colored silks and satins worn by those who gather in Beihai Park to sing old songs: they are expressing their cosmopolitan good taste and modernity in the present, even as they sing to recover the moments of their youthful years when they wore dark, padded-cotton jackets and cloth shoes, worked to build socialism, and studied Mao Zedong Thought. These days, confidently embodying a mixed temporality, yangsheng enthusiasts such as these singers assert their coevalness with moderns everywhere. But this is a coevalness that includes having a past.

Nevertheless, we have sustained a sense of urban Beijing's social and historical distinctiveness. Chinese people all over the world are turning up in urban parks to practice taiji and qigong, to jog and do calisthenics. But Beijing, and especially its old downtown neighborhoods, recommended itself to us as an especially good site for yangsheng research. We felt we knew the city well (though we discovered otherwise), and we had witnessed there a growing popular enthusiasm for "self-health" (ziwo baojian) activities that everyone classified under the heading of yangsheng. The neighborhood in which we did most of our fieldwork included both large and small parks, around which much of the housing was low rise, overcrowded, and occupied by retirees. These older residents had lived there for a long time, at the heart of several cultural revolutions, one of the most dramatic having been a radical turn toward global capitalist participation in the early 1990s. Their enthusiasm for a little-commodified, constitutively local, pleasurable way (or, perhaps, Way?) of crafting lives impressed us as both responsive to historical experience and a way of making history, crafting an urban culture for a present and future Beijing. This study is not about China or Chinese people exactly, though surely Beijing urban life much resembles that of other Chinese cities and Chinatowns around the world; it is, rather, searching in one place for those specificities that can nuance our sense of the common ground—time, space, embodiment—we all must try to occupy.

These reflections on pleasure and power lead us back to an even fuller appreciation of the literature and daily practice of yangsheng. The vision of health and pleasure these materials offer can ground civil, rich, and enjoyable lives in the activity of an individual, but one who is inseparable from an unbounded collective while demanding little from others. No wonder so many in Beijing are practicing the arts of yangsheng.

When people describe their daily activities, they may not be telling the literal truth about what they actually do every day. When they give us advice about diet or exercise, this may not be advice that they themselves follow. We can be fairly certain, however, that they are at least trying to make sense of, and communicate about, their daily lives. They report particular approaches to crafting significance and offer particular insights about why life should be lived in certain ways. The materials from which this common sense is crafted are not invented by individuals; rather, they are first and foremost a shared heritage of language and lore, education and experience, limiting conditions and imaginable freedoms. But each individual has connected the sense-making resources of a language, a mediascape, a physical and economic environment, to his or her own life in unique ways.

It is this craftwork, this linkage of common resources with personal aims, this concern for achieving, in the present, a particular well-lived life, that impressed us most during the interviews about yangsheng that we conducted. We interviewed thirty-five Beijingers at length, and they rewarded our historical and cultural interest in yangsheng mainly by being interesting people, each facing her or his own situation with courage, creativity, and activism. Sometimes they surprised us with unusual opinions or especially penetrating insights, but more often they echoed the kind of lore we found in our reading of popular literature. The particular combination of interests and concerns was unique to each person, of course, and every interviewee seemed intent on educating us about a personal synthesis of yangsheng practice. As we listened, we marveled at the self-confidence of these Beijingers, their certainty that they had worked out in their experience some correct principles of long life and happiness. Certainly they were aware of what the experts had to say, and in many cases could use technical language well, but as we sat by the lakeshore or in teashops or in family sitting rooms, talking, we realized that these were the experts on life. Or at least their own lives.

Longevity in Theory and Practice

The recent Chinese enthusiasm for life-nurturing theory and practice owes much to the presence in Chinese cities of a large aging population. Though retirement age tends to be early by US standards, and many who practice yangsheng are not weak or ill, it is nevertheless widely felt that the culture of nurturing life is a particular specialty of older people. As a consequence, there are many self-health works that (like the "successful aging" literature discussed in the introduction to this volume) directly address the topic of "long life" (*changshou* 长寿).

Scanning bookstore shelves, for example, one sees titles such as the following: *Good Health and Long Life Are Up to You*; *Ninety Tips for Good Health and Long Life*; *How to Use Yangsheng to Live 100 Years*; *How to Cultivate Self and Nurture Nature to Live 100 Years*; *The Yangsheng Way of Long-Lived People*; and, a personal favorite, *The Everyday Happy Way to Live 100 Years*. The rhetoric used in these works to speak of long life is predictable for a self-help genre: if you regulate your life in wholesome ways, then you will live long. Good personal habits may or may not actually defer death (many environmental hazards are unavoidable, and the causes of many deadly diseases are unknown), but the popular literature is unanimous in its promises: you can take charge of your own health, you can prevent disease, and thus you can live long. To live long is, moreover, unquestionably a good thing.

The idea of changshou/longevity has a long and humble history in Chinese discourses, predating the recent demographic tilt toward senior generations, the shift in modern populations toward the "diseases of civilization," and the privatization of health care. Folk imagery, for example, offers the ubiquitous vision of three auspicious old men representing wealth, prolific fertility, and longevity. To see what elements of the good life are most obvious for Chinese people, even today, it would only be necessary to consult the New Year's prints that proliferate at Spring Festival time: along with the goldfish that symbolize surplus, the flowers and old coins that symbolize wealth, and the many-seeded pomegranates that symbolize fertility, one often sees "Grandpa Longevity." Unlike his companions, the tall and rather austere gods of family blessings and profits, the god of longevity is short, round, and cheerful. He leans with one hand on a long staff shaped like a *ruyi* scepter, indicating both his advanced age and his position as a lordly patriarch. The name for the ruyi carving means "everything as you wish." In his hand he often holds a large, ripe peach, recalling the peaches of immortality cultivated by the gods in the orchards of paradise. The god's broad, wrinkled face, thick lips, and long ears are said to be modeled on the looks of the sage Laozi, traditional founder of Daoism (whose name, incidentally, means "the old one"). And invariably his forehead bulges with accumulated wisdom, reflecting the surplus stored up from a life lived well.

In 2003 our group interviewed a retired Daoist monk in his eighties; he was a yangsheng theorist, and we were particularly interested in his sophisticated system of teaching health habits for long life. At first, however, Judith Farquhar thought of him as quite debilitated by old age; he could not move around his apartment very well, and he initially appeared fatigued and inarticulate. But once he got going on the technicalities of Daoist yangsheng, displaying his active intellect and warm engagement with students and colleagues, his liveliness was much more marked. Even so, in the United States he would have been seen as an ill old man, well "down" the path of decline. But as we walked away, Zhang Qicheng and our Beijing graduate students all agreed that this old Daoist was quite youthful: his skin was "that of a sixty-year-old," and his intellectual passion demonstrated ageless good spirits (*shen* 神), the sign of a life well lived.

A Morning Walk

Let's take a walk around some of Beijing's parks, beginning early in the morning, at first light. It doesn't matter what the season of the year is, some of the same life-nurturing scenes are visible everywhere and every day. In the coldest months of the winter, some activities cease for a few months or take place only in the middle of the day, when the winter sun has warmed the parks a bit. In the hottest days of the summer, everything is done either in the early morning or late in the day to avoid the heat. But whether bundling up in the winter or rising well before sunup in the summer, a lot of Beijingers daily head for the parks to nurture their lives in public.

One very popular form of yangsheng is calisthenics, and no matter which park we start our walk in, we will find groups of middle-aged and elderly people doing group exercises. Calisthenics is a form of yangsheng that is usually done in groups. In the wide plaza at the south end of the Houhai lake system, for example, seventy-five to a hundred people routinely gather to do their morning exercises, guided by one or several leaders who call out each exercise in turn, counting off the repetitions.

Calisthenics groups tend to be large, so some leaders use a microphone or an amplified tape recorder to reach everyone with their directions. Touching toes, twisting at the waist, pounding fists on the lower back and legs, rotating outstretched arms, rolling the head, swiveling the hips—all these and many more separate actions are built into a comprehensive regime that gets bodies moving and keeps joints limber.

Most of those who join daily calisthenics groups are past the age of their greatest vigor. Though they have sought out a public place for this physical activity and join large numbers of others to do it, exercisers do not seem to perform for an audience. The visual aesthetics of calisthenics in Beijing parks has nothing to do with elegance, and for the American who watches, it is odd for something as personal as an exercise regime, with all its unavoidable awkwardness, to be unselfconsciously performed in such a public place.

Moreover, most of the exercises people perform seem so minimal and gentle as hardly to qualify as a physical discipline. Those who prefer this form of yangsheng, however, emphasize not physical rigor but regularity and repetition. Getting out into the fresher air of parks, being around other people, and moving and stimulating all parts of the body for a sustained period (half an hour to forty-five minutes) every day are all activities considered to be good for nurturing life and maintaining health in the course of aging. They are also felt to be enjoyable, not just a technique or a means to a healthy maturity, but an intrinsic element of the pleasure one can take in life after retirement.

It is, after all, retired people who can best devote time to nurturing life. No longer required to get up early and send young children to school or to catch an early bus for a long ride to work, retirees can seek out their own pleasures when they rise early, the result, they say, of long custom. Often combining a daily trip to a street-corner vegetable market with a regular exercise regime or having chats with yangsheng acquaintances during a long walk or a bus ride that takes them a distance from home, older Beijingers have more control of their own time than their hard-working grown children or grandchildren. The relatively young mandated retirement age of forty-five for many women and fifty to fifty-five for most men (at least in Beijing's center city) makes for a cohort of healthy urbanites with time to spare. Yangsheng culture provides these Beijingers with meaningful, pleasant, and inexpensive pastimes.

Yangsheng Common Sense: Two Exemplary Beijingers

Two interviewees presented us with the ideal image of the healthy and cheerful practitioners of garden-variety yangsheng. Both were enjoying their liberation in retirement from onerous duty and stress, and both actively crafted their health and happiness through a variety of life-nurturing practices. They said they were content with their lives, and as we got to know them (in both cases, beyond the interview context), we became persuaded that they were indeed happy, satisfied people.

Zhu Hong is a widow, sixty years old at the time of our interview, who had spent many years nursing her ill husband; he had been hemiplegic for twelve years as a result of a work injury. He died in 1998. She lives on a few hundred yuan a month supplied by her two sons, and we believe she was the "poorest" (in economic terms) of our thirty-five interviewees. She came to the interview with her good friend, Chen Zhihong, and the two of them joked and laughed throughout the several hours we spent together.

She told us:

> I think the significance of yangsheng is that it's good for your body. For example, after I started exercising my body, my urinary tract problems didn't recur. Also, my spirits are good. Now I can't afford to see a doctor, even for an examination, so I have to nurture my own life well—yangsheng is better than everything else. If you don't get sick, on the one hand, you

can avoid medical costs, and on the other hand, it's good for society. Having more long-lived elderly people is good for a society's image, and it's also good for the nation. In our neighborhood, we have two people over ninety years old. . . . Yangsheng makes you happier, and this is very good. Plus, if you save medical costs, that's more money for other important things.

You should find your own happiness, and don't go looking for reasons to be sad. Don't work too hard. My work is light. Don't get mad. This advice is good for body and health, spiritual enjoyment, elevating mood, and extending life. Watching TV is good, too.

ZQC Comment

Zhu Hong's way of talking about yangsheng makes little distinction between happiness and physical well-being, between the rationality of avoiding doctor bills and the hedonism of feeling good by cultivating happiness or "finding enjoyments" (*zhao le* 找). For her, this is all one package. The good life includes freedom from worry about the future, for example, the concern that one's children might have to take on a heavy burden of nursing care for her, similar to the care she provided for her disabled husband over many years. Her good life included finding many small pleasures in the present; indeed, it had been her enthusiastic endorsement of daily foot soaking and her description of how to cook the Beijing specialty *hutazi* (a vegetable crepe) that first charmed us. And she also expressed a concern for the public good and for the "image" of her society and nation. Though Zhu Hong, unlike some of our interviewees, was not actively involved in collective work, she still had strong views about the nature of a civil community and the ways in which the quality of individual lives contributes to it. For example, she admires the long-lived neighbors she mentions and wanted to introduce us to them for an interview. In general, then, she has a rather holistic view of health that includes pleasure, personal responsibility, avoidance of medical care, and a sense of the broader social good.

JF Comment

It is also interesting to note that in her way of talking about these life virtues, Zhu Hong speaks of yangsheng, health, and the good life as a personal *project*. She feels that she can actively cultivate her life, successfully banish anger, refuse to think about unpleasant things, and—one senses from this optimistic way of talking—successfully guarantee an old age free of illness. An American reading this material notices an interesting absence, especially when we consider that these comments come from a sixty-year-old widow with a very low income. There is no sense of being or becoming a helpless victim of an inexorable aging process or of social forces beyond one's control. Zhu Hong shows no sign of fearing the process of aging, nor does she seem to turn to a language of lack or loss, grief or anxiety, subjugation or powerlessness. Of course, to speak of the dark side of getting older and facing illness and death would run counter to Zhu Hong's policy: "Don't go looking for reasons to be sad," and "Don't get mad."

One might suppose that she does have some secret worries, nighttime terrors, and feelings of grief as older friends and relatives drop off. But we should also take seriously her insistence that this is the best time of her life: now that her ill husband has died, she is free to nurture her own life and enjoy her own gratifying pastimes, including her neighborhood and her friends. Put another way, now that her freedom to craft a life is no longer limited by the needs of her husband, she is confident that she can actively make her own health, her own happiness, her own social goods.

This sense of project is consistent with the theme of activism that emerged in other interviews. Ultimately, if we are to understand the kind of personal and collective agency imagined—and thus mobilized—by contemporary Beijingers, we will have to turn to metaphysical questions. In a cosmos characterized by unceasing change, constant generation and regeneration, every level of reality is at all times open to intervention. When nothing about life is carved in stone, the imperious external and internal structures that appear to limit the "agency" (in a narrow sense) of the human actors conceived by Euro-American social theory can appear as just more arenas for tinkering. We are not here proposing that yangsheng practitioners either seek or find some ultimate plane of freedom. Beijing's city dwellers are quite well aware of the limits of their powers to change their environment and improve their conditions. But these limits are not seen as utterly fixed; because the constraints on daily life are always shifting, ordinary activity can find ways to redefine, bypass, or leapfrog the most immediate confining structures. At the very least, many believe, one can always craft a positive everyday life for oneself. Zhu Hong refuses to be victimized by worry or anger, and she does not see her body as subject to inevitable "natural" decline. She has confidence in the efficacy of her own activist outlook to keep difficulties at bay.

Zhu Hong's understanding of yangsheng is consistent with that of many others who emphasize exercise, fan dancing, climbing in the hills, seeking out simple pleasures (*zhao le* 找乐), living on a regular schedule, and avoiding anger. But we think it is important that she pointed out spontaneously that the value of yangsheng is not confined to the individual but also benefits the nation and society. "Having more long-lived elderly people is good for a society's image, and it's also good for the nation." Her comments are fairly representative, typical of the approach of many older Beijing residents to the relationship between their own lives and public duty and civic life. Again and again we have heard Beijingers speak of the simple achievement of living long as a public contribution, and most of her contemporaries would agree with her. This way of thinking is founded on the assumption that the nation is not a separate entity from its people, and perhaps in it there are echoes of the difficult challenges that have been met and overcome by the Chinese people. Having survived so much in good health, people imply, is not only an index of a sound nation, but the very substance of national soundness.

Our second "model" yangsheng practitioner is Li Jianmin, a sixty-one-year-old retired factory worker who brought samples of his calligraphy and painting to our interview, as well as his sword to demonstrate taiji swordplay, his equipment for water calligraphy, and his choral-singing songbook.

"Now that I'm retired," he said,

> I'm taking up a lot of hobbies that I have always loved but didn't have time for. From a young age, I always loved to sing. I would always sing at home while I was doing housework, but while working at the factory, I never had time. From last year, because it's convenient when I take my grandson to school at Jingshan Primary and meet him there at the end of the day, I have been participating in the Beihai Wulongting Retired People's Choral Group. Tuesdays and Thursdays, 9:30 to 11:30. I usually go both days every week; when it's most crowded, there are as many as three hundred people, everyone sings together, it's really rousing for the spirit [jingshen zhenfen], the mood is totally happy and worry free [xinqing shuchang], it's an extremely good feeling. The first time I went and heard so many older people singing at the top of their lungs, I felt an upsurge of emotion, and tears came to my eyes. I brought a book [here today], a selection of 100 years of twentieth-century Chinese songs. . . .
>
> The significance of yangsheng is: if your body/health is good, you can do everything, and there are benefits for your family and the society. Without body/health, you can't do anything. Nowadays, seeing a doctor is too expensive, but if you pay attention to yangsheng, you can minimize illness and lessen the burden on your children. Yangsheng includes taiji, regulation of food and drink, sports and exercise, mountain climbing, and so on.
>
> When I exercise, I feel that my body is healthy, my mood is carefree, my life is happier and healthier, my energy is charged up, and I am saving medical costs. . . .
>
> I think for people who live in the world, if you can move, you should exercise. With exercise, you definitely have to keep it up; if you're not steady, then it will certainly be useless, so to keep doing it, you have to

have willpower. In the winter, I, too, like to nestle in my warm quilts, but as soon as I think that it is for my health, for my body, I then climb out and go do my exercises.

JF Comment

Even though he's retired, Li Jianmin is a busy man. During the school week, he and his wife look after one of their two grandsons; their two-room apartment in the Gulou area is closer to the child's school than the apartment near the airport where his parents live, so he stays with them during the week. Every morning, Li Jianmin takes his grandson to school on his bike or his motorbike and then goes on to a nearby park for yangsheng activities such as singing, pavement calligraphy, and taiji. He also seems to do much of the shopping for the household while he's out, bicycling long distances to find good bargains, and he finds time for calligraphy and painting on paper, as well. On our first interview, he brought catalogs from art shows he had visited—he is particularly fond of the Europeanized ink paintings of Xu Beihong.

These artistic activities were not new to him, as he told us. Even while working as a heating-and-cooling technician, he had joined in the calligraphy and taiji clubs organized by his factory work unit. With his relatively long experience of yangsheng skills, one might expect him to adopt the air of a master and become a local leader of some kind. But this is not his style. In speaking of his pavement calligraphy, for example, he was more interested in telling us about a particularly skilled practitioner in Beihai Park whose work he liked to observe than he was in claiming any particular ability for himself. And he was attracted to the large singing group in Beihai because of the feeling of merging together with others in song. I came to think of Li Jianmin as an everyday collectivist, comfortable in social groups, serving the people (and especially his immediate family) in whatever way comes to hand, and claiming no special virtues for himself. This kind of humble approach to getting through life, combined with an obvious capacity for taking great enjoyment in little things, seems the very picture of health.

American readers may find it odd that such an apparently generous and pacific person should take pleasure in singing martial songs. One song that Mr. Li noted as a favorite is the following:

GREAT BROADSWORD MARCH

The great broadsword sweeps off the heads of the demons,
Twenty-ninth Army brothers, the Anti-Japanese War is here today.
The guerrilla army of the Northeast ahead of us, the people of all China
    behind us,

Our Twenty-ninth Army is not alone.

Pick out the enemy, then wipe them out, wipe them out!

Charge!! The great broadsword sweeps off the heads of the demons—Kill!!

I was at first a bit shocked by this anti-Japanese rhetoric, and on several occasions I asked Li Jianmin whether singing such songs could "have a bad influence on China-Japan friendship." At times he insisted, "These are just songs, fun to sing, and they remind us of our youth." At other times, especially when influenced by 2005 commemorations of the end of the Anti-Japanese War, he saw these lyrics as important ways of remembering Japan's crimes against the Chinese people. But in understanding his tastes and those of the many other retirees who sing such songs in the parks, it is important to bear in mind that these are *songs*. The tune, the meter, the ring of the lyrics, all combine to make up their charm. They are also the music of a bygone era, when Li Jianmin and his age-mates were young, idealistic, and vigorous. Even I, a more or less pacifist foreigner, when singing along with the "Great Broadsword March," wholeheartedly enjoyed shouting out "Charge" and "Kill!"

Perhaps the release involved in these songs is also a form of yangsheng. It is in any case a way of exercising little-used parts of the self. Particularly charming was Li Jianmin's remark, "For people who live in the world, if you can move you should exercise." In this respect, he, like Zhu Hong, seemed committed to making a project out of life, to carrying life to a higher level, both more disciplined and more joyful. Just being able to move is not enough: one should dance and sing. Just being able to read and write is not enough: one should read culture and write calligraphy.

ZQC Comment

Choral singing is a common yangsheng activity in Beijing. Those who participate in it are mostly retired people, though there are also a number of middle-aged participants. This is not only a kind of exercise (*yundong*), it is even more a form of nostalgia; it is a deeply felt remembrance and arousal, and it is also a powerful way of sharing the fellow feeling (*ganqing*) of a generation. Laozi said, "He who wants to live long should 'return to infancy.'" I am reminded of the phrase "return to spring" that is often heard in the world of Chinese medicine. As winter turns to spring, trees and grass come back to life. Thus, the phrase "a return to spring at the clever hands [of the doctor] [*miaoshou huichun*]" is a figure for the highest level of medical skill, allowing a return to life even from the brink of death. It also figures yangsheng and its ability to reverse aging and return youth. Many of the older people we spoke with in Beijing had experienced this "return to spring" phenomenon and become "like elderly children."

In practice, these phrases mean two things: one is that the body is returned to health. If in the past there was some illness, it is either cured or the symptoms are much lessened. The other sense of the term is that the spirits are improved, morale is improved, and one feels happy in his or her heart/mind. These "elderly children" are thought of as resembling actual children, at least in that they have returned to a kind of spontaneous wisdom that allows them to get over any small frustrations in their daily lives quickly. There are none of the negative connotations of a "second childhood" in English; rather, it is an achievement of age to recover spontaneity and uncomplicated pleasure.

Among Li Jianmin's interests is a practice worthy of some attention, and that is his use of writing and calligraphy as a form of yangsheng. Though he says he had long been interested in calligraphy, earlier in his life he had not thought of calligraphy as a form of yangsheng. While still working, he wrote mainly because there were calligraphy contests sponsored by his work unit. But now he speaks of his writing as good for yangsheng. Note, though, that he chooses to practice calligraphy in public, with water on pavement, even though he does have space in his house to spread out and ink words on paper in private. He often goes to a plaza near Wangfujing to practice his pavement calligraphy. At the time of our interview, he demonstrated at our spot by the edge of the lake. Dipping his large sponge "brush" into the water of the lake, he wrote "The Red Army fears no extremity or hardship" in cursive script on the stone pavers. He also showed us a piece of calligraphy he had done earlier on paper, listing the four characters "fortune, longevity, health, stability," as well as some poems by Chairman Mao and a painting of a horse in the style of Xu Beihong. Judging from his manner as he shared these things with us, he was a person who enjoyed much inner satisfaction. But in addition, because this kind of calligraphy and painting takes energy and engages movement of the hands, feet, and the whole body, it certainly is a form of exercise. Without doubt, many famous calligraphers and painters in China have lived to a ripe old age.

JF and ZQC Comment

Reflecting on the lives and attitudes of these two interviewees, Ms. Zhu and Mr. Li, we remain impressed with their optimism, their enjoyment of simple daily pleasures, and their active crafting of the times and spaces of life. They were both in their early sixties at the time, which may be too young to worry much about a bleak future of true old age and illness. Perhaps they feel that this stage of their lives, while they are still fairly vigorous, is meant to be an enjoyable interlude: onerous duty is in the past, and uncontrollable physical or economic pressure has not yet become a problem. Perhaps their most obvious characteristic, however, is their ability to conduct the good life with such simple and inexpensive tools. They rely on their own resources, and even though neither of them speaks much of spiritual life, it is clear that they understand the meaningful depths of yangsheng in practice. The ways in which these two Beijingers talk about yangsheng and everyday life may sound rather banal; but it is in the living of this common sense that we can perceive a real achievement, one that is both unique to each person and understandable to anyone. Common sense, indeed.

Conclusion

Our research has taken a variety of routes into the large and diverse phenomenon that is life nurturing, or yangsheng, in contemporary Beijing. It has emphasized the ways in which yangsheng activity fills and transforms the space of the city. It has read some of the popular literature that has given shape to an ongoing yangsheng movement. It has made acquaintance with the daily lives and values of the postrevolutionary generation that most enthusiastically embraces life nurturance. And it has offered for reflection some of the philosophical resources and challenges that make more lasting sense of yangsheng phenomena. Throughout, the aim has been to hear, echoing through the streets and parks of Beijing, the voice of a distinctly modern activism chartered by a protean ancient metaphysics; to read the tastes, pleasures, and disciplines of contemporary urbanites as deliberate and deliberative; and to allow cultured Chinese bodies to resonate with concerns of human embodiment anywhere. The theme has been life, but not life itself—rather, it has been modern life, Chinese life, park life, social and political life, the life of the mind, spirited liveliness, the life of healthy or ailing bodies, family life, lives well nurtured. As the life-nurturing literature keeps telling us, drawing on an ancient metaphysics that tells how the world with its myriad phenomena comes into being, the shapes and currents of the myriad things number ten thousand upon ten thousand: birth upon birth, transformation upon transformation. The meaning of any particular thing—as long as it lasts, and with considerable luck, skill, and determination—is gathered, centered, and harmonized with the Way things go.

NOTES

1. The Chinese Law Assuring the Rights and Interests of the Aged went into effect in July 2013. See http://www.gov.cn/flfg/2012-12/28/content_2305570.htm. Also see http://www.cncaprc.gov.cn for the activities of the new agency tasked with services for the elderly.

2. The passages that follow are adapted, with permission from Zone Books, from *Ten Thousand Things: Nurturing Life in Contemporary Beijing* (Farquhar and Zhang 2012, 17–18, 21–22, 27–28, 16, 23, 174–175, 144–145, 64–67, 176–185, 292–293, in this order), while deleting most endnotes and other references that appear in the book.

3. For more on these ideas, see Farquhar and Zhang 2005.

REFERENCES

Farquhar, Judith, and Qicheng Zhang. 2005. "Biopolitical Beijing: Pleasure, Sovereignty, and Self-cultivation in China's Capital." *Cultural Anthropology* 20 (3): 303–327.
———. 2012. *Ten Thousand Things: Nurturing Life in Contemporary Beijing.* Brooklyn, NY: Zone Books.
He, Henry Yuhuai. 2001. *Dictionary of the Political Thought of the People's Republic of China.* Armonk, NY: M. E. Sharpe.
Jullien, François. 2007. *Vital Nourishment: Departing from Happiness.* Brooklyn, NY: Zone.

12

Depreciating Age, Disintegrating Ties

On Being Old in a Century of Declining Elderhood in Kenya

JANET McINTOSH

There is an old oracle still recounted by the Mijikenda people of the Kenya coast. It was first delivered in the nineteenth century, they say, by the famed prophetess Mipoho, as she stood in the middle of a circle of beating drums. Mipoho predicted that a people as white as butterflies would soon arrive, bringing craft that soared across the sky and great traveling machines that would roll across the land. Mijikenda youth would scorn their elders and abandon their old ways. Mipoho turned out to be right. The white people arrived from Europe and brought with them not only the Mombasa railroad and tarmac roads, but many other things as well: a paper bureaucracy that took land out from under ancestral guardianship and put it into privately held title deeds; a taxation system that would force young men out of their homesteads in search of wages; new religious creeds that damned initiation ceremonies and traditional ritual knowledge as "witchcraft"; and schools that claimed the best and most important learning would come from Westerners, not the tribal elders. Mijikenda homesteads were partially dispersed through the centripetal forces of the market economy and the new individualism. And youth began to look over the heads of their elders for the new possibilities and forms of authority appearing on the horizon.[1]

While many aging people in the United States and Europe struggle to preserve the appearance of youth and independence, some older people in sub-Saharan African societies lament instead the decline of elderhood. To be precise, older generations in certain rural areas of Kenya—not only Mijikenda of the coast, but others, too, such as Meru in central Kenya—are nostalgic for an era when cohorts collectively worked their way through stages of the life course, or "age grades," until reaching a revered position as an elder (defined as much by social seniority as biological age). In gerontocratic societies, the role of elder typically includes social and spiritual potency and knowledge keeping, with male elders usually having political and economic primacy. As the body declines, furthermore, elders expect to be cared for by extended networks of kin—to be desirably interdependent, in other words—even as they remain highly useful, orchestrating matters such as local governance, land use, marital patterns, and rituals, while dispensing valued knowledge. Upon their death, elders join the company of ancestral spirits, often propitiated by the living in hopes of continuing reciprocity. But in some communities today, elders cannot be guaranteed of their own authority, or of reciprocal care from their kin. Says an older Meru man to anthropologist Samuel Thomas, "Youth today have little [respect]. They no longer listen to the advice of the old. They may say, 'You are wasting my time. You didn't even go to school. How can you advise me?'" (Thomas 1992, 188). An elderly Mijikenda man on the Kenya coast tells me, "Youth today are neglecting their ancestors—they forget to pour palm wine for them. And they hoard the money they earn in town to buy clothes and prostitutes. Why would they send money to take care of their elders if they don't even fear their ancestors anymore?"

How has this sense of loss come to pass? In this chapter I describe some of the forces of change in Kenya and elsewhere in sub-Saharan Africa that have shifted many gerontocratic political economies on their axes, compromising age-grade systems and precipitating a loss of authority and social security among many older people. These forces include twentieth-century colonial administration and the permeation of market economies, as well as other "modern" institutions and now globally circulating values. To make this case, I draw mostly (though not exclusively) from scholars' work on male elders in rural Meru near the center of the country and my own long-term fieldwork on rural coastal Mijikenda.[2] I was not primarily focused on elderhood, but its losses stared me in the face in my day-to-day contacts and in public and media-based discourses in Kenya. Walking through villages, I could see male Mijikenda elders gathered sometimes in circles under large trees, sharing palm wine in small, hollowed-out gourds, their clothing a semiotic profusion—Mijikenda *shuka* (white cotton cloths, secured at the waist), threadbare t-shirts from the secondhand clothing trade from the West, sometimes even a tweed jacket in the equatorial heat, a sort of holdover from colonial hegemony. They would lament the corruption of local politicians and the loss of young kin seduced by the lure of towns and cities, such as Mombasa and Nairobi, and occasionally prepare for a village tribunal, where they would adjudicate some matter—a charge of adultery or witchcraft, for example—under the radar of the state. But the authority they retained was tenuous, and their social roles often unclear. The material I furnish may not say anything particularly new to Africanists (indeed, it will probably feel quite abbreviated), but in the context of this volume it offers a counterpoint to the widespread Western models of "successful aging" described in other chapters, throwing their strangeness into relief.

Authoritative Age and Desired Interdependence

Gerontocratic power, especially patriarchal power, has been a powerful organizing principle across sub-Saharan Africa, but it has taken distinctive local forms (Aguilar 1998). Although the patterns I describe are variations on a historically widespread theme, the reader must bear in mind that no sweeping claim will apply to all; Kenya alone, for instance, is home to more than seventy—depending on how they are counted—ethnolinguistic groups living today in highly diverse circumstances: pastoralist, subsistence agriculturalist, urban cosmopolitan, and beyond. Nevertheless, generally speaking, in many Kenyan societies a person's life course was customarily—and in some cases still is—marked by a series of elaborate initiation rituals with their cohort. As each "age-set" or "age grade" moved into different stages of seniority, they took on distinctive social roles.

A few examples of elders' responsibilities follow, drawing on Meru and Mijikenda histories. Meru adult males would go through a stage of being a "ruling elder" before entering the senior-most "ritual elder" stage; a select group of these became members of Njuri Ncheke, the supreme council of elders that customarily holds sway over the entire Meru community.[3] Among Meru girls and women, marriage was often a key marker for entering an upper age grade, and with seniority would come the power to organize female initiation ceremonies, common feasts, and sometimes female disputes (Fadiman 1994; Thomas 1992). Among coastal Mijikenda, as female elders entered their postreproductive years, they accrued power over girls' initiation ceremonies, as well as fertility and marital rituals—and some, such as Mipoho, became widely influential ritual leaders. Mijikenda boys and men went through a new series of rituals about every three years, as elders gradually introduced them to more (and often secretive) knowledge about governance, law, and land use; the many intricate rules of clan and marital organization; supernatural potencies, including supernatural prohibitions upon certain kinds of sexual contact; the social role of the young warrior; and so forth. As they moved into elderhood, they could proffer livestock, palm wine, and other goods in exchange for privileged access to sacred spaces, medicinal trees and plants (*mitishamba*), and ritual instruments, including the protective charm known as *fingo* and the sacred *mwanza* friction drum used during rituals. Elders could intercede with the ancestors during ceremonies designed to prevent bad luck and sickness, purifying contaminated spaces and healing the community; they were often credited, too, with the arrival of rain. Until the mid-nineteenth century, each of the nine Mijikenda subgroups had its own *kambi*, or ruling council of male elders, with a ritual center in a forest known as a *kaya*. These elders played vital roles in village legislation and political economy, serving as middlemen in the trade between coastal towns and the interior, adjudicating the distribution of land and bridewealth, arbitrating disputes and imposing fines, and redistributing cattle and agricultural surplus (Brantley 1981; Willis 1993). Though Mijikenda dispersed from the kaya over time, senior men from particular lineages and clans retained political, ritual, and other authority.

As older generations had clear seniority, they earned respect and reciprocity from younger generations. Meru youngsters, for instance, shadowed their grandparents to learn from them and internalized the idea that elders were to be esteemed and cared for. Young Meru were expected to show respect and dedication toward their elders through an attitude known as *giteo*, which included being well mannered, refraining from jokes and vulgarity, giving way to elders on the path, serving elders first, obedience, and generally "making yourself small" in the elders' presence. A crucial aspect of giteo is also the willingness to undertake labor for them, "obedience . . . without questions," as one old man put it. This often meant "going when sent" by elders; that is, performing tasks at their behest, such as harvesting elders' yams, furnishing grass or water for their cattle, and tending their beehives. One respondent told Thomas that "the most important measure of giteo is how often a person is willing to be sent and how quickly they perform the task. In the past, if a youth was given a task to perform for an elder, they did it in the shortest time possible" (Thomas 1992,183, 187). Similarly, among Giriama it was presumed that as elders required material support, their younger kin (who typically would have lived nearby, some on the same homestead) would provision them without question. In these societies, then, senescence was not an embarrassment but rather a phase of life that evoked reciprocal care and respect even as one maintained status.[4]

So far, the portrait I am painting of "successful aging" in these communities looks strikingly different from those common in the United States and Europe. In many Western contexts, a common anxiety about getting older is the fear of losing one's youth while becoming "dependent" or burdensome. Westerners thus strive to maintain their vigor with a frenzy of self-improvement, hoping to maintain youthful looks while "keeping active" and "self-reliant." But because aging for many rural Kenyans has customarily involved a succession of life stages in which elders' role is not supposed to be the same as that of youth, growing and looking old is not embarrassing, and "successful aging" (should such a phrase even be in circulation, which it generally is not) does not look like the pretense of enduring youth. Rather, it takes the form of a valued interdependence, because even as the aged may depend on the resources and labor of younger generations, they bring to bear a lifetime's accumulation of valuable leadership, expertise, and knowledge, some of it secret and privileged. Furthermore, while Western ideologies of personhood tend to be individualistic, most rural Kenyans (and most rural Africans, generally) have placed a priority on communitarianism and interdependence. To be successfully old, then, is to be ensconced among extended kin and at least partially dependent upon their assistance, but, simultaneously, needed for the community's functioning. The ability to continue one's physical labors is valued, to be sure, but complete "self-reliance," in this context, would feel more like abandonment and disrespect.

Changing Times: The Attrition of Elders' Power

Yet a very real weakening of communal support is increasingly a source of anxiety among older Kenyans. One could see glimmers of it in the satirical newspaper column "Whispers," written by beloved humorist Wahome Mutahi between 1983 and 2003. By the late 1980s, "Whispers" was centering on a Kikuyu family in Nairobi, including a patriarchal Mzee, or honored male elder, who feels he deserves reverence on traditional grounds, yet fears it is slipping from his grasp. Mzee, says scholar George Ogola (2006, 574–575), allegorizes the changing nation and "personifies the old male face of power in Kenya." In one passage from 1997, Mzee describes how five wives would have come running to tend his patriarchal ancestor, and he waxes nostalgic about a time when he himself could count on the obedience of his younger kin. But, he laments, these days "I am being told I can sneeze if I want. I can even cough my lungs out if I wish but nobody will even take notice of me in the house." The loss of elder male authority is twinned, here, with the loss of caretaking in the event of his physical frailty. Inasmuch as the authority of father figures resembles the authority of male elders, Mzee's frustration reveals a broader shift in elderhood.

The greatest threat to customary elderhood in sub-Saharan Africa arrived when Europe's "scramble for Africa" culminated in an imperial take-over of most of the continent by the early twentieth century. Between the incursions of European colonialism and the influence of global modernity since Independence, elderhood has been damaged along numerous lines.

One such line is political and juridical. Colonial administrations had mixed feelings about elders' authority; on the one hand, they needed to establish their own governance, but on the other hand they recognized they could not instantly supplant preexisting structures (indeed, some British administrators in East and Central Africa feared that rapid cultural change could lead to a sort of collective insanity). The result, often, was an awkward and complex compromise; in parts of East Africa, for instance, male councils of elders were retained as part of the colonial structure of "indirect rule" but lost some power over time nevertheless as, for instance, new government courts handled criminal cases. In

Kenya civil cases were often handed over to native tribunals that were loosely modeled after elders' councils—but over time these tribunals were increasingly reformed in a European model. Although elders all over Kenya found creative ways to articulate with these new systems, the very assumptions of European law detracted from elders' authority; the personal, contextual knowledge of the elders, for instance, seemed less relevant in the face of the supposedly impartial written code of law.[5] Meanwhile, as part of indirect rule, colonial authorities often instated "chiefs" of their own choosing, arrangements that sometimes had no basis in the precolonial structures of authority elders inhabited.

In some Kenyan societies, councils of elders continued to operate under the radar of the colonial authorities and, subsequently, on the fringes of the fragile postindependence state, but they frequently struggle for potency. With so many social structures changing or destabilized, furthermore, it has been harder for elders to cohere. Among pastoralist Orma in northeastern Kenya, for instance, one elder lamented the deterioration of his community's grazing policies and the way some elders had turned to the state in desperation for help with enforcement. "In the old days," he said, "even if the elders lied they lied together. Even if they made a mistake, they made it together. [Today] we cannot agree" (Ensminger 1990, 691). Although community leaders in some areas have argued vociferously that elders should have more authority and rights, the implementation of this idea has been unevenly felt.

The market economy further damaged elders' power. The British in Kenya began to collect "hut taxes" in the early twentieth century, forcing households to participate in the colonial economy and produce cash. The colonial administration organized around the idea of a male labor pool, an ideology with long-term repercussions for women, who lost out in the new allocation of cash and ultimately education and opportunity. Young men went in search of wages, sometimes to work on European-owned plantations, and their migration and new ability to accumulate wealth fragmented homesteads, weakening elders' control over marital and reproductive practices and destabilizing the organizing principle of age-grades. Since Kenya's Independence in 1963, the market economy has continued to foster conflicts between generations. Among Mijikenda, for instance, the rising market in coconut meat transformed what had been a relatively egalitarian and reciprocal economy by injecting cash and fostering high demand for land and trees. By the late 1960s, a small group of middle-aged men began to accumulate land and wealth at the expense of the elders (Parkin 1972). The flow of money has affected elders' control over who marries whom; one fifty-something Mijikenda man I knew bent my ear repeatedly about the fact that his son was renting an apartment in town, working as a store manager, and wooing *wazungu* (white people, most of them European tourists) rather than letting his seniors identify a suitable girl from the village. Other young men, it should be said, have found themselves facing the rigors of poverty and inflation, unable to pull together the resources (in cash, cattle, or other commodities) for bridewealth, thus curtailing their ability to rise into social maturity, let alone elderhood, with a suitable network of kin and descendants.[6]

In the transaction of land, too, elders' authority and knowledge have been sidelined. Customary land use often hinged on communal rights and sharing, adjudicated by elders' knowledge of land's social history and ecology, but colonial administrations partially gutted this structure. European powers seized vast amounts of land from Africans, and as the decades unfolded, brought possessive individualism through title deeds, surveyed plots, and registered records. In many areas male elders lost the power to allocate land rights, and older women were disenfranchised in various ways; Meru widows, for instance, lost their customary rights to use their husbands' land once title-deed inheritance laws resulted in the passing of land from father to son (Thomas 1992, 120), and without gainful employment, such women were at terrible risk of impoverishment. (The skewing of literacy in favor of men, too, has compounded women's losses in the arena of title deeds.) The individualism encouraged by the market economy took root quickly, and it has escalated as more Kenyans have become landowners since Independence. According to Thomas (1992, 67), his Meru informants insist that "when separate land titles are granted, nearly all joint decision-making and economic interdependence ceases. . . . Once someone obtains a title to their land, they basically depend on themselves, except in times of crisis." On the coast, Mijikenda elders feel that land alienation has added insult to injury by compromising the spatial loci of their authority, for land-grabbers have seized some of the sacred kaya forests that historically served as ritual centers.

If elders lost power and status with the changes brought by Europeans, their once-prized knowledge gained competitors. For several centuries, Christian missionaries from Europe fanned out across sub-Saharan Africa, and almost wherever they landed they dismissed the traditional medicine of the elders as backward superstition and quackery. Mission schools offered simultaneous education and salvation, alienating many young people from their extended families and the knowledge of both male and female elders. Today's elders, if influenced by Christian missionaries in their youth, may be reluctant even to discuss the older ways of their clan or tribe, having been taught to construe them as "ways of the Devil" (Thomas 1992, 116). Traditional healing, too, was disparaged, and while it lives on, it is often relegated to the shadow of the biomedicine introduced by missionary and state hospitals. The European educational systems established by colonial states further disrupted indigenous lifeways—as District Commissioner H. E. Lambert wrote in 1939 of Kenya's colonial-era schools: "[Their goal] is to cram the individual to climb out of his class and his age-grade, out of his tribal environment, and so out of his tribe. So that every academic success is a tribal failure" (quoted in Thomas 1992, 118).

The repercussions of such changes are vivid among Mijikenda. On the one hand, male elders do retain social importance, perhaps especially in the realm of ritual knowledge about protecting and cleansing the community. This role was evident in, for instance, the case of two terrible road accidents that claimed many Mijikenda lives in 2011. Many suspected witchcraft within the community, and male elders were asked to step in to ritualistically reassert customary morality (Ciekawy 2015). On the other hand, I found that Mijikenda living near the coastal town of Malindi report a drastic decline in the number and frequency of initiation rites. Although the women's *kifudu* fertility cult lives on in some communities, in others organized societies of female elders are dwindling. And while male elders are still recognized, one senior Mijikenda elder says that a few decades ago he was approached by at least twenty young people per year seeking initiation into elderhood, but today the number is closer to five—and some of these abandon the sequence of rites after they've begun them, leaving them more confused than not about Mijikenda custom (Brantley 1981; McIntosh 2009). Meanwhile, with so much competition from state governance, formal schooling, and beyond, elders complain that youth favor "book learning" over the kinds of education they could provide; as one elder put it to me, "When we die, no one will remain as a living archive for traditional knowledge."[7] Some younger Mijikenda mourn the loss; as one man in his twenties frames it, "The community's expertise is grounded in the old men and as you can see, all the [Mijikenda] youth are living in towns and have no time to learn the work. This is too bad. . . . I think it would be good if the youth would come back . . . and learn some skills which can help the community." (Meru elders have described a similar shift; according to Jeffrey Fadiman [1994, 6], by the 1960s many were keenly aware that younger people alienated by schools no longer wished to seek them out.) Noting the role loss of many elders as I traveled through numerous villages in the late 1990s and mid-2000s, I was struck when my research assistant recurrently pointed out solitary old men sitting on a stool or weaving slowly down a path, clutching a gourd or bottle of palm wine. "No purpose, no money," he would tsk, and tell me of a rise in alcoholism among the elderly. Ironically, palm wine has a long and respectable history in Mijikenda society as a libation with tremendous ceremonial importance, often used to consecrate important social and ritual moments, and routinely splashed on the ground to honor the ancestors. Apparently this drink that marks the elders' authority has also, in some cases, medicated their decline.

Ironically, life expectancy in Kenya has lengthened, from about forty-seven at Independence to about sixty today—accompanied by diseases of modernity, including heart disease, stroke, diabetes, and cancer, as well as HIV/AIDS (indeed, sadly, some elders find themselves taking care of their orphaned grandchildren as a result). People live longer on average, but not necessarily in good health, and often without the reliable life course trajectory that once would have clarified their role as they aged. Kenya thus has a population of older people in great need of support from younger kin, without the social structure to furnish it reliably.

Reoriented Youth

Today, in fact, the alienation of youth from elders is palpable in Kenya's urban centers, with their disproportionate population of young people. The global circulation of imagery, ideas, and celebrity culture on the internet, television, and glossy magazines has turned the heads of young people; many are increasingly reluctant to be governed through traditional law or held to customary rites of passage. They listen to loud, often foreign, music; their dress creatively borrows from Western closets; they are encouraged by NGOs into ever more creative forms of micro-entrepreneurialism and self-help. As they contest customary marriage, they give new shape to family structures. Young women may eschew marriage altogether, live as single mothers or childless by choice, and turn to feminist texts as they contest child marriage and customary female social roles. These youth are far more likely than their elders to have some formal education and literacy—symbolic capital that in some contexts trumps the seniority of elderhood. And while the symbolism of elderhood—including, for instance, the fly whisk and honorifics such as "Mzee"—is widely used among Kenyan politicians, it has been striking to see younger and younger politicians wielding it, suggesting that the authority associated with elderhood has been abstracted. Political authority has been steadily decoupled from age and mapped onto a generalized, metaphorical notion of elderhood, at the same time that the *imagery* of gerontocracy has been used to give politicians legitimacy (Robert Blunt, personal communication, 15 September 2015).

The ideological clashes between generations can be seen in a recent anecdote from anthropologist Beth Brummel (2015, 114–116). Brummel had a ringside seat during a verbal conflict between a young man named Oti and an elder man in a bar in western Kenya. Both men were Luo, and they did not know one another, but when the older one spied Oti lighting a cigarette in the company of the American anthropologist, he used the Luo language to request that the younger extinguish it. Oti declined in English, saying repeatedly that he was a paying customer and a full citizen with the right to smoke in a restaurant that allows it. Oti's English, says Brummel, framed the disagreement in terms of "democracy, rights, and modernity," while his elder's insistence on using the Luo language implicitly insisted upon "a gerontocratic model of authority

with its expectations of ethnic allegiance and consequent obedience to elders."
Oti refused to play along; no wonder elders complain repeatedly about lack of
respect.

Variations on the same theme play out across Kenya; says one elderly Meru
woman interviewed by Thomas (1992, 249): "They claim this is a new Kenya
and they have no time for traditions. . . . I try to give advice . . . but no one
seems to take it very seriously." Giteo—both its large, life-sustaining gestures
and its small matters of etiquette—is in decline, as children have gone to
school and spent less time learning at their elders' knees. Dynamics like these
across sub-Saharan Africa have added up to the perception that, in the words
of one Senegalese journalist writing a headline for UNESCO, "African youth are
staging a takeover bid" (Bop 1999, 31).

Productivity and Independence: New Evaluations of Aging

If customary African elderhood has come to seem a dwindling institution
whose faintly antiquated expertise on matters such as rainmaking, land, adju-
dication, and traditional medicine has been marginalized by weather reports,
title deeds, government courts, hospitals, and schools, the question remains:
what work is left for the elders? In many postcolonial African societies, "work"
is increasingly construed in terms of labor that makes money, and contributions to society tend to be calibrated in an undifferentiated fashion, according
to economic productivity. The ruthless calculus of the market thus reduces
many elders' efforts to an inferior version of youthful productivity, rather than
a life stage with distinct powers and social contributions. Thomas's statement
captures this perfectly; by the early 1990s Meru elders were widely thought to
have "the same essential life task [as younger people]: that of having a family
and providing for them" (1992, 161). Certainly many elders engage in labor until
late in life, stopping only with death or severe disability, but nevertheless, since
they may not be able to meet all their own needs, they are at an increased risk
of being seen as "dependent" and hence burdensome—particularly in a weak
Kenyan economy where many millions of younger people already struggle with
the expenses of daily life.

In their contexts of declining elder authority, sometimes-absent youth,
compromised interdependence, and poverty, Meru and Mijikenda elders fret
about provisioning for themselves. To be sure, goods still flow between generations, sometimes across long distances, but the structures of provisioning are
now more uncertain. By the late 1960s, says historian Jeffrey Fadiman (1994,
6), "No longer did [young Meru people] appear in respectful bands of learners,
bearing the gifts required by tradition: the gourds of milk and beer and the
meat and snuff and honey that not only sweetened the lives of many elders but

also permitted them to live out their final years in economic dignity." Today, although some young Meru furnish some support to their elders, others decline or even leave home when struggling elders request assistance with resources. Daughters-in-law may refuse to provision for their mothers-in-law; sons in the city may be struggling in their own right and can barely send remittances back to older kin in rural areas. Reports one elderly man to Thomas (1992, 197): "My son refused to help me buy iron sheets to complete the roof on my house after I had given him land. This is negligence. This is disrespect." Mijikenda elders, similarly, are widely known to be at risk of hunger, in part because of the loss of their authority and disintegration of kin support. At a recent gathering of Mijikenda elders in Kwale and Kilifi counties, the charismatic among them issued a call for the elders to "reclaim past glory," including a voice in governance—but meanwhile attended to the most pressing issue among their fellow elders: providing rice and maize flour to those at risk of malnutrition (Mwachiro 2015).

As elders have faced such challenges, they have, of course, come up with some creative solutions. Some, such as some elder Tiriki (an Abaluyia group in Western Kenya), have discovered that as youth head for wage labor in the cities, they open vacancies in local economies that elders can fill (Sangree 1986). A few male Mijikenda elders have turned entrepreneurial, selling customary ritual knowledge to tourists. And elders across the nation vie for influence on elected politicians, sometimes helping to mediate their disputes or issuing denunciations of politicians' behaviors. A particularly controversial practice among Mijkenda elders has been bolstering their prestige through symbiotic relationships with politicians, who compensate elders for a ritual "blessing" of sorts that garners publicity for both parties (McIntosh 2009). Between 2003 and 2006 there was a flurry of such activity, as one politician after another appeared in the Kenyan newspapers, garbed in feather headdresses, seated on Mijikenda stools adorned with customary red, white, and black or blue cloths, or receiving ceremonial staffs, sometimes claiming they had been installed as an honorary elder. Yet many were cynical about these transactions; elders complained that the superficial incorporation of politicians cheapened their customary authority, hard earned during a long life of recurrent ritual training and community involvement. A couple of older men who sold such favors to politicians were accused of fraudulently anointing politicians without themselves having the proper ritual or social qualifications. And some elders were cynical about politicians' motives: "The politicians are using us. They don't need our expertise. They only want us during the political season." Even some younger Mijikenda expressed nostalgia for the era when elders were perceived as having more moral probity and social influence. Entrepreneurial though these events were (and are, as they continue to take place), it seems many perceive these maneuvers as hustling rather than anything resembling "successful aging."

The Kenyan state today recognizes that many elders are poor, ailing, and neglected by their children, but it still offers an inadequate safety net. Its meager elder-support welfare policies typically focus on financial resources (such as the monthly stipend Kenya's new 2010 Constitution says elders should receive) rather than a century's worth of social upheaval that has devalued elders' special resources while disembedding them from customary sociality and care. In fact, to some degree, Kenyan policy work is informed by hegemonic Western assumptions about what ideal aging should look like. In 1982 Kenya became one of the signatories of the International Plan of Action on Aging adopted in Vienna, Austria, and in so doing the government officially committed itself to United Nations principles. These stipulate "the rights of older persons to independence, participation, care, self-fulfillment, and dignity." A state report on the elderly for the UN Department of Social and Economic Affairs, prepared in the early 2000s, focuses on such matters as poverty, the risks and burdens of HIV/AIDS, poor health and nutrition, tenuous housing, and the lack of income generating projects for older persons (Olum n.d.). It applauds a prominent nonprofit called HelpAge Kenya, which, in its Strategic Plan for 2002–2005, allocates money toward "sensitizing older persons on their rights," training older people in business skills, and furnishing medical care (25). But aside from a few lines about the importance of educating younger people in their role in caring for older persons, the report sidesteps the fact that entire systems of meaning and value have shifted with the loss of older economic systems and age-grade organizations, and that successful aging was once founded on the twinned notions of elders' irreplaceable authority and the reciprocity of youth.

Kenya is hardly alone in being influenced by global hegemonic notions of aging. Medical anthropologist Julie Livingston, for instance, finds that global rehabilitation programs in Botswana "stress independence and individualism in ways that do not always resonate with elderly women" (2007, 169). Rehabilitation planners assisting elderly women (whether caretakers of disabled grandchildren or themselves disabled) tend to focus on "empowerment" and autonomy, including bodily autonomy. These workers, influenced by global rehabilitation rights movements, tend to presume that "maximum independence and self-determination" are "fundamentally desirable modern projects." But, says Livingston, for her Tswana respondents ideal personhood is intersubjective, and bodies cannot be separated from the social networks they're embedded in. Elderly women vex the aims of these programs by attempting to "reinforce interdependencies" with their daughters and (to a lesser extent) their sons, reminding both of their sacrifices while reminding in-laws and husbands of their work in building the family and lineage. Rehabilitation workers are sometimes surprised to find that for these older women "regaining various bodily functions and resisting or disrupting the aging process is not necessarily a goal" (170–172, 179). But with Botswana experiencing social disruptions somewhat related to the ones I have described in Kenya, younger women sometimes resist the efforts of these elders to prevail over them.

Conclusion

I have described wrenching changes in social structure, in Kenya and beyond, that challenge elders who seek the status and interdependencies they might have counted on a few generations earlier. But this is hardly to say that elders' authority is dead. Elders are still called upon in matters of suspected witchcraft and community healing, and some seek to galvanize their power and potential influence on the state. Article 159 of Kenya's 2010 Constitution includes new phrases promoting traditional dispute-resolution mechanisms; what this means has been subject to interpretation and wrangling, but some elders have argued they should be allowed greater public influence. Meanwhile, young people in cities have told me of reconfiguring their lives when an ancestor appeared to them in a dream; they may yet fret about how disrespectful their current way of life might seem to elders; they may still send remittances back home when they can—a process made easier by mobile phone banking (known as *m-pesa*). Nor, indeed, are communalism and interdependence gone; they remain powerfully felt as a counterpoint to the possessive individualism encouraged by some quarters. Maria Cattell (1990), for instance, has argued that in spite of widespread Kenyan discourses about the attrition of the extended family, she sees good evidence of the endurance of intergenerational reciprocity, however imperfect, among aging Samia (an Abaluyia group) of Western Kenya. The older ways of life have not altogether dissolved; they are transfigured, existing in an uneasy tension with newer ideologies of individualism, independence, the valorization of youth, and state power.

A century ago, though, aging looked different in many parts of sub-Saharan Africa. The signs of physical decline were often accompanied by a clear rise in stature for men and women alike. One aggregated authority over the life course, and one could generally expect to be tended to by kin and community as one's body declined. Today, as older persons' authority is imperiled, they have lost not only social stature and clarity of meaning but also social security, aggravating the danger of impoverishment and hunger. In parts of Kenya—and indeed in many parts of sub-Saharan Africa—many aging people wish most fervently not to be young again but to be properly treated as *elders*: revered and desirably interdependent, offering a history of sacrifice and a lifetime's worth of knowledge and expertise in exchange for the care they receive.

NOTES

1. Meru, Kikuyu, and Kamba prophets were said to have made similar prognostications about the arrival of Europeans and their technology (see, e.g., Fadiman 1994, 101–102).
2. A full discussion of female elderhood would expand this chapter beyond its word limit. See Cattell and Udvardy 1992 for compelling discussions of complex gender dynamics across sub-Saharan Africa, including issues of older women's authority and elders' agency.
3. Whereas the elders' authority among most other East African groups was more locally bound, Njuri Ncheke's centralized influence extended across the wider Meru community since at least the seventeenth century. In recent years, Njuri Ncheke has been wracked by infighting, particularly as its members struggle to sort through their relationship to politicians and national politics.
4. I don't wish to suggest there was no structural tension between generations in the precolonial era. At times, for instance, fathers seeking younger wives would even find themselves competing for bridewealth with their older, marriage-eager sons (Celia Nyamweru, personal communication, 21April 2016).
5. For a detailed discussion of some of the articulations between Mijikenda elders and the Kenyan state, see Ciekawy 1998.
6. The tension between generations can be acute; Mijikenda and other elders, for instance, are at risk of being accused of witchcraft and killed for it. Some attribute this phenomenon to the greed of younger family members wishing to inherit land, but aged women are also subject to such accusations (Celia Nyamweru, personal communication, 21 April 2016).
7. See Cattell 2008 for similar discourse among the Abaluyia of Western Kenya.

REFERENCES

Aguilar, Mario I., ed. 1998. *The Politics of Age and Gerontocracy in Africa: Ethnographies of the Past and Memories of the Present.* Trenton/Asmara: Africa World Press.

Bop, Codou. 1999. "African Youth Stages a Takeover Bid." *UNESCO Courier* (January): 31–32.

Brantley, Cynthia. 1981. *The Giriama and Colonial Resistance in Kenya, 1800–1920.* Berkeley: University of California Press.

Brummel, Beth. 2015. "Youth for Life: Language, Narration, and the Quality of Youth in Urban Kenya." PhD diss., University of Chicago.

Cattell, Maria. 1990. "Models of Old Age among the Samia of Kenya: Family Support of the Elderly." *Journal of Cross-Cultural Gerontology* 5: 375–394.

———. 2008. "Aging and Social Change among Abaluyia in Western Kenya." *Journal of Cross-Cultural Gerontology* 23: 181–197.

Cattell, Maria, and Monica Udvardy, eds. 1992. "Gender, Aging, and Power in sub-Saharan Africa: Challenges and Puzzles." *Journal of Cross-Cultural Gerontology* 7 (4): 275–399.

Ciekawy, Diane. 1998. "Witchcraft in Statecraft: Five Technologies of Power in Colonial and Postcolonial Coastal Kenya," *African Studies Review* 41(3): 119–141.

———. 2015. "Distinctions in the Imagination of Harm in Contemporary Mijikenda Thought: The Existential Challenge of Majini." In *Evil in Africa: Encounters with the Everyday*, edited by William C. Olsen and Walter E. A. van Beek, 157–175. Bloomington: Indiana University Press.

Ensminger, Jean. 1990. "Co-opting the Elders: The Political Economy of State Incorporation in Africa." *American Anthropologist* 92 (3): 662–675.

Fadiman, Jeffrey A. 1994. *When We Began There Were Witchmen: An Oral History from Mount Kenya*. Berkeley: University of California Press.

Livingston, Julie. 2007. "Maintaining Local Dependencies: Elderly Women and Global Rehabilitation Agendas in Southeastern Botswana." In *Generations and Globalization: Youth, Age, and Family in the New World Economy*, edited by Jennifer Cole and Deborah Lynn Durham, 164–189. Bloomington: Indiana University Press.

McIntosh, Janet. 2009. "Elders and 'Frauds': Commodified Expertise and Politicized Authenticity among Mijikenda." *Africa* 79 (1): 35–52.

Mwachiro, Anthony. 2015. "Mijikenda Elders Root to Claim Lost Glory." *Habari Kilifi*, February 8. http://habarikilifi.com/news/mijikenda-elders-root-to-claim-lost-glory, accessed 9 October 2015.

Ogola, George. 2006. "The Idiom of Age in a Popular Kenyan Newspaper Serial." *Africa* 76 (4): 569–588.

Olum, Gondi Hesbon. N.d. "Report on Status and Implementation of National Policy on Ageing in Kenya." Prepared for United Nations Department of Economic and Social Affairs (UNDESA). http://www.un.org/esa/socdev/ageing/documents/workshops/Vienna/kenya.pdf, accessed 1 October 2015.

Parkin, David. 1972. *Palms, Wine, and Witnesses: Public Spirit and Private Gain in an African Farming Community*. San Francisco, London: Chandler.

Sangree, W. H. 1986. "Role Flexibility and Status Continuity: Tiriki (Kenya) Age Groups Today." *Journal of Cross Cultural Gerontology* 1 (2): 117–38.

Thomas, Samuel P. 1992. "Old Age in Meru, Kenya: Adaptive Reciprocity in a Changing Rural Community." PhD diss., University of Florida.

Willis, Justin. 1993. Mombasa, the Swahili, and the Making of the Mijikenda. Oxford: Clarendon.

PART IV

Medicine, Morality, and Self

Lessons from Life's Ends

13

Successful Selves?

Heroic Tales of Alzheimer's Disease and Personhood in Brazil

ANNETTE LEIBING

On December 19, 1997, one of Brazil's first public specialized units for older people with mental health problems—a center for care, teaching, and research with a clear focus on dementia—was inaugurated in Rio de Janeiro. This center formed part of the Institute of Psychiatry, which was located within the beautiful old campus of the Federal University of Rio de Janeiro, with its majestic trees and colonial architecture. The CDA, the Portuguese acronym for Center for Alzheimer's Disease and Other Mental Disorders of Aging, quickly assembled a multidisciplinary team. The photos taken at the inauguration show the staff laughing into the camera—a motivated team, fascinated by the challenge of working with patients suffering from this "new disease" (Leibing 2005, 2006).

The beginning was not easy. Some therapists abandoned their new positions, finding the task of working with affected individuals too depressing. They felt anxious because patients could not remember them from one session to another and because they associated these patients with decline and imminent death. It was a time of trial and error. In the early stages of the CDA almost no teaching material was available in Portuguese, and not everyone read English. Many of the therapists, some of them following psychoanalytical theories, had to adapt their approaches to more modest interventions, while others discovered, by chance, some strategies that worked. The music therapist, for instance, was surprised by the ability of many group participants to sing along to old songs, even to remember the words, when they were not able to tell whether and what they had eaten for lunch. The clinical director, a psychiatrist specializing in old age psychiatry, had access to international literature and was invited to national and international conferences, but he found it impossible to treat the core symptom of dementia itself: cognitive decline. He instead evaluated older people, diagnosing Alzheimer's disease and treating concomitant conditions such as psychotic symptoms, depression, and sleeping problems. Other therapists, including psychologists, occupational therapists, and physiotherapists, strove to provide interventions for suffering family caregivers and, increasingly, for the patients themselves—especially after the question of personhood became an issue.

During a trip abroad, I had bought the bestselling autobiographical book *Living in the Labyrinth* by Diana McGowin (1993), who wrote about the difficulties of getting a diagnosis in the 1980s United States when Alzheimer's, and especially the early onset form she thought she was suffering from, was still not well known.[1] McGowin described in a moving way how, after finally being diagnosed, she became a nonperson, and was ignored even by her family: "If no longer worth holding, why do I crave for it? . . . My every molecule seems to scream out that I do, indeed, exist, and that existence must be valued by someone!" (114). During the weekly study groups at the CDA, McGowin's account was discussed intensively. The team became mobilized by her suffering and, as a result, was more aware of signs of personhood among their own patients—such as continuity, agency, and connectedness with others.

Successful aging is simultaneously one of the most popular and criticized concepts in the wider field of gerontology. Scholars have questioned the decontextualized, individualizing, and some would say neoliberal messages underlying discussions on how to age well (see the *Gerontologist* 2015 for an overview). The life of individuals suffering from dementia, including its most common form, Alzheimer's disease, is often conceptualized by both gerontologists and the public as an antithesis to the ideal of successful aging, which, in its most general terms, posits continuity with one's middle-age performances and activities (Havighurst [1963] 2009; Rowe and Kahn 1987, 1997; see also Lamb 2014). People with dementia, who experience increasingly severe physical, psychological, behavioral, and cognitive loss of capacities, are easy to blame for being unsuccessful, especially in the context of a "new public health" emphasizing continuous preventive measures and self-care (e.g., Bell 2011), and even more so given the recent turn toward prevention of dementia itself (see Leibing 2014a, 2015; Leibing and Kampf 2013).

A lot has been written about the tragic "loss of self" that can accompany failing memory and difficulty connecting with others in a shared world. However, the "personhood movement" (Leibing 2006) strives to rescue the nonperson of early accounts of Alzheimer's disease, as social scientists, caregivers, and health professionals endeavor to recognize the enduring "person within." In this sense, the "rescued self" can be seen as a niche of successfulness within the general framing of dementia as unsuccessful aging—a point I want to discuss using the concept of heroism.

A hero is the main character of a tale, someone who is admired for doing or living something that is positively valued as exemplary and above the average. Heroes, following philosopher Peter Sloterdijk (2008), live a life of honor and sacrifice, or as Mike Featherstone (1992, 160) argued, a life "in which the everyday is viewed as something to be tamed, resisted, or denied, something to be subjugated in the pursuit of a higher purpose." The different types of heroes in this chapter, each one representing a kind of successfulness regarding dementia care, linked to a specific period of time, not only show the virtues of honor and sacrifice but also reveal visions of the good and bad, and of moral quandaries surrounding love, loss, and solidarities.

Studying dementia in Brazil is not only about local or cultural forms of the disease. Brazil is strongly connected to the international consumption and production of geriatric and gerontological knowledge (Leibing 2009, 185ff). To research and understand Alzheimer's disease in Brazil thus requires a "glocal" perspective, heeding the local grounding and production of internationally circulating knowledge.

Wider notions about aging in Brazil form one of the local backdrops of this investigation. Although the Brazilian population is undergoing one of the fastest aging processes worldwide, Brazil maintains the image of a "youthful country" (Veras 1994), partially as a result of an obsession with performance of the perfect body: Brazil is well known for its leadership in plastic surgery, an intervention that is available not only to the rich elite (Edmonds 2014). Brazilians are also one of the highest consumers of medications worldwide: for instance, the national Viagra market is estimated at US$114 million per year (Agarwal et al. 2012). Older people can be strongly stigmatized, perhaps more so than in many other countries. At the same time, seniors in Brazil have been encouraged by the "third age" movement (*terceira idade*) to occupy public spaces—a global trend promoting the empowerment of (consuming and active) seniors (Debert 2002; Robbins-Ruszkowski this volume), especially in big urban centers. Older Brazilians have also been found by politicians and marketing firms, who increasingly value their roles as consumers and voters.

In the mid-1990s I had the rare opportunity to observe how knowledge of the increasingly globally circulating category of Alzheimer's disease began to emerge and spread in urban environments in Brazil (Leibing 1997, 2005), changing local landscapes of aging. This resulted in new perceptions of the typical symptom clusters of dementia, which had earlier been thought of either as normal aging—as a gentle sliding away into another world—or when there was aggressive and disruptive behavior, or an early onset, as a highly stigmatized form of madness.

Amid such local and global contexts, this chapter focuses on one of the most popular topics among social scientists and the caregiving professions studying dementia: the question of personhood. With its strong humanistic appeal, the personhood movement is about sustaining continuity in dementia, about enhancing someone's capacities and skills, and about looking beyond symptoms and losses. My aim is to add some further nuance to the discussion, especially as pertains to two issues: first, I argue that personhood needs to be seen in its sociohistorical context (e.g., personhood in the mid-1990s Brazil is not the same as today); second, discussions of personhood in Brazil reveal differences from, even while referring

to, models of personhood abroad. Most notably here, Brazilian discussions emphasize a less individualistic understanding of personhood than found within North
American and northern European debates.

Discoveries: The Heroic Caregiver (around 1997)

As in North America a decade earlier (see Gubrium 1986), Brazilians started
to become aware of the existence of Alzheimer's disease in the 1990s—more
or less at the same time as aging in general became increasingly thematized
as a national problem. The 1990s saw the creation of institutions, laws, and
movements for older people, as well as polarized media accounts of both the
abandonment and exclusion of elderly individuals in need of help, and of heroic
physically, socially, and sexually active seniors (Debert 2002). Alzheimer's disease, once described in the media as a disease affecting people elsewhere,
started to be portrayed as a "Brazilian disease." It was a time of astonishment.

In an interview with Jacob Guterman, then president of the Rio de Janeiro
Alzheimer's Association, I was told that the reason for founding the group was his
desire to help and educate other Brazilians who knew so little about the disease.
He described his story of difficulty in finding a diagnosis for his wife's symptoms in
the 1980s as similar to Diana McGowin's. After observing several group meetings, I
was struck by the insistence on what one could describe as sustaining personhood,
the message repeated by group members that "you can still do something, and
that is loving the person with dementia." This hopeful-sounding message, which
in reality meant that nothing could be done in terms of slowing down the disease,
was also a key slogan among the CDA's therapists and the growing consensus in the
international literature. S. B. Wilen, S. M. Harman, and D. Alexander-Israel (1997,
44) articulated the state of the art at that time: "Alzheimer's disease has no specific
treatment; care often must be directed to patient behavior. . . . The more caregivers
know, the easier it is to ensure the Alzheimer's patient is comfortable and secure."

Under these circumstances, what does it mean to preserve or sustain someone's personhood in dementia? At the CDA, the staff slowly began to routinize
their therapeutic practices; for example, they found that their patients were
able to enjoy certain activities at the day center or at home, thanks to family
counseling in combination with pharmaceutical interventions.

I remember an older woman of Portuguese origin, Dona Eliza, who was considered a "difficult patient" because she hardly engaged in any activity or communication with others and could become quite grumpy when someone insisted
on having her participate. She arrived every afternoon at the day center and spent
most of her time lying on the brown sofa in the main room we called the living
room. One day I sat close to her, asking her whether she liked it there, at the CDA.
She slowly opened her eyes, smiling at me just a little bit, and whispered: "Here I

like it, at home I only watch TV." The discovery that she appreciated a detached way of engaging with a community, combined with their increasing certainty that other participants at the day center did, in fact, react to certain activities (as well as to the staff's great warmth and cordiality), reinforced the professionals' opinion that their approaches were starting to have positive effects. Some of these interventions were addressed to a conception of the person more akin to a child than to an adult who might continue to be herself despite cognitive decline (whereas a "continuity of self" would be the central point in a personhood philosophy). For instance, one participant, Sr. Moisés, described his daily visits to the day center as going to the "school for small children" (a escolinha).

This anecdote reveals the difficulty of translating personhood philosophy into practice. There are two main reasons for this. First, signs of agency, continuity, and connectedness were sometimes difficult to detect because many affected individuals were already in an advanced stage of the disease when they arrived at the CDA. Alzheimer's disease had only started to become better known in Brazil, and therefore patients were generally diagnosed after a long history of searching for an explanation for their symptoms and decline. Second, signs of personhood were easily overshadowed by the general negative image of Alzheimer patients, both locally and abroad. The most general prevailing image in the 1990s was that of an apparently homogeneous group of persons who were not merely childlike but almost gone—the glocal metaphor of the "living dead"—and for whom little could be done.

The other international bestselling book of that period, The 36-Hour Day (Maze and Rabins 2012 [1981]), now in its fifth edition, and also a reference in Brazil, captures that early period of dementia awareness. In it, the individual with dementia is a source of suffering for the caregiver, who appears as the real victim of the disease, since the affected individual is thought to be unaware of her condition. "Caregiver burden" was a highly discussed topic in the international literature, and the "caregiver burden inventory" (Novak and Guest 1989) was a central instrument for measuring the degree of strain placed on caregivers by the work and responsibility of providing "total care" over the metaphorical thirty-six-hour day.

For those in the CDA, personhood emerged haltingly from discovering fragments of continuity amidst varied and often severe symptoms characteristic of advanced stages. In one interview, for instance, a woman told me of how she took care of the husband from whom she had been divorced, feeling that her former marriage was a bond for life, but that he was no longer "there": "He is my husband, but he is not my husband anymore. I take care of him, I love him, but I love what he was; he is not there anymore." Within this context of perceiving the individual as a nonperson, discovering and nurturing elements of personhood meant undertaking an archaeology of their self, which was often more of a guessing game than real continuity. As one woman said about her husband: "I don't know what he wants every time he gets angry. Sometimes I make him watch soccer; and sometimes he says 'Flamengo' [a famous team]. Then I know he is still there."

The heroic person of early accounts of Alzheimer's is glocally—in Brazil and beyond—the caregiver who provides total care. To some extent, the caring individual, who had to put in "thirty-six-hour days," was also transformed into a nonperson, having had to give up her own life and almost fuse with the helpless and dependent dementia victim. Although I do not have data on exact numbers, the need for total care could also lead to violence and desperation. We heard stories about individuals with dementia being locked in or even chained at home, in order to not turn on the gas or leave the house and get lost, when the other family members had to work. Some individuals were neglected or only minimally cared for, although I had the impression that the majority of those who made it to the CDA had a dedicated family. Exactly because of the high ideal and the unquestioned desirability of heroic acts, it might be that researchers easily portray too much of the good side of dementia care: it is a difficult task to observe or make people confess attitudes that do not reflect these ideals.

Continuities: The Heroic Individual with Alzheimer's (around 2005)

Ten to fifteen years later, by around 2005, Alzheimer's disease had become a very well known issue in Brazil through TV programs, regular articles in the print media, and intense public discussion of cases of dementia among famous people and soap opera characters. These accounts were still pessimistic and generally referred to a depressing loss of self. At the same time, hope emerged through pharmaceutical interventions that targeted dementia itself. This hope was perceptible in both media coverage and among health care professionals I interviewed around 2005, even though the specialized literature increasingly circulated the conclusion that existing dementia medications had minimal effects on dementia, especially in the advanced stages (e.g., Royall 2005; also Leibing 2009). Nonetheless, Luiz E. Garcez-Leme, Mariana D. Leme, and David V. Espino (2005) described Brazil, for geriatrics, as "a big country with big opportunities" in which the pharmaceutical industry invested heavily (see also GaBI online 2011) and the number of psychogeriatric health professionals steadily grew.

Internationally, but also in Brazil, personhood had become a salient issue in both specialized and popular literature. A number of researchers exploring innovative and beautiful projects, many of them using art, showed that signs of selfhood—creativity, humor, and personal preferences—persisted long after a diagnosis of Alzheimer's disease, fighting the medicalizing of symptoms and behaviors (e.g., Basting 2014; McLean 2006).

In fact, because of the awareness raised by numerous national and international campaigns, many more people than before with symptoms of

Alzheimer's were searching for recognition. These individuals were not help-less victims anymore. Some, at least in the United States, spoke up for them-selves even in advanced stages and participated in self-help groups, published books, and became leading characters of films and novels. It was not only love that could be given to these individuals, as was the case in earlier accounts; these were people who could respond to therapeutic interventions and lead a relatively independent and fulfilling life. The negative side of dementia had little place in these accounts. There was, of course, still a lot of suffering involved, but as the late Richard Taylor—a well-known Alzheimer's activist who suffered from the disease himself—stated, people were sitting in a "cognitive wheelchair." They were handicapped, but the wheelchair—a combination of caregivers' help, medications, self-help groups, and personal willpower—could compensate for much of the loss.

This brighter outlook on dementia gave hope to many and, to a certain extent, contributed to a destigmatization of the condition, although some also called attention to the limits of optimism. For example, Eva-Marie Kessler and Clemens Schwender (2012), in a study of the growing number of photos showing individu-als with a dementia in news magazines between 2000 and 2009, argued that—at least in Germany—the portraits of these patients might have become "too positive," highlighting "characters with dementia . . . living an autonomous as well as social integrated life" (267) and therefore did not adequately prepare individuals for the challenges of living with the syndrome. They concluded that positive images can result in a decline of taboos and stigma surrounding Alzheimer's, but at the same time they might reduce efforts made by society to create better living conditions for people affected by dementia. Further, not only do approaches that humanize dementia care rarely deal with advanced stages, but when they do, researchers in most cases only emphasize signs of enduring personhood and ignore the some-times dramatic co-occurring symptoms—such as psychotic incidences, inconti-nence, and aggressive behavior—individuals can experience due to dementia.

The ambiguities surrounding the heroic person with Alzheimer's were also true in Brazil, although in some slightly different ways. The daily work with the elderly I observed at the CDA in Rio de Janeiro produced enthusiastic accounts of continuity and agency but also called attention to the limits of the personhood movement. Just as direct contact with patients a few years earlier had revealed signs of personhood and therefore relativized the then generally negative image of the nonperson in Alzheimer's disease, now the relationships health professionals established with their patients challenged the prevailing optimism of the personhood movement in the 2000s. Patients got worse, and there often came a moment when the CDA could no longer take care of them—a painful decision, since it was extremely difficult to find public care for individu-als in advanced stages who had difficulty communicating or performing basic activities of daily living. At such moments, signs of nonpersonhood became in fact more important than searching for continuities in self, because of the urgent need to deal with the tangible problem of care. The CDA professionals wove back and forth between spotting signs of the former person and interpreting disturbing new symptoms as signs of a non- or no-longer (full) person in need of care. Focusing on the need for help rather than on signs of normalcy might, in fact, be a better way to reach what Janelle Taylor (2008) has called "keeping the cares together."

In Brazil the concept of personhood in dementia is also in general less individualistic than in North America (although this is, of course, a generalization that does not uniformly apply). The first time I became aware of this distinction was when projecting the American documentary film *Complaints of a Dutiful Daughter* by Deborah Hoffmann (1995) during a class on the social aspects of psychogeriatrics at the CDA. Some of the students were visibly shocked by the long time the mother in the film stayed alone in her apartment, even though the daughter called and visited regularly. The daughter's claim that maintaining her mother's independence was her highest goal resulted in a lively discussion in class. Without resorting to a dichotomy of dividual/individual or egocentric versus sociocentric societies, and thinking instead in terms of a spectrum, it seems important to consider that the dominant ethos in Brazil values a life connected to others and devalues "keeping to oneself" (DaMatta 1989). Although, as elsewhere, there have been cases of elder abuse and violence, families are generally very protective of their elders, and personhood is less strongly associated with independent living than in North America. Of course, this image might be partial; it is difficult to say who was not able to come to the CDA because he or she lived alone.

The sociocentric aspect of personhood also emerged as an important feature in the observations I and my colleague Daniel Groisman made during a one-year ethnographic fieldwork project in a shantytown (*favela*) in Rio de Janeiro in the early 2000s. The professionals at the local health post told us that they knew of some cases of Alzheimer's disease in the favela but had never met these people. We finally attended group meetings of older women with hypertension (see Leibing 2014b), in which we tried, among other topics, to explore what dementia, loss of memory, decline, and the need for help might mean in the women's lives. What the group members told us was that there was no such thing as Alzheimer's where they lived. And when we reminded them that two famous personalities in the community had been recently diagnosed (news we had gleaned from the daily papers), the women disdainfully described these individuals as antisocial and crazy but not suffering from a "disease." They complained about a famous samba singer who once was a *bohème* and very well liked but who now did not even look at them. They continued their account by mocking some older people they knew who displayed bizarre behaviors. When we later visited one of the group members on the hill, she invited a woman of a very advanced age to meet with us as a paradigm of vitality, wit, and strength in old age. She was introduced to us with the words, "We do not have this Alzheimer's here on the hill."

Reading symptoms of dementia in the environment of the favela rested on a question of deservingness—memory loss without negative symptoms meant care, if someone was there for the person who was *caduca* (forgetfulness as a normal part of aging). But when disruptive behavior was the issue, a double exclusion was at work: the condition was interpreted as craziness resulting in shame, stigma, and accusations. This might have been the reason why the health professionals we spoke to never met dementia patients; they were hidden from the public. Additionally, the incapacity to maintain social relations became a primary sign, not of a pathology of the brain but of a condemnation of the social person herself.

At the CDA, the framing of the symptom cluster as a disease of individual memory led to insisting on forgetfulness as the core symptom of Alzheimer's, even though behavioral symptoms were by far the most disturbing ones for families. The paradox was that the social conception of dementia led to isolation of the individual who was cut off from community, while the individualized conception of brain pathology, once it was recognized as a disease category, resulted in community and a certain recognition of the individual, including the search for continuities with one's former self.

In other words, although the hero in the favela was the vital, witty old woman challenging all stereotypes of aging, in the CDA, and even more so in the international literature, the hero was the individual who continued to live a relatively autonomous life, even though she suffered from Alzheimer's disease.

Total Care 2.0: The New Heroism

In this last section, I want to describe an intriguing trend that I first noticed recently in the Brazilian media and that I then became aware of in other contexts—for instance, in the German film *Honig im Kopf* (*Head Full of Honey*). This new phenomenon describes a further type of heroism in dementia care: the one of grandchildren taking care of their grandparents.

"The saga of the grandson who abandoned everything in order to take care of his grandmother"[2] is the headline of an article telling the story of a woman from southern Brazil, Nilva de Lourdes Aguzzoli, who passed away in 2014 as a consequence of her Alzheimer's disease but who had a "joyful and eventful end of her life. Joyful thanks to her dedicated 22 year-old grandson.... And eventful because he decided to share the moments they spent together on Facebook" (Terra online 2014). The same story is told under the headline of "Student abandons everything and becomes the 'father' of his grandmother with Alzheimer's" (Saúde Plena 2014)—a story that was also turned into a book.

Another tale bears the headline: "Young woman changes her routine in order to dedicate herself to her grandmother with Alzheimer's—The disease changed the lives of granny and grandchild who even sleep together in the same bed" (Globo.com 2015). In the article one reads that after learning of her grandmother's diagnosis, "the young woman, Christiane, moved in with her grandmother and abandoned all activities young people do at her age. She does not go anymore to the gym and can't even remember the last time she traveled. Even the *forró* [a popular Brazilian dance], once her passion, she put aside. All this for taking care of her grandmother who needs constant attention. . . . The only moment the two are not together is when Christiane works [and the grandmother stays at a day center], so that she can pay for her grandmother's treatment." The article continues: "Since Alzheimer's disease has no cure, the treatment consists of medications that slow down the progression of the disease. 'I learned . . . that the disease does not hurt the sick person, but the caregiver. She does not know what is happening to her,' . . . [Christiane] laments. Christiane created a page on Facebook in which she shows everyday life with her grandmother and especially the moments in which the two are having fun together. 'It is as if she is my daughter,' says Christiane."

Finally, a last Brazilian example: A chapter of a popular *telenovela* (soap opera) is discussed in an online newspaper with the headline "Benjamin cries because . . . Izabelita (Nicette Bruno) received the diagnosis of Alzheimer's and, in order to avoid the asylum, the architect [grandson] moves in with her" (Tribuna Hoje 2015).

When relating these three examples to the other accounts of heroism in this chapter it is striking to see that, once again, the heroic person here is the caregiver, albeit of a new kind: Instead of the suffering, depressing image of the overwhelmed, isolated, and burdened caregiver (who was previously usually an adult child or spouse), the new heroes are youthful grandchildren smiling into the camera and making their dedicated carework visible through social networks. These tales of a publicly exposed heroism and of a certain fame also highlight a sense of continuity and personhood; the individual with dementia is being sustained, but not through the North American ideal of independent living. It is rather through an intense, almost fusional connectedness ("They even sleep together in the same bed") that resembles again the famous "thirty-six-hour day." In this new heroism, it is accepted that the person with dementia becomes a child again, and personhood is understood as sustained through a benevolent paternalism, love, and ongoing intimacy in the everyday spaces of a well-known environment. Different from the early accounts, there is joy and continuity in the childlike state and in connectivity; the image of the nonperson is only marginally evoked.

I recommend following the links of the Brazilian articles and looking at the photos of the smiling heroes[3]—images that both inspire and, once again, could transmit too much optimism, as was the case when focusing on personhood alone. Sloterdijk related heroism to sacredness. It is exactly the saintly attitude of sacrifices ("the grandson who abandoned everything") that make these stories so special but, at the same time, so unreal for people who are not able to give up everything to provide such a total care. These tales have an exemplary character and seem to invite others to become a hero, with the additional gain of a certain notoriety displayed in the news and social networks.[4] However, the moments in which the protagonists are not smiling—for instance when diapers need to be changed, and when sundowning, confusion, and restlessness interrupt sleep at night—are totally absent in these articles on the altruistic grandchildren.

In the international literature, several authors have written about the fusional relations involved in ideal dementia care settings; Judie Davies (2011), for example, writes about a "collaborative venture" and an "us identity," while David Karp (2002) argues that couples have a "joint career" into memory loss after the diagnosis of a dementia. This profound ethos of being there for the other is also at the core of the accounts about caring grandchildren, although these stories curiously leave out the figure of both the spouse and the adult child. Grandchildren might have fewer conflicts with their grandparents than one might find between generations who are directly connected with each other (Joshi et al. 2015), but I think that there is more involved in this new phenomenon.

The Brazilian stories do not even mention the generation between grandchildren and grandparents, while the older individuals seem to be either widowed or divorced. Where are the parents in these stories, and the spouses? Wouldn't parents tell the architect to pursue his career instead of giving it up for his grandmother, and wouldn't worried parents recommend their daughter Christiane to get some distractions for her mental health, as in the often-heard recommendations for traditional caregivers offered by Alzheimer's associations and self-help groups? The astonishing absence of the middle generation seems to indicate that these heroic acts are happening because the traditional caregivers were overwhelmed by the task, unable to build a dyad of care.

In the above-mentioned German film *Honig im Kopf*, the middle generation is present, but both parents are unable to understand and sustain the increasingly confused grandfather, for different reasons: While the father diminishes the losses, his wife only sees the negative and disturbing symptoms of dementia. The granddaughter's taking over is an act of desperation, in order to save the beloved grandfather from institutionalization, just as in the third example from Brazil. Maybe because of the generational distance, the grandchild is more easily able to acknowledge her grandfather as the person he was before. However, it cannot be concluded that from now on grandchildren should provide dementia care; in my opinion, these stories can be seen as parables showing that both distance and fusion are ideally needed for accompanying individuals with dementia (cf. Markell 2002).

Finally, we might consider how single persons, even single families, are rarely able to provide complex care by themselves—a call for a rethinking of care solidarities among families and health care professionals. In times of financial cuts in many health care systems, it might make sense to think also about "state heroism," about what kind of policies are exemplary for sustaining those who deal with the complex task of caring for an individual with dementia.

In closing, there are four points I want to highlight emerging from this discussion: First, changing understandings of dementia in Brazil reveal the intersecting of local and global processes, as the emerging biomedical category of Alzheimer's disease interpenetrates with evolving Brazilian ways of envisioning aging, care relationships, and personhood. Second, within the framework of heroism we should ask what it is that we define as sacred, since this might show that heroes all over the world share a lot of characteristics but that, ultimately, they are deeply connected to local ways of reading symptoms and the constantly changing social relations among vulnerable and less vulnerable people. Third, what all these examples show is that heroism is about exceptions and should not be expected to be the norm. Finally, the personhood-in-Alzheimer's movement, in both Brazil and abroad, shares a striking similarity with successful aging ideologies, in that disease, decline, and dependency get excluded from the propagated ideals of the continuity of the person in Alzheimer's disease. The examples explored here indicate that even negative symptoms—such as memory loss and dependence—need to be taken seriously and not be excluded from public images of dementia and dementia care. These symptoms *are* part of personhood. If we are to really view the person with dementia as a "person," this must include acknowledging both needing care and providing care as central to many people's experiences of what it is to be human.

ACKNOWLEDGMENTS

I am grateful to the Social Sciences and Humanities Research Council (SSHRC; grant no. 430–2015–01165), for financing my current research on Alzheimer's disease.

NOTES

1. Diana McGowin found out later that, in fact, she was not suffering from early-onset dementia, as some specialists had suspected (Peter Whitehouse, personal communication).
2. All translations from Portuguese to English are mine.
3. See, for instance, http://g1.globo.com/sao-paulo/sorocaba-jundiai/noticia/2015/07/jovem -muda-rotina-para-se-dedicar-aos-cuidados-da-avo-com-alzheimer.html and http://sites .uai.com.br/app/noticia/saudeplena/noticias/2014/04/28/noticia_saudeplena,148451/ estudante-larga-tudo-e-vira-pai-de-avo-com-alzheimer.shtml, accessed 27 January 2016.
4. Interestingly, the story of the heroic grandson (example number one above) has also been used by the pharmaceutical industry. Libbs Pharmaceuticals, which produces the cognition-enhancing medication galantamina in Brazil, has distributed high-gloss folders in private geriatric clinics, in which examples of the grandson's care strategies are

paired with photos of grandson with grandmother, without ever mentioning directly the medication; only the label "Libbs" can be read on each page.

REFERENCES

Agarwal, Sanjeev, Joao d'Ameida, and Tracy Francis. 2012. "Capturing the Brazilian Pharma Opportunity." *McKinsey & Company: Insights and Publications* (April). http://www.mckinsey.com/insights/health_systems_and_services/capturing_the_brazilian_pharma_opportunity, accessed 8 February 2016.

Basting, Anne. 2014. "The Arts in Dementia Care." In *Excellence in Dementia Care: Principles and Practice*, 2nd ed., edited by Murna Downs and Barbara Bowe, 132–143. Maidenhead, UK: Open University Press.

Bell, Kirsten, Darlene McNaughto, and Amy Salmon. 2011. *Alcohol, Tobacco, and Obesity: Morality, Mortality, and the New Public Health.* London: Routledge.

DaMatta, R. 1989. *O que faz o Brasil, Brasil?* Rio de Janeiro: Rocco.

Davies, Judie C. 2011. "Preserving the 'Us Identity' Through Marriage Commitment While Living with Early-Stage Dementia." *Dementia* 10 (2): 217–234.

Debert, Guita Grin. 2002. "O idoso na mídia." *ComCiência*–Velhice (September). www.comciencia.br.

Edmonds, Alexander. 2014. "Surgery-for-Life: Aging, Sexual Fitness, and Self-Management in Brazil." *Anthropology amd Aging Quarterly* 34 (4): 246–259.

Featherstone, Mike. 1992. "The Heroic Life and Everyday Life." *Theory, Culture and Society* 9 (1992): 159–182.

GaBI Online. 2011. "The Pharmaceutical Market in Brazil." GaBI Online: Generics and Biosimilars Initiative. http://www.gabionline.net/Generics/General/The-pharmaceutical-market-in-Brazil, accessed 8 February 2016.

Garcez-Leme, Luiz E., Mariana D. Leme, and David V. Espino. 2005. "Geriatrics in Brazil: A Big Country with Big Opportunities." *Journal of the American Geriatrics Society* 53 (11): 2018–2022.

Gerontologist. 2015. "Special Issue: Successful Aging." *Gerontologist* 55 (1): 1–168.

Globo.com. 2015. "Jovem muda rotina para se dedicar aos cuidados da avo com Alzheimer." http://g1.globo.com/sao-paulo/sorocaba-jundiai/noticia/2015/07/jovem-muda-rotina-para-se-dedicar-aos-cuidados-da-avo-com-alzheimer.html, accessed 8 February 2016.

Gubrium, Jaber F. 1986. *Oldtimers and Alzheimer's: The Descriptive Organisation of Senility.* Greenwich, CT: JAI Press.

Havighurst, Robert J. 2009. "Successful Aging." In *Process of Aging: Social and Psychological Perspectives*, edited by Richard H. Williams, Clark Tibbits, and Wilma Donohue, 299–320. New Brunswick, NJ: Aldine Transaction.

Hoffman, Deborah, director. 1995. *Complaints of a Dutiful Daughter* [Motion picture]. Women Make Movies.

Joshi, G., S. Gezan, C. Stopka, M. Pigg, and M. Tillman. 2015. "College Students as Informal Caregivers and Their Attitude toward Their Older Relatives." *International Journal of Aging and Society* 5 (4): 47–60.

Karp, David. 2002. *The Burden of Sympathy: How Families Cope With Mental Illness.* New York: Oxford University Press.

Kessler, Eva-Marie, and Clemens Schwender. 2012. "Giving Dementia a Face? The Portrayal of Older People with Dementia in German Weekly News Magazines between the Years 2000 and 2009." *Journals of Gerontololgy*, ser. B 67B (2): 261–270.

Lamb, Sarah. 2014. "Permanent Personhood or Meaningful Decline? Toward a Critical Anthropology of Successful Aging." *Journal of Aging Studies* 29: 41–52.

Leibing, Annette. 1997. "Narrowing Worlds: On Biography and Alzheimer's Disease in Brazil." In *The Medical Anthropologies in Brazil*, edited by Annette Leibing, 221–242. Berlin: VWB-Verlag.

———. 2005. "The Old Lady from Ipanema: Changing Notions of Old Age in Brazil." *Journal of Aging Studies* 19 (1): 15–31.

———. 2006. "Divided Gazes: Alzheimer's Disease, the Person Within, and Death in Life." In *Thinking about Dementia: Culture, Loss, and the Anthropology of Senility*, edited by Annette Leibing and Lawrence Cohen, 240–268. New Brunswick, NJ: Rutgers University Press.

———. 2009. "Tense Prescriptions? Alzheimer Medications and the Anthropology of Uncertainty." *Transcultural Psychiatry* 46 (1): 180–206.

———. 2014a. "The Earlier the Better: Alzheimer's Prevention, Early Detection, and the Quest for Pharmacological Interventions." *Culture, Medicine and Psychiatry* 38 (2): 217–236.

———. 2014b. "Heterotopia and Illness: Older Women and Hypertension in a Brazilian Favela." *Anthropology and Aging* 34 (4): 225–237.

———. 2015. "Dementia in the Making: Early Detection and the Body/Brain in Alzheimer's Disease." In *Popularizing Dementia, Public Expressions and Representations of Forgetfulness*, edited by Aagje Swinnen and Mark Schweda, 275–294. Bielefeld, Germany: Transkript.

Leibing, Annette, and Antje Kampf. 2013. "Neither Body nor Brain: Comparing Attitudes to Prostate Cancer and Alzheimer's Disease." *Body and Society* 19 (4): 61–91.

Markell, Patchen. 2000. "The Recognition of Politics: A Comment on Emcke and Tully." *Constellations* 7 (4): 496–506.

Maze, Nancy L., and Peter V. Rabins. 2012. *The 36-Hour Day: A Family Guide to Caring for People Who Have Alzheimer Disease, Related Dementias, and Memory Loss*. Baltimore: Johns Hopkins University Press.

McGowin, Diana. 1993. *Living in the Labyrinth: A Personal Journal through the Maze of Alzheimer's*. New York: Dell.

McLean, Athena. 2006. *The Person in Dementia: A Study of Nursing Home Care in the US*. Toronto: University of Toronto Press.

Novak, Mark, and Carol Guest. 1989. "Application for a Multidimensional Caregiver Burden Inventory." *Gerontologist* 29 (6): 798–803.

Rowe, John, and Robert L. Kahn. 1987. "Human Aging: Usual and Successful." *Science* 237 (4811): 143–149.

———. 1997. "Successful Aging." *Gerontologist* 37 (4): 433–440.

Royall, Donald R. 2005. "The Emperor Has No Clothes: Dementia Treatment on the Eve of the Aging Era." *Journal of the American Geriatric Society* 53 (1): 163–164.

Sloterdijk, Peter. 2008. "Philosopher Peter Sloterdik on the Tour de France." *Spiegel Online* (July 10). http://www.spiegel.de/international/europe/philosopher-peter-sloterdijk-on-the-tour-de-france-the-riders-are-just-regular-employees-a-565111.html, accessed 8 February 2016.

Taylor, Janelle S. 2008. "On Recognition, Caring, and Dementia." *Medical Anthropology Quarterly* 22 (4): 313–335.

Taylor, Richard. 2014. *Richard Taylor: Alzheimer's from the Inside Out* [video file]. Dementia Alliance International. https://www.youtube.com/watch?v=EU_aeOqdKIQ, accessed 8 February 2015.

Terra online. Saga de neto que largou tudo para cuidar da avo vira livro. http://noticias.terra.com.br/brasil/saga-de-neto-que-largou-tudo-para-cuidar-da-avo-vira-livro,b35cad2487d86410VgnVCM3000009af154doRCRD.html, 14 June 2014, accessed November 2015.

Tribuna Hoje. 2015. "Paraisopolis! Benjamin chora por doença da avó e decide morar com ela." July 17. http://www.tribunahoje.com/noticia/148556/entretenimento/2015/07/17/paraisopolis-benjamin-chora-por-doenca-da-avo-e-decide-morar-com-ela.html, accessed 6 February 2015.

Veras, Renato P. 1994. *País jovem com cabelos brancos*. Rio de Janeiro: UnATi.

Wilen, S. B., S. M. Harman, and D. Alexander-Israel. 1997. "Home Care and the Alzheimer's Disease Patient: An Educational Imperative." *Caring* 16 (1): 44–46.

14

Comfortable Aging

Lessons for Living from Eighty-five and Beyond

MEIKA LOE

On warm days, Florence leaves the front door of her suburban ranch-style home open so that the mail carrier can walk in and hand her the mail. Several years ago, when I was conducting research for my book, *Aging Our Way*, I approached her front door for the first time and saw and heard her through the screen, waving me in. "Come in, hon."[1]

I walked into a large living room and greeted a tall, bookish-looking nonagenarian, or elder in her nineties, who was sitting in her recliner, the spot where she spends the better part of each day, wearing comfortable clothing and sensible shoes. She was in the most agreeable place she could be, and rather than haphazardly making do, Florence had designed a user-friendly space that kept her occupied and connected and met her changing health needs.

Florence surrounded herself with the essentials of her life. Pictures of her husband and family surrounded her on all sides. On a side table to her right sat a lamp, a transistor radio, and telephone. A cane leaned against the table. Slightly below that (perched on an ottoman) were two plastic containers, one that held mail and a calendar and one that she called her "medicine cubby" for about ten prescription bottles and a large container of Rolaids. To her left sat her walker, which doubled as a storage shelf, complete with flashlight, checkbook, and a Lifeline alert necklace draped over the side. And on the floor next to her recliner were a blanket, a pillow, and her purse. This small area symbolized relative self-sufficiency for Florence.

Florence told me, "I'm content to sit here [in the recliner]. My back aches most of the time. And I have everything here that I need. I've got my addresses, my checks, letters to answer. My TV remote. My chair remote. See, my legs are up like they are supposed to."

It was Florence who really taught me about comfortable aging. Because she valued rest and relaxation over busyness, she was content to concentrate her life around her most comfortable place, her reclining chair. There she had her family pictures, her cubbies, and her television. By contracting most of her daily activities into a small space, she had set up a central command center from which she could manage phone calls, deliveries, medical needs, and entertainment, or just zone out.

For three years I shadowed thirty elders like Florence, wanting to know how they approached the project of aging in place, or aging at home in Upstate New York. They were a diverse group geographically, living in suburban, urban, and rural settings, who varied in terms of religion, ethnicity, gender, and socioeconomic backgrounds. When I met them, all thirty lived at home alone or with their life partners. Few had family members living locally, but many had children living several hours away who made intermittent visits. I wanted to know what quality of life looked like for them in old age and what they did to achieve comfort and meaning. I watched, learned, and listened, while accompanying them in their daily routines (Loe 2011).

Visits with Florence and others helped me to recognize that elders, like all of us, are creative problem-solvers, aging and adapting as circumstances shift. I noted that they created comfortable, user-friendly spaces and systems to meet their needs, many times with the help of others.[2] I watched as they learned to scale back; ask for assistance; interview, hire, and fire aides; tour care facilities and weigh the options; or mobilize a wide array of resources for support (many of them free), including family and friends. Ironically, it was by relying on such a newfound safety net of friends, family, and public support that elders were able to retain a sense of autonomy and control, and in most cases to increase their quality of life.

If my research had focused solely on "successful" or "productive aging," or the media-friendly "new old" with active and healthy lifestyles, I would have missed meeting an elder like Florence, who spends much of her daily life in her recliner, relaxing her back, watching classic movies, and taking care of herself and others while in this seated position. Florence is not focused on being a productive member of society. She does not eat a particularly healthful diet, nor does she have an exercise routine. She is not in optimal health, nor does she believe that is possible at her life stage. Instead, she accepts her limitations, rests her aching body, and works toward achieving personal comfort and continuity. She takes each day as it comes. Personal aides cycle in and out. At times she is bored, lonely, and in great pain. Other times she is content to watch movies, take phone calls from family members, and make excursions to the local diner, where she is treated as a VIP. At ninety-five Florence was just being herself. In fact, simply being herself—persistent, prudent, and responsible (and not particularly cheery)—likely contributed to her long life (Friedman and Martin 2011).

In many ways, Florence is not unlike many of the oldest old, a term scholars have used to refer to the segment of the population aged eighty-five and older, the fastest-growing segment of American society. She and others I followed represent how aging is changing. First of all, Florence is a woman, like almost 70 percent of elders in her age group. Second, many of us know nonagenarians like Florence who are mostly able-bodied, relatively healthy, active decision-makers, resilient, and multifaceted. As the so-called active life span (or life stage without significant disability) expands, today's elders are helping craft what it means to live into the eighties, nineties, and beyond. Third, most of the oldest old who survived the Great Depression and two World Wars, a cohort commonly referred to as the Greatest Generation, continue to value the American ideal of rugged individualism but recognize they cannot do it alone. And fourth, while Florence will not make any headlines for her daily feats of survival, she models what it looks like to establish lifelong continuity, to create an enabling living space, to protect autonomy while also asking for help, to seek opportunities for human contact, and to prioritize comfort. These are lessons for living, at any age.

Most important, Florence allows us to identify and expand upon a new paradigm for aging well: comfortable aging. On the face of it, Florence's daily life is devoted to physical ease. Dig deeper and one quickly realizes how physical comfort is deeply tied to financial security, location, health, and relationships, as well as personal acceptance of vulnerability, disability, and mortality.

A New Paradigm: Comfortable Aging

A recent New York Times piece entitled "Giving Alzheimer's Patients Their Way, Even Chocolate," discusses how a dementia care facility in Arizona emphasizes therapy based on comfort. Patients are allowed anything that brings them comfort, from chocolate to perfume to baby dolls. Caregivers, who are encouraged to scour patients' biographies and "find their strengths," offer activities related to the ones patients once enjoyed, from filling photo albums to snapping beans to sitting and chatting. The results of this care experiment are clear: less moody and belligerent, more active and content patients. And with less needy patients, caregivers get breaks and the facility saves money. It turns out that emphasizing comfort and continuity can be a healthy thing for all involved (Belluck 2010).[3]

The vast majority of the oldest old in my research study prioritize aging comfortably, which directly contrasts with the popular "successful" or "productive aging" paradigms. As Margaret Cruikshank points out in Learning to Be Old (2003, 3), the latter can be simplistic and youth focused, while missing the complex multidimensional and structural components of aging. Furthermore, in our highly medicalized world, we tend to lose sight of the social and relational aspects of health. A comfortable aging paradigm can reveal new ways of thinking about well-being and new paths for preventative health. Comfortable aging emphasizes ease and subjective health, as opposed to external signs of success and functionality. Comfortable aging emphasizes learning to "be" in a culture of doing.[4] Most important, comfortable aging is attainable across health status; while we can fail at being "successful" or "productive," personal comfort is subjectively defined and attainable. As such, comfortable aging has financial, social, psychological, physiological, and policy-based dimensions unique to each elder. That said, there are some common threads. This chapter will explore three key threads: accepting the care of others, embracing vulnerability, and coming to terms with mortality.

Four years after the publication of *Aging Our Way* (Loe 2011), I have attempted to contact all of my original study participants to see how and if they are managing to age comfortably. Eight of the thirty are still living, and half are into their hundredth year. These members of the Greatest Generation, many of whom have scrimped and saved their whole lives, are now somewhat financially comfortable. Most own their own homes and rely on social security checks to pay the bills. These eight use their resources to age in their communities, with assistance. One, Mary, has moved to a care facility. As I visited with Johanna, Glenn, Florence, Seymour, Mary, Ruth, and Margaret, once again I asked about comfortable aging. I wanted to know if their strategies for comfort have shifted, and if so, how. So, as I checked in and asked about their lives now, I paid attention to how they discussed comfort. One of the first lessons that came through was how, for them, comfort is tied to social capital, or relationships, and the ability to ask for help.

Comfortable Aging Requires Interdependency

For many, comfortable aging requires giving up on some autonomy and accepting the care of others. Shana is a perfect case of this; for most of her life she was a devoted mother who delighted in entertaining, caring for her extended family, and hosting countless international exchange students. Five years ago, when I rang Shana's doorbell she came to the door apologizing. She was deboning a chicken so her hands were greasy. She could still handle standing in the kitchen and prepping a kosher meal for her family, but she admitted that she had a hard time gardening; she kept falling forward into the plants. Solving this problem involved nieces, who set up a raised garden in the back. They set Shana up in a chair where she could reach to pull weeds. In this way she was able to continue her lifelong love of gardening. In fact, Shana repeatedly said she wanted to die in her garden: her favorite place.

This time Shana's daughter answered the door. She led me into the TV room, where Shana sat in a large padded chair eating a peanut butter and jelly sandwich and sharing bites with her son's dog, Hermes. This was her second breakfast, she said with a smile. She also told me that most of her friends had died and she now had around-the-clock care, with four hours midday to herself. After breakfast, we moved outside to the garden. Shana's daughter helped her out of her recliner, and then Shana used a walker and cane to get outside to her favorite patio chair. From there she was able to view the flower garden and the pool. Her daughter walked around pulling weeds, loudly pointing out the plants they put in last year (one had done well; it had five hot pink flowers) and pulling Swiss chard for dinner. She says her mother taught her well. Shana reminded her about a few plants she had recently purchased to put in that afternoon, including tomatoes. It seemed clear to me then that Shana is still the garden manager, and this is still her favorite place, but she knows her limits. Luckily she has a care team, including paid careworkers, family members, and a dog, who dote on her.

When I asked Shana if she misses cooking and gardening and anything else, she replied no. She relies on a small community of helpers. She calls for her aides in the morning, and they help bathe and dress her. She described how they pick "just the right clothing," like the lightweight pants she was wearing that hot summer day. In the four hours a day when she does not have formal help, she can call her son who runs a business just blocks away. He can always come and help her to the bathroom. Her friend Ethel calls many times a day to check in. Her nephew and daughter cook for her and keep the home kosher. And then she takes care of the things she has always done, like reading the paper, caring for her son's dog while he's at work, caring for her itchy dry skin with her well-placed tubes of Cortisone, and eating a whole lot of raw onions, her secret for living a long healthy life. With all of this help, Shana is able to age in place and stay comfortably in her home.

Aging in place, or not having to move from one's present residence in order to secure necessary support services in response to changing need, sounds like it is about autonomy (Mahmood et al. 2008, 105). In reality, aging at home, for those in their advanced years, may work only in a social context of interdependency, or "socially inclusive independence." In the United States we emphasize individualism and independence, sometimes to our own detriment. At eighty-five and beyond, most of one's peer group is gone, and the potential for isolation, loneliness, and depression is strong. The antidote to loss is new and old connections. In fact, sociological research shows that the loss of a spouse is more likely to immediately intensify social relationships than attenuate them, and social participation rates increase a few years after the death of a spouse (Ferraro 1984). Social connections provide much-needed buffers and supports in the context of changing bodies, as well as personal loss and hardship. They also help us to grow. Many elders know this, and they focus on making new friends, or on keeping existing connections going.

While US-based elders might talk more often about independence, I have observed that many are simultaneously leaning toward interdependence. As I watched elders in their respective environments, I found some reaching out at church, networking with neighbors, caring for grandchildren, doting on pets, and caring for plants. When asked specifically, these elders admit to depending on others, and some are quite strategic about it. For example, Seymour emailed to report that as he crept toward ninety-eight years of age, he was gradually depending more and more on his wife, age eighty-nine, whom he describes as his personal "gofer." Glenn tells me he doesn't know what he would do without his weekly "coffee klatch," a group of retired scientists and state workers who discuss all things over breakfast. And even Florence, who spends most days resting her back, admits that visiting her favorite diner on Fridays is worth the physical discomfort, because seeing familiar faces, experiencing human contact, and feeling respected boosts her mood considerably. In these ways, comfortable aging is relational and interdependent.

Comfortable Aging Is about Accepting Vulnerability and Limitations

As long as I have known Margaret, she has been nervous about her knees giving out on her. Denial didn't work for her, so she eventually learned to rely on a series of walkers (covered by Medicaid) to navigate the small subsidized apartment where she lives alone. She stations one at her bedside to help her get to the bathroom at night and leaves her three-wheel folding model near the front door so she can take it downstairs (via elevator) to play Bingo. Additionally, knowing her physical limits, she positioned a small eating table just steps away from her kitchen, and she stopped washing dishes to avoid standing too long. For her, living alone confidently and comfortably has required accepting and accommodating her vulnerabilities. Her only complaint in life is weak knees. So she carefully choreographs her daily routine and relies on a series of tools in a familiar space to support her.

Knowing Margaret's reputation as a technology savvy elder, or technogenarian, I should not have been surprised, then, to hear about Margaret's latest technological intervention to ensure her comfort at the age of 102. On the phone, she described it as a chair that lifts her, so she avoids the pain of getting up on her own. With the help of her son, this was her latest investment in the continuity of comfortable aging, and she wanted me to come by so she could show it off.

With time, bodies become less resilient and increasingly unreliable. This is not a disease; it is a normal process of aging. Rather than deny age and health concerns, many of the oldest old accept and anticipate some loss of health and control. As Doris Grumbach recounts in her memoir, *Coming into the End Zone* (1991, 3), "We may feel eighteen years old sitting in the park, but eighty when we rise." Similarly, Edwin Shneidman, a thanatologist or scientist who studies death, admits that at ninety he is just "wearing out like an old Oldsmobile: one of my headlamps is broken, my differential isn't differentiating, my muffler has become muffled, my distributor won't distribute—and I can't buy replacement parts at Pep Boys" (2009, xv).

Stiff joints, balance issues, decreased energy, vision problems, and general weakness serve as reminders of aging that the oldest old actively negotiate. In almost a decade of following these elders, I have watched many of them come to fuller acceptance of vulnerability and disability, particularly as their bodies have changed. Margaret has come to accept that weak knees are just another stage of life and learning. Over time, as her acceptance of this weakness has grown and the risk of falling has intensified, she and her family have invested in more and more mobility devices for support. Similarly, Florence accepts her disability, pain, and lack of mobility. When we first met, Florence would sacrifice pain for sociability (by rising to meet visitors or taking trips to the local diner), but now she opts for comfort twenty-four hours a day. "It is what it is, and that's the story," she likes to state, especially now as she is into her hundredth year.

Glenn is one of many who views physical limitation in terms of opportunity. For him, a restricted physical lifestyle has opened up potential for more internal (memory) exploration and reminiscing. For years Glenn has chuckled about the saliva that drips from the corner of his mouth, a small exception in his overall good health. But now he also adopts a serious tone when acknowledging that he is "not entirely comfortable" since his yearlong bout with shingles. He says he has become dependent on pain medication at night, and he begrudgingly accepts favors from friends (e.g., rides, mail delivery, and personal care visits). These examples reveal how difficult accepting change can be. Those complaints aside, Glenn stresses over e-mail, perhaps a bit ironically, "I am happy to be alive and I enjoy my somewhat restricted lifestyle. . . . [I have] reduced energy and mobility, 'ass-bound,' so-called. But I do a great deal of reading and reminiscing. I find myself thinking quite a bit about my first wife and our life together."

In sum, perhaps more than any other life stage, old age can be about vulnerability, honesty, and growing into oneself. Accepting age can be a healthy process, as noted by sociologist and cultural critic Martha Holstein, who emphasizes, "Denial [of aging] is self-defeating and threatening to our integrity" (2013, 315). Thus, as Shana and others reveal, comfortable aging can be about physical and psychological acceptance.

Comfortable Aging Is about Coming to Terms with Mortality

At nine o'clock on a summer night, the lights are all on downstairs in Ruth's home, and the front door is wide open. Ruth seems to be wanting visitors. So I decide to ring the bell. I hear the low hum of a television program. Maybe five minutes later, I hear a slow shuffling from the back of the house. Ruth is coming to welcome me. Next week, Ruth turns 102, so her living room table is filled with flowers. She says even the life insurance company has sent along an arrangement. Ruth and I have had many conversations about death and dying. Ruth is highly organized, and she is constantly preparing herself and her family for her death. Last time I visited, Ruth showed me a letter she had written to her family in the event of her death. She kept it on her shelf for them to find. But since then, someone had moved it to the outside of her refrigerator with her DNR (do not resuscitate) paperwork. Now I see a jar of marbles on the shelf. "That's in case I lose my marbles," Ruth says.

Ruth tells me that she's thinking more about death these days. She reads quotes, and a book called *Let Evening Come* by Mary C. Morrison (1998), before she goes to bed. I get the sense that it calms her to read, think, and prepare, just as she has done as the wife of a professor of philosophy for so many years. She mentions that her late husband Steve has been communicating with her recently. Twenty-five years after his death, he told her, "It is okay," when she was worried. Sometime recently he said, "I'm going to see you soon."

Death is something that Ruth has to think about. It surrounds her. She has outlived almost all of her peers. She tells me of a friend who had "no quality of life"—she had lost the ability to read and to hear. She committed suicide, and Ruth understood that completely. Amid this focus on mortality, I get the sense that Ruth might be treating our visit as our final chance to see one another, truly living each day as if it is the last. Near the end of my visit, Ruth looks at me sideways. "I am memorizing your face," she explains.

Many of the oldest old have learned to accept death. They have watched many of their contemporaries die, and they know their own death is not far off. Like Ruth, Margaret and Glenn are organized and communicative when it comes to death preparations. They have completed living wills and advance directives. Margaret has also created a file with her favorite hymns and psalms. She believes that whenever God is ready, she will go. Glenn jokes about purchasing his own cremation for $800 twenty-five years ago. Then, on a serious note, he says he has instructed his children, "I want no obituary notice over two inches in length, . . . just: He came this date and left that date." So many conversations such as these have helped Glenn come to terms with death. He says, "My fear and unease about death has abated, and I no longer think it is such a terrible event."

With all of this planning and anticipation, however, many still find mystery in death. Unlike Ruth, Glenn, and Margaret, Shana and Seymour rarely discuss their mortality. They are uncomfortable when the subject is raised. When pressed, Seymour says, "I am still afraid of dying and am fully aware that it can happen at any time. I still have the desire to keep on living as long as I still have all of my 'buttons.' When the inevitable ravages of time do finally catch up to me, I would very likely think differently." Shana also seems anxious about dying. Her daughter, in the background as we chat, echoes this, saying, "I certainly don't want to be there when Mom dies." Shana says, "I don't think people leave this world without something happening. I mean, there's an event of some sort. It might be a struggle. I don't know. But I do think about it. I'd like to be at home and by myself when it happens."

For the oldest old, their own sense of mortality and the anticipation of death can animate their lives. Some imagine their own demise, wondering where the death will take place, who will discover them, and how long it might take to discover their body. For example, when Johanna, at age 101, found herself with a nosebleed that would not stop, she called both a friend and 911. She said, "I was certain the end was near." After several days in the hospital, she returned home surprised once again at her body's resilience, and maybe even a little frustrated. This wasn't the first time she was fooled.

Philosopher and psychiatrist Viktor Frankl (2000) has said that death gives value and meaning to life; without it, we would postpone what is most important. It follows that denying death does not allow us to truly live in the present. Those who are most comfortable with death seem to live actively in the here and now, while preparing themselves and others for death. Perhaps if more of us accepted mortality and vulnerability, we could be more comfortable with foregoing extreme end-of-life care. There is no doubt that Americans are rethinking our relationship to death denial and expensive life extension; these are key messages in physician Atul Gawande's bestselling book *Being Mortal* (2014) and medical anthropologist Sharon Kaufman's *Ordinary Medicine* (2015).

Is US Society Ready for Comfortable Aging?

As I write this, the 2015 White House Conference on Aging is streaming live on my computer. The meeting is an all-day affair, with panels focusing on caregiving, elder justice, health, and technology. "Successful aging" is a catchphrase that is repeated regularly by speakers, as well as words like "vitality," "productive," and "active." President Barack Obama asks what it will take to protect quality of life and help older Americans to thrive. One speaker captured my attention when he talked about asking his college students to design a personal longevity plan. He tells students to expect to live to one hundred, and then asks, "How will you map out your life? Your finances? Your health?" This is a question with an agenda; the key is to accept the normalization of longevity and then think through what late life might look like. The elders in my study help us to see what it might look like to live one hundred years or even more. I wonder, will students have enough wisdom to know that quality of life and personal comfort are directly related to so many factors, including finances, physical health, psychological health, and perhaps most important, relationships and the ability to accept change?

As I reflect on what I have learned from elders, it is clear that while attitudes and relationships are crucial, they don't tell the whole story. Openness to change and availability of social capital must be complemented by structural factors for comfortable aging to be achievable in society. Thus, Florence's comfort can be achievable with a sense of adaptability and acceptance, *and* the right chair technology, presence of loved ones, financial resources, and other forms of assistance in old age. For all of us, comfort is ultimately linked to these more structural realities.

Countless social barriers impede elders' chances of aging comfortably. While Glenn may be facing obstacles linked to physical health, he has resources to help him through these challenges. As a veteran, he has access to generous health benefits. He is fortunate to have five children who care deeply about him and who check in by phone every night, as well as younger friends to visit with. Glenn is also financially comfortable; he owns his own home and years of investment in personal care insurance is now coming in handy in paying for a daytime personal assistant. Margaret's situation is slightly different. While she may be more fortunate than Glenn in terms of her healthy or "pain free" existence, she is one of many women elders in the United States who has less of a financial cushion; she relies on free or affordable mobility technologies, a government-subsidized apartment, and gifts from her family members (like her new chair) to help her achieve personal comfort. That said, Margaret is fortunate to have access to affordable housing in a country where access to such opportunities is quite limited.

Over the years I have seen all of the elders in my study confront obstacles, whether it be ageism, lack of in-home care, or overcare at the end of life. Importantly, most structural issues linked to comfortable aging are not age specific—social respect, affordable housing, community-oriented neighborhoods, access to transportation, dependable services, and care that honors all stages in the lifecycle—these are universal needs. Thus, it has become clear to me that a society that enables comfortable aging is one that benefits us all.

Conclusion: "It Is What It Is"

Two months before her hundredth birthday, I called Florence. On the phone, Florence's aide Linda warned me that Florence has been bedbound and uncomfortable sitting. She was concerned. "I'm worried that there isn't much to live for now. She doesn't even watch movies." She wants me to visit next week. "Maybe then we'll have the special cushion so she can sit in her recliner pain free."

When I visit a few days later, Florence is sitting in her recliner. The cushion had arrived. I greet Florence and ask how she is doing. She says, "At my age, I'm pretty good. What's the point of complaining? It is nice to see you." Linda jumps in to say that they tried four different kinds of cushions, and finally found one that works, sent by her daughter in Israel. That magic cushion has returned Florence to her chosen lifestyle—to quality of life. She is back in her command center and feeling good. She is surrounded by many of the same things as last time I visited. In plastic cubbies I can see her mail, pictures of grandchildren, a container of Tums, a telephone, a box of raisins, and some new stuffed animals and chocolates, things that were put there by someone else, she thinks. Over the course of our conversation she repeated that she was in a good place. "I like it here. I like it here in this house. And if I had a choice, I'd choose here instead of Israel [with my daughter]. That's the story, my dear."

There, in her recliner, she faces the same shelf with framed pictures of her family, the electric candle she lights on May 20th, her late husband's birthday, and a tapestry of Jerusalem. When I ask if she likes being alone, she says, "No, but I have the television to keep me company." These days Florence's Lifeline call button is worn as a bracelet, not slung loosely over her walker. Florence also has had twenty-four-hour aides ever since she took a fall and her grandson found her on the floor. "They don't want me to be alone." She shrugs her shoulders as if to say, "Whatever they want." When she mentions her late husband, I ask her about death and dying.

ML: Do you think about dying?

FLORENCE: Nothin' to think about; I'll be dead. If I die, I die. . . . It is what it is. There is nothing we can do.

ML: Do you believe you will see your husband someday?

FLORENCE: I don't think so. But I will be next to him. They'll probably put me next to my husband.

These days Florence doesn't make most of the decisions, nor does she want to. Her birthday party is being planned by her daughters, and she mostly nods and supports their efforts. Her daughters brought several outfits home for her to try on, and she chose one in her favorite color, purple. Her family members coordinate her care, and she has accommodated their twenty-four-hour care demands. She has befriended her aides and seems to appreciate their company. At one hundred, her doctor has agreed to make house calls. Her beloved diner is closing, so Friday trips no longer take place. The command center surrounding her recliner is less her doing, and perhaps most objects in her life placed there are less meaningful. She's willing to go along with all of this, as long as she is comfortable. In her recliner, with her special cushion, things are very matter-of-fact. "I'll be here until I die. What else can I do?" This sentiment, shared by Florence in a reclined position, sums up comfortable aging for her. Florence accepts her disability and mortality and has found a physical place and chair where she can be comfortable passing her days, and just be.

Listening to the oldest old helps reveal new ways of thinking about well-being and new paths for preventive health. These elders emphasize ease and subjective health, as opposed to external signs of success and functionality. As such, I see elders like Florence as proponents of a new paradigm for well-being across the life course, comfortable aging. While we can fail at being "successful" or "productive," personal comfort is subjectively defined and attainable. However, comfortable aging is not as simple as installing recliners in all elders' dwelling

places. On a macrolevel, it requires paying attention to and enabling resources, location, health, and relationships. On a microlevel, comfortable aging requires personal
acceptance of vulnerability, disability, and mortality. For those of us caring for elders,
comfortable aging requires listening to elders and their desires. One does not have to
be one hundred years old to start to focus on comfort. We are all aging now.

NOTES

1. Portions of this chapter have been adapted from Loe 2011.
2. All of the elders in this study designed a physical place to age comfortably. Such adap-
   tation fits with German developmental psychologist Paul B. Baltes's (1990) theory of
   selection, optimization, and compensation, which emphasizes how elders alter and
   adapt their environment to fit their current needs.
3. For research on staff satisfaction in a care facility, see also, e.g., Loe and Moore 2011.
4. See also Corwin (this volume) for an exploration of how nuns in a US convent also
   emphasize "being" rather than "doing" as they approach older age.

REFERENCES

Baltes, Paul B and Margret M. Baltes. 1990. "Psychological Perspectives on Successful Aging:
    The Model of Selective Optimization with Compensation." In *Successful Aging: Per-
    spectives from the Behavioral Sciences*, edited by Paul B. Baltes and Margret M. Baltes,
    pp. 1–34. New York: Cambridge University Press.
Belluck, Pam. 2010. "Giving Alzheimer's Patients Their Way, Even Chocolate." *New York
    Times.* December 31.
Cruikshank, Margaret. 2003. *Learning to Be Old: Gender, Culture, and Aging.* Lanham, MD:
    Rowman and Littlefield.
Ferraro, Kenneth. 1984. "Widowhood and Social Participation in Later Life." *Research on
    Aging* 6 (4): 451–468.
Frankl, Viktor E. 2006. *Man's Search for Meaning.* Boston: Beacon Press.
Friedman, Howard, and Leslie R. Martin. 2011. *The Longevity Project: Surprising Discoveries for
    Health and Long Life from the Landmark Eight-Decade Study.* New York: Hudson Street Press.
Gawande, Atul. 2014. *Being Mortal.* New York: Metropolitan.
Grumbach, Doris. 1991. *Coming into the End Zone: A Memoir.* New York: W. W. Norton.
Holstein, Martha. 2013. "On Being an Aging Woman." In *Age Matters: Realigning Feminist
    Thinking*, edited by Toni Calasanti and Kathleen Slevin, 313–333. New York: Routledge.
Kaufman, Sharon R. 2015. *Ordinary Medicine: Extraordinary Treatments, Longer Lives, and
    Where to Draw the Line.* Durham, NC: Duke University Press.
Loe, Meika. 2011. *Aging Our Way: Lessons for Living from 85 and Beyond.* New York: Oxford
    University Press.
Loe, Meika, and Crystal Dea Moore. 2011. "From Nursing Home to Green House: Changing Con-
    texts and Outcomes of Elder Care in the U.S." *Journal of Applied Gerontology* 31 (6): 755–765.
Mahmood, Atiya, Toshiko Yamamoto, Megan Lee, and Carmen Steggell. 2008. "Perceptions
    and Use of Gerotechnology: Implications for Aging in Place." *Journal of Housing for the
    Elderly* 22 (1): 104–126.
Morrison, Mary C. 1998. *Let Evening Come: Reflections on Aging.* New York: Doubleday.
Shneidman, Edwin S. 2009. *A Commonsense Book of Death: Reflections at Ninety of a Lifelong
    Thanatologist.* Lanham, MD: Rowman and Littlefield.

15

Ageless Aging or Meaningful Decline?

Aspirations of Aging and Dying in
the United States and India

SARAH LAMB

On a recent fieldwork excursion to West Bengal, India, a region I have studied as a cultural anthropologist for the past twenty-five years, I was struck by how elders so readily spoke of their readiness for death. Virtually every older person I encountered talked about being ready to die, or remarked that they were going to die soon, or queried, "Who knows if I will still be here the next time you come back?" I had noticed this way of speaking for years, but this time it caught my attention more keenly, as it seemed a striking contrast to what I was hearing in my concurrent research with elders in the United States, where death rarely came up unless I specifically asked about it.

Bengali elders' ready-for-death remarks tend to be uttered in a lighthearted, matter-of-fact way. That is, such remarks are not limited to those who are ill or depressed but are voiced regularly by those in excellent physical and mental health. These remarks seem to express a commonly held cultural perspective that human life is transient, that no body can last forever, that it is best to die while one's "hands and feet are still working," and that it is inappropriate in one's later years to cling unduly to life.

Purnima Banerjee was one who spoke often of her readiness for dying. A retired English professor in her early seventies, she had never married and lived now alone in her natal home instead of in a multigenerational household with children, the more common arrangement for elders in India. Purnima-di¹ had been very attached to her parents and brother, as well as engrossed in her career and students, and she gave these as her reasons for not marrying. Her brother had passed away as a younger adult, and then her parents died, leaving Purnima-di living alone for the past twenty years. Although she often told of feeling lonely, she had an active social network of friends and neighbors who dropped in frequently for tea and conversation. She also volunteered in an Alzheimer's day care center and as a visitor to homebound elders, did all her own shopping and cooking, enjoyed listening to the radio, and was one of my own best interlocutors and fieldwork companions over many years. She had begun in her late sixties to speak of some aches and pains, mentioning that she is not as strong as she used to be, but she remained in general good physical and mental health.

In her cheerful and reflective style, Purnima-di spoke of death and dying almost every time I saw her. She voiced: "I am not afraid of death, because it is inevitable. Because I am born, I know I have to die. No one born can escape death," and "A machine also has retirement. When clothes are worn out, you just take them off and wear new ones. The body is also like that," and "We have to accept decay. I have accepted." Once after she mentioned that she would likely die soon, I commented, in perhaps an American style, that she looked great and healthy to me and might live a good ten years more. Purnima-di exclaimed, "No, don't say that! I don't want to keep living. I am ready to die."

Sometimes Purnima-di emphasized wishing to die while her hands and feet are still working, a common refrain among Indian elders. Although it is normal for older Indians to depend on their junior kin in later life, as part of a valued system of lifelong intergenerational reciprocity (Lamb 2000, 42–69), many older people nonetheless express a wish not to be completely bedridden or full burdens on their families (Vatuk 1990). Purnima-di remarked: "I say to God, whenever you are ready, take me; just please don't have me be bedridden." When I was departing for the United States, she said nostalgically, "When you come back again next time—I am thinking that this is the last time I will see you." She paused to look at me lovingly. "Because I want to die while my hands and feet are still working and I can walk and move around. If it is God's grace, he will take me while my hands and feet are still moving. I can still walk now—that's a great thing!"

Purnima-di also underscored her vision of eternal life, articulating a widely held Hindu view common even among more secular Indians and those of other faiths,[2] that the soul or self moves on to some form of ongoing life after the body has died, such as by reincarnating or joining God. Purnima-di said, "The body will die, but the soul will not die. Wherever I go, I will go *somewhere* else. Those dear ones who have died, why should I cry for them? There is no use crying for a departed soul. God is a giver and a taker. Today is mine; tomorrow I will go and the day will be someone else's. I should not be sorry for that."

Over my years of fieldwork in West Bengal, Purnima-di and others have offered such ready-to-die remarks, while also speaking of interdependence and dependence as normal and valued parts of life and the impermanence of the person as a fundamental part of being human.[3] The attitudes expressed by

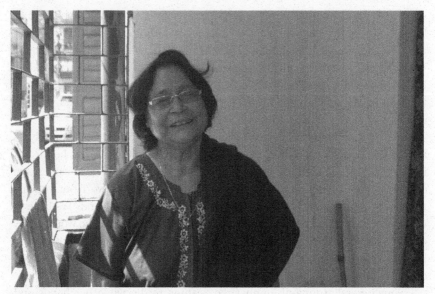

FIGURE 15.1 Purnima-di: "I am not afraid of death, because it is inevitable." (Photo by Sarah Lamb)

Bengali elders have made me wonder about our own North American emphasis on permanent personhood, agelessness, and independence explored in this volume's introduction. Consider, for example, the remarks of physician Henry Lodge, coauthor of *Younger Next Year: Live Strong, Fit, and Sexy—Until You're 80 and Beyond*, quoted in the introduction. He describes the ailments and deteriorations of normal aging (the implied opposite of successful aging) as an "outrage," "intolerable and avoidable" (Crowley and Lodge 2007, 29). Bengali perspectives spur me to ask, however, if it is not possible to view normal aging as something other than "intolerable," "avoidable," and an "outrage." Can we not accept signs of aging—even if they include declines, vulnerabilities, and ephemerality—as in some ways a meaningful part of life? Shouldn't it be possible to regard old age and death not as intolerable outrages, nor as failures of medicine and self, but rather as inevitable facets of life, defining in part what it is to be human?

Many older Americans are seeking answers to such questions as well. Although the successful aging discourse—with its emphasis on independence, agelessness, and permanence of the person—does inspire many Americans in ways that feel positive to them (as I examine further below), others are seeking alternative visions. This chapter explores how elders in India and the United States varyingly contend with the transience of the human condition that the successful aging discourse strives to deny. I use the voices and experiences of elders to help me argue that we need to incorporate meaningful images of aging and oldness, transience and decline, into our views of life, rather than simply pursuing a dream of prolonged middle age grounded in an aversion to aging, oldness, and decline.[4]

My fieldwork materials come from twenty-five years of research in West Bengal in both urban Kolkata and rural villages, primarily with Hindus of a range of social classes and castes. I also draw on two years of more recent research with Boston-area elders. In Boston my research subjects have been largely white, well educated, and middle or upper-middle class; Jewish, Christian, and agnostic or atheistic; and experiencing a range of health conditions (from very fit to near dying) and living situations (from independent homes, to co-residence with children and grandchildren, to retirement communities and assisted living facilities).[5] In both nations, the ages of my older interlocutors have spanned from about sixty (or, in India, some begin to define themselves as old in their fifties) through to one hundred.

"I Am Successfully Aging!" Embracing Active, Healthy, Ageless Aging in Everyday Life

I had expected when beginning fieldwork in the United States, after years of researching aging in India, to find people critical of the successful aging paradigm, as I had been. Yet I was quickly struck by how many seemed to delight in the idea of successful aging; and why not? The elders I was growing to know were members of the same cultural milieu that produced the successful aging paradigm, so it might make good sense for them to embrace its ideals. Further, for those with the physical, mental, social, and economic resources to succeed in aging well according to the paradigm's criteria, then certainly all the positive imagery of successful aging can be very inspiring.

Often my interlocutors ask me to tell them a little about my own research interests before or after we conduct a formal interview. If I get to describing the successful aging movement, with its emphasis on being physically, mentally, and socially active and independent, my interlocutors not uncommonly interrupt to chime in with "I am successfully aging, then! I do all that!"

Ellen and Max smiled at each other when I asked them what successful aging means to them. "Our lives! Aren't we the poster boy and girl for successful aging?" The two had known each other in childhood and reconnected in their sixties and seventies after both had become widowed, marrying several years later and very much in love. Eighty-three-year-old Max went on: "We're both relatively healthy, which I think is really prime. We both have our minds still—which is also prime. We are economically comfortable, so we can do pretty much what we want. We are both active in various ways. We're quite happy! One reason is that we really enjoy each other. We have a light touch. Some of our friends are, oh, so serious. 'Oh, life is hard'—which of course it is! But it's better to have fun!"

One-hundred-year-old Alice Rosenthal attributes her long life and good health partly to fortune—she feels very lucky not to be poor—but also to her own individual efforts, including eating well, exercising physically (such as walking rather than taking a wheelchair), and most importantly engaging in daily mental exercise, including reading books and the *New York Times*, and taking classes where she will "learn new things—learn a lot."

Marie Lawrence voiced the value of productive activity in later life, after describing all her activities postretirement—exercise, a second part-time job, and volunteering as a fundraiser and secretary for a nonprofit organization: "I want to be busy, busy, busy. I absolutely want to be. I have to get up and go. . . . I'm happier when I'm really busy." She articulated her vision of successful aging: "Being able to do everything I can do now."

For many of my interlocutors, these practices of active, successful aging are pursued as a self-conscious, self-disciplining project. Betty Rowe acknowledged that "it takes a lot of energy" to be upbeat all the time, to exercise every day, to stay active, and to not let on to one's family that one feels needy at times. Edna Feldman commented: "I do think you have only yourself to blame if you don't use whatever body you have left, to upkeep it." Marjorie Newman, at age seventy-six, declared, "I had two knee replacements and I'll do anything I have to, to just be very active. . . . I have aches and pains and I try not to focus on it. But if it stops me from doing what I want to do, then I am going to do something about it! I'll have the parts replaced one by one until I have a whole new bionic body!"

Ideals of agelessness and longevity are common themes in my interview materials. After learning that I was a professor studying aging, Barbara Winters approached me at a gathering at her retirement home, dressed in a lively, black-and-turquoise satin dress with a matching bright turquoise necklace and a nicely coiffed halo of white hair. She professed to be in her nineties, expecting to turn ninety-three in June. She asked eagerly, leaning in toward me, "Tell me! Tell me! Do you know?—Have they discovered the mystery of life?" I stalled. "Umm, I'm not sure—uh, what do you mean?" "Oh, I mean, have they figured out how to live forever? I would like to live forever! I am looking for the mystery of life!" I told her that, indeed, people are working on this very issue.[6] She was excited: "Tell me—what have you learned?" I had to acknowledge that I found this to be an impossible quest. Impatiently she agreed, "Yes, yes, the earth wouldn't be large enough and all that—but still, I would *like* to live forever! . . . I don't want to miss anything! I've already lived longer than I ever expected to, of course, but still I would like a lot more!"

The majority of US elders in my study have not brought up death and dying unless I raise the topic myself. If I do raise the topic, it is often quickly dismissed—as in one man's response: "I'll cross that bridge when I come to it," or another's: "No, I don't think about it"—or answered only in terms of the practical details of having one's wills and trusts in order (a sign of the comfortable class status of this group).

If, curious about the contrast between Indian and US views, I raise the possibility of moving in with children, most have dismissed the idea out of hand, some saying while laughing, "No way!" or exclaiming, "I would hope not!" Common themes are that they do not want to be "burdens" on their children and that they value their independence. The few in my study who do live in multigenerational households with children and grandchildren make sure to specify that they, the elders, are helping their juniors at least as much as the juniors help them, such as by having been the ones to pay the down payment for the duplex home or by providing childcare for the youngest generation. That is, they make an effort to present themselves not as elder dependents but as active, productive, agentive participants in a mutually beneficial situation.

Listening to the voices of Boston-area, middle-class elders, I have thus found that many eagerly pursue the ideals prevailing in our wider US society—of successful aging as an individual project entailing independence, busy activity, and agelessness as valued aspirations.

"People Don't Die in Our Society" and Other Critiques

Yet fieldwork with intelligent, thoughtful elders in the United States has also highlighted to me the need to critique the successful aging paradigm for insufficiently grappling with the normal human conditions of decline, dependency, change, and mortality. Some of my US research subjects, who have expressed their disgruntlement with our wider US society that denies the realities of death, dying, and decline, are eager to hear from me about alternative Indian perspectives.

I was chatting with Max and Ellen Stemmer, the couple introduced above who had remarried after each becoming widowed, and Max commented: "Our society shuns death, pretends it doesn't happen. . . . The Baby Boomers haven't quite accepted that they're mortal. Yet isn't the whole process of living a gradual acceptance of: Hey, I'm really going to die?" I mentioned that I welcomed his speaking about death and dying, because it's a subject people don't seem to acknowledge or talk much about in our society. "Certainly they don't!" Max replied. "People don't die in our society; they pass away." We all laughed. Ellen rejoined, "No, now they just pass." Max concluded with a broad smile, "Or, one could say they failed."

Max and Ellen had both had close encounters with death, making death an undeniable reality, in that each had lost a first spouse to death, and each had also lost a parent at the age of fourteen. About their parents' passing, Max described: "None of our families talked about it at all. Ellen found out that her mother was going to die just the day before, and I never knew my father was going to die until he was already dead."

Shirley, a cancer survivor in her sixties, commented: "I hate the way that death is viewed in this culture; it's just viewed as something that's bad." She offered a saying she admires, attributed to Justice Louis D. Brandeis and that had helped her during her cancer ordeal: "If you would only recognize that life is hard, things would be so much easier for you."

Emilie Seiler declared in a similar vein that she wished her mother hadn't made it all look so easy. Emilie described herself as someone who had once been "delighted" by aging but who was now "terrified" by the same prospect. She felt completely unprepared for how difficult aging had become after she and her husband both became increasingly frail after they had passed age eighty-five, and she eventually lost her beloved husband and lifelong companion to death. Our rosy vision of successful aging, Emilie remarked, is utterly contingent on certain things beyond individual control, such as good health.

Eighty-year-old Dorothy commented regarding the successful-aging public discourse surrounding her, "It's a lot of pressure." Always a highly active person who loved dancing, walking, socializing, spending time with her grandchildren, and working (she had taken up a second job as a boutique sales clerk after retiring), Dorothy had recently had to give up almost all such activities due to severe back spasms impairing her mobility. She hoped this problem would resolve itself, but in the meantime felt not only frustrated to miss out on activities she loves but also bewildered and embarrassed by her incapacities.

In a lifelong learning program, I once showed the class the cover of a *New York Times* Sunday magazine from January 30, 2000, featuring two older people riding scooters as they cheerfully wave, with the headline: "Racing toward Immortality (Or at Least Your 150th Birthday)." I commented that such images imply that successful aging is to maintain as much as possible one's active, independent adulthood. One woman, who had come to class in a wheelchair, retorted: "That almost makes become disabled a crime! I mean, this is designed to make people who can no longer do those things feel bad." Another: "It's a fantasy." I was curious: "A fantasy. Is it, you know, a sort of pleasurable fantasy to pursue, or is it scary because you know you can't achieve it?" The reply, "It makes you feel like something's wrong with you."

Frances Brooks was one who accepted the fact of her own coming mortality but began to weep when imagining the possibility of becoming very dependent on her children before dying. She had been diagnosed with terminal cancer shortly after her eighty-fifth birthday, and she spoke with peace and conviction about not wanting any "heroic attempts" to extend her life. She told of the bright pink DNR (do not resuscitate) paper taped onto her refrigerator, commenting, "Don't do a darned thing but let me go." She believes that she has lived a long and wonderful life and feels certain that she will rejoin her long-deceased husband, elder sisters, and parents after dying—convictions that, she agrees, certainly make thinking about one's own dying easier. "The last great experience or adventure you can have is to die," Frances reflected. Her real concern is that "I don't want to drag it out too long and become totally incapacitated. . . . It's not the suffering—I can stand anything I have to stand. It's that someone will have to do for me the things I did for [my sister when she was dying]. I can't stand the thought that they—." She broke off, weeping. "I just hope it doesn't happen."

I myself also wanted to be able to see dying and vulnerability as OK and normal, rather than embarrassing or tragic conditions, when dealing with my own sudden ovarian cancer diagnosis at age fifty-one, after my oncology surgeon announced that I had only eighteen to twenty-four months to live. I was hungry for more positive, realistic, yet meaningful models of dying and vulnerability in our society.[7] If every human being must die, then is it best to regard dying as a tragedy or failure or embarrassment? I am now enjoying glorious good health and pleased that I get to live longer. But whenever my time comes, I prefer not to think of my own dying as a tragedy. And if I am fortunate to live long enough to experience frailty in old age—perhaps walking slowly from my front steps to pick up the morning paper, bending down only with difficulty, or needing to accept some bodily care—then I prefer not to think of those bodily signs of ripe old age as a tragedy or failure either.

John Robbins, author of one of the few popular successful aging books drawing on cross-cultural data to offer alternative perspectives to those prevailing in the United States, reflects toward the end: "In the modern West, on the other hand, we are conditioned not only to deny death but to view it as a failure" (2007, 303). He continues: "If we think of dying people as a separate group, we can imagine that we are not dying. We can pretend that it isn't happening to us" (204). The same could be said for aging. Robbins goes on: "But every day that passes brings us steadily closer to our death. It is happening to each of us, and it is happening to everyone we know and everyone we love" (304–305). This knowledge already exists in our society, but we don't generally recognize it without experiencing a serious illness or debility.

Meaningful Decline? Returning to Perspectives from India

Models of aging well in India can look quite different from those in the United States. Accepting death and dying and the ephemerality of the human condition are ideals commonly held up as appropriate to older age. Just as rice plants grow, drop their seeds, and then wither away, so does the human body. One Kolkata businessman in his fifties quoted from the Ashtavakra Gita when learning of my research interests: "The body comes, it lingers awhile, it goes. But the Self neither comes nor goes. So why grieve for the body?"[8] Interdependence within an intimate family setting and seva—respectful care for and service to elders—are also central to prevailing visions of aging well in India.

The classic Hindu vision of the four stages of life (asramas) foregrounds the meaningfulness of old age. In this religious-cultural paradigm, persons move through a series of four life stages—as a student, a married householder, a disengaged forest dweller, and finally a wandering ascetic renouncer. In this schema, fully half of the life course—two of four stages—constitutes older age. When a man sees the sons of his sons and white hair on his head, he knows it is time to enter the forest-dweller phase—departing from his home to live as a hermit, either with or without his wife, or remaining in the household but with a mind focused on God.[9] The final life stage as a wandering ascetic is conceptualized as a time of complete renunciation of the phenomenal world and its pleasures and ties. Few Hindus actually move to the forest or become wandering ascetics, but many do speak of late life as an appropriate and valuable time for focusing increasingly on spiritual awareness even while living at home, as part of preparing for the transitions of dying and grappling with the reality of human transience (Lamb 2009, 39–40, 161–169).

National aging policies also reflect local cultural ideals, here emphasizing the family as the most appropriate site of elder care. The government of India enacted in 2009 the Maintenance and Welfare of Parents and Senior Citizens law stipulating that families—specifically adult children or those in a position to inherit—are not only morally but also now legally obligated to provide care for their elders. Under "Need for the Legislation," the lawmakers declare straightforwardly: "It is an established fact that family is the most desired environment for senior citizens/parents to lead a life of security, care and dignity."[10] The National Old Age Pension Scheme, similarly resting on a vision of appropriate dependence within families, limits pensions to elders who can document that they have no support from family members (Lamb 2013).

In everyday talk, elders and juniors often state that it is precisely what parents once gave to their young children—including co-residence, food, material support, love, time together, assistance with daily routines, and toileting—that adult children will later reciprocate to their parents.[11] One group of older ladies in the village of Mangaldihi commented together: "When we grow old, we live right with our sons and daughters-in-law!" "Yes! We receive care from them, love from them. If we are sick or weak, they tend to us, just like we tended to them." Narayan Sarkar, a retired Kolkata engineer, narrated: "In our families, we raised our children—why? Our idea, our dream, was that when we grew old, our sons and daughters-in-law would serve us [seva karbe]. And it is our dream, and a natural thing, to hope for this, to want this. We did this for our parents, and they for theirs." One morning I came across a middle-aged man washing his bedridden mother's bedsheets in a village pond. He reflected to me: "As parents raised their children, children will also care for their parents during their sick years, when they get old. For example, if I am old and I have bowel movement, my son will clean it and he won't ask, 'Why did you do it there?' This is what we did for him when he was young. When I am old and dying, who will take me to go urinate and defecate? My children will have to do it."

In fact, too much independence is commonly regarded as the worst thing that can befall one in old age, rather than the ideal celebrated in US successful-aging discourse. The phenomenon of elders living alone is depicted by the Indian media as a serious problem of modern society, with headlines such as "Alone and Insecure in the Winter of Life," "Loneliness, the Other Name for Old Age," "Ageing Parents Home Alone," and "Death from Loneliness at Eighty" (Lamb 2009, 176; see also Cohen 1998). A retired widowed math professor who lives alone in Kolkata, her two professional daughters having settled abroad, commented: "Human beings have always lived together. It is not part of human nature to live alone." Rather than living alone, in fact, some in urban India are choosing residence in the old-age homes or elder ashrams springing up around the nation as a result of globalization (Lamb 2009). If for a variety of complex reasons one has no children with whom one can live, opting for a communal institutional setting where respectful care is offered—even if by hired staff rather than kin—can feel much more familiar and welcome than living independently.

However, despite widespread acceptance of forms of dependence in later life, it would be too simple to suggest that Indian elders unequivocally embrace bodily and other declines. Recall Purnima-di's hope to die while her "hands and feet are still working." Most do not wish to lose all sense of independent functioning before dying. In fact, this can be one of the main reasons many do not wish to cling excessively to life. Further, despite widespread ready-to-die talk, elders also reflect on the difficulty of facing dying. Choto Ma of Mangaldihi village, an aged widow living with her sons, daughters-in-law, and grandchildren, commented to me often of her readiness to die, as on one occasion: "I don't still have any wish to live. But what will I do? I am being compelled to live. When God takes me, then I will go." After a short pause, though, she went on, "But there is always a fear of death. Let a snake come. If a snake comes, will I be able to say, 'Bite me'? No, I won't. If a snake comes, will I be able to pick it up and stand with it right by my head? No, I'll run away. That's what life is like. I'll say, 'No, no. I won't die! There's a snake, I'm going to run away!' That would happen, wouldn't it?" Retired professor Vijay Bhatia reflected to me by email from New Delhi, after sending me an essay he had written on the Hindu philosophy of *iccha mrtyu*, or self-willed death: "I feel that people are attached to physical objects, to their memories, to their children and loved ones. This feeling of attachment has been well discussed in Indian philosophy. . . . In this sense we are also attached to our physical being–self and fear that this will end with death. I feel that we are deeply attached to our life."[12]

Further, some in India compellingly point out that one reason people forgo life-extending medical treatments in their nation has less to do with a distinct cultural philosophy than with the lack of economic and technological resources in India, compared to the United States, where "most of us want [and expect] the miracles of medicine to extend our lives" (Kaufman 2015, 2). Even so, some older Indian immigrants to the United States, although impressed by the grandness of US medical technology, are at the same time reluctant to prolong their own dying hooked up to machines (Lamb 2009, 228).

Accepting frailty and death is not simple, easy, or unambivalent. Nonetheless, one can find within India a widespread acknowledgment of human vulnerabilities and transience helping many elders accept changes to their bodies and selves as they age.

Concluding Remarks

Around a year after I had taken the photograph of Purnima-di appearing in this chapter's opening pages, I returned again to Kolkata. On the bright February morning after my arrival in the city late the night before, I walked through the familiar busy lanes between my residence and Purnima-di's. Her home looked eerily locked and shuttered, and an unopened old bill lay faded on the front verandah. I wasn't sure why I hadn't phoned first. On the way over, I had imagined Purnima-di asking me teasingly, "Is it because you thought I might be dead?" Seeing me ringing the bell and shaking the padlock, a neighbor came over to tell me that Purnima-di had passed away. She had ended up dying suddenly from ovarian cancer just a few months before. Her friends reported that she had been comforted by the fact that I had had the same disease as she. She tried to reach me by phone in America after her diagnosis, they relayed, but she had misplaced my phone number or could not get through. She died swiftly after being admitted to the hospital just a few days before her passing, and she was surrounded at the time of death by friends who had gathered to sing Tagore songs.[13] As she had wished, Purnima-di's "hands and feet were still working" until the end.

I cried when I heard the news. Yet I cannot help but be heartened by the fact that Purnima-di had said again and again that she was ready to die and had offered as a premonitory consolation: "Those dear ones who have died, why should I cry for them? There is no use crying for a departed soul. God is a giver and a taker. Today is mine; tomorrow I will go and the day will be someone else's. I should not be sorry for that."

One tactic in fighting ageism and Western society's conventionally negative views of aging and old age has been—through the contemporary successful aging movement—to argue that old people do not decline, and are not subject to disease, frailty, dependence, and dying—because they can be ageless in their so-called successful aging.[14] This seems to me a limited goal. Another tactic could be to challenge broader assumptions about personhood and value in North American society—striving to envision that the normal human experiences of frailty, dependence, and mortality can, in fact, be OK. Our personhoods need not necessarily be permanent or ageless to be meaningful and valued.

People in North America with their own intimate experiences with illness and mortality are surely already living with such knowledge, but this knowledge is not reflected in our prevailing cultural models. Those in North America might do well to take up some insights from South Asian traditions and contemporary dialogue, learning to temper our overemphasis on positivity and individual autonomy and coming to better terms with the normal human conditions of decline, interdependence, and death—so that not all situations of dependence, debility, and even mortality in late life will be viewed and experienced as failures in living well. Such an acceptance of the natural limits of the human condition need not be incompatible with living a vibrant late life.

ACKNOWLEDGMENTS

Some of the ideas and fieldwork examples in this chapter were first published in Lamb 2014. I thank my interlocutors from the United States and India for sharing their insights and experiences. I am also grateful to the Theodore and Jane Norman Fund for Faculty Research at Brandeis University, which made possible some of my research in India.

NOTES

1. Bengalis commonly use "di," short for "older sister," and "da," short for "older brother" (or other terms for "uncle," "aunt," "elder-sister-in-law," etc.), as signs of respect as well as closeness when addressing those senior to one.
2. Hindus make up about 80 percent of India's population (and Purnima-di herself is Hindu), while the secular state of India is also home to Muslims (about 13 percent), Christians, Sikhs, Buddhists, Jains, and others (http://censusindia.gov.in/Census_And _You/religion.aspx, accessed 30 June 2015).
3. I explore these attitudes further below and also in Lamb 1997 and 2000.
4. Other recent works offering related arguments include Cruikshank 2009, Lamb 2014, and Rudman 2015.
5. In the United States I have conducted formal interviews with thirty-four individuals and participant observation research in a neighborhood aging-in-place organization, a lifelong learning institute, and a retirement community.
6. I was thinking of the surge of anti-aging science and organizations such as the American Academy of Anti-Aging Medicine (http://www.a4m.com/) (Fishman, Binstock, and Lambrix 2008).
7. I had in fact been interested in critiquing the successful aging paradigm long before the cancer diagnosis, but the experience, I felt, added new insight to the project.
8. The Ashtavakra Gita, or Song of Ashtavakra, is a classical Hindu Vedanta text.
9. The classic Hindu ethical-legal texts, the Dharmasastras, devote little explicit attention to defining the stages or asramas of a woman's life, which are determined by her relationships to the men upon whom she depends: her father in youth, her husband in marriage, and her sons in old age (Manu 1991, v.146–151).

10. The text of the 2007 bill preceding the 2009 law is available at http://www.prsindia.org/uploads/media/1182337322/scr1193026940_Senior_Citizen.pdf, accessed 8 June 2016.

11. Although Bengalis often speak of "children" providing care, conventionally it is sons and daughters-in-law who care for elders, while married daughters take on obligations to their husbands' parents.

12. Bengalis speak of a paradox in the human condition: One's emotional and bodily attachments (called *maya*) naturally grow stronger and more numerous as life progresses, but at the same time it is in old age when one must cut the ties of maya to prepare for the myriad leave-takings of death (Lamb 1997).

13. Rabindranath Tagore's songs, also known popularly in Bengali as *Rabindra Sangeet*, are beloved to many Bengalis.

14. For more on these ideals, see the introduction to this volume.

REFERENCES

Cohen, Lawrence. 1998. *No Aging in India: Alzheimer's, the Bad Family, and Other Modern Things*. Berkeley: University of California Press.

Crowley, Chris, and Henry S. Lodge. 2007. *Younger Next Year: Live Strong, Fit and Sexy until You're 80 and Beyond*. New York: Workman.

Cruikshank, Margaret. 2009. *Learning to Be Old: Gender, Culture, and Aging*, 2nd ed. Lanham, MD: Rowman and Littlefield.

Fishman, Jennifer R., Robert H. Binstock, and Marcie A. Lambrix. 2008. "Anti-Aging Science: The Emergence, Maintenance, and Enhancement of a Discipline." *Journal of Aging Studies* 22: 295–303.

Kaufman, Sharon R. 2015. *Ordinary Medicine: Extraordinary Treatments, Longer Lives, and Where to Draw the Line*. Durham, NC: Duke University Press.

Lamb, Sarah. 1997. "The Making and Unmaking of Persons: Notes on Aging and Gender in North India." *Ethos* 25 (3): 279–302.

———. 2000. *White Saris and Sweet Mangoes: Aging, Gender and Body in North India*. Berkeley: University of California Press.

———. 2009. *Aging and the Indian Diaspora: Cosmopolitan Families in India and Abroad*. Bloomington: Indiana University Press.

———. 2013. "In/dependence, Intergenerational Uncertainty, and the Ambivalent State: Perceptions of Old Age Security in India." *South Asia: Journal of South Asian Studies* 36 (1): 65–78.

———. 2014. "Permanent Personhood or Meaningful Decline? Toward a Critical Anthropology of Successful Aging." *Journal of Aging Studies* 29: 41–52.

Manu. 1991. *The Laws of Manu*. Translated by Wendy Doniger, with Brian K. Smith. New York: Penguin.

Robbins, John. 2007. *Healthy at 100: The Scientifically Proven Secrets of the World's Healthiest and Longest-Lived Peoples*. New York: Random House.

Rudman, Debbie Laliberte. 2015. "Embodying Positive Aging and Neoliberal Rationality: Talking about the Aging Body within Narratives of Retirement." *Journal of Aging Studies* 34: 10–20.

Vatuk, Sylvia. 1990. "'To Be a Burden on Others': Dependency Anxiety among the Elderly in India." In *Divine Passions: The Social Construction of Emotion in India*, edited by Owen Lynch, 64–88. Berkeley: University of California Press.

Epilogue

Successful Aging and Desired Interdependence

SUSAN REYNOLDS WHYTE

In the 1970s the matron of a county council home for the elderly in rural England summed up the disposition of the people in her care in this way:

> Most of the old people I have helped have gotten used to being old. It is ordinary to them and they hardly ever discuss it. You don't often find anyone demoralized by his collapsed body, or anything like that. You must give the old credit for understanding the facts of their kind of life. They are acceptors in the main. You accept being near death and having no strength, and your face all funny. You accept because you have no other option, that's all there is to it! So there is really not much point in dwelling on these things. You have got several diseases because you are wearing out and coming to a stop. (Blythe 1979,143)

Four decades on, this disposition seems remote for many who live in the Global North. Being near death, having no strength, living with a collapsing body and your face all funny are not conditions to be accepted. Instead, aging has become a site of intervention. Or in the words of Nikolas Rose, "Biology is not destiny, but opportunity" (2007, 51). Nowhere is this principle more pronounced than in the discourse on successful aging, which admonishes us to tend our bodies and minds carefully so as to avoid the deterioration of age.

This volume's introduction issues a clear call to critically examine this paradigm. The chapters respond to this challenge with thoughtful analyses and ethnographically rich variety. As an afterthought, I offer a perspective from African experiences of aging. I suggest that the conditions upon which the paradigm of successful aging rests hardly exist in Uganda—the African country I know best. More pronounced is the paradigm that Janet McIntosh (this volume) calls "desired interdependence." The contrast between desired interdependence and successful aging may be considered in the light of three of the volume's more or less explicit themes—biopolitics, moral personhood, and inequality.

Nikolas Rose, one of the major contributors to current discussions of bio-politics, uses the term to refer to "strategies involving contestations over the ways in which human vitality, morbidity, and mortality should be problematized" (2007, 54). To look at *contestations* is to introduce a focus on tensions, conflicts, alternatives, doubts, and disagreements. This is not always the spirit in which biopolitics are studied. There is a tendency simply to recognize and confirm the workings of biopower, to show how power flows through expertise, commerce, and technology to effectively shape the dispositions of subjects. Thence come generalizations about prudent citizens of advanced liberal democracies, like those ideal subjects about whom Rose writes. This book offers a welcome alter-native by avoiding simple affirmation and addressing biopolitics in the sense of contestation—examining skeptical reflections and other ways of aging.

Current discussions of biopolitics and biopower, inspired by the work of Michel Foucault, assume a particular historical conjuncture: well-developed, heavily institutionalized biomedicine; increasingly sophisticated biomedical technology; and widespread convictions about the importance of maintaining population and personal health. These conditions do not exist in Uganda, where I work, nor in most African countries. There are some exceptions in areas where donors have been heavily involved, such as HIV/AIDS and child immunization. But despite increasing longevity, there is little political priority given to chronic conditions such as cardiovascular and metabolic diseases, let alone mental problems, that affect older people. The Uganda Health Sector Strategic Plan only included noncommunicable diseases in 2005 and the portion of the Ministry of Health budget allocated to noncommunicable disease efforts is miniscule at 0.01 percent (Schwartz et al. 2014). Policy attention is directed toward child and reproductive health, not toward that of older people. Health care for the elderly is not taken for granted; it is a possibility about which there are struggles and doubts. A few NGOs, like HelpAge Uganda, are beginning to advocate for greater attention to the situation of older people, but their influence is very limited.

In contrast to the Global North, there is no hegemonic discourse about suc-cessful aging in the sense of remaining healthy and independent. The notion that individuals can take an initiative to tend their own bodies in order to avoid the chronic diseases and weaknesses of age has little cultural resonance. For many, decline is expected and accepted. But that is not to say that it is unprob-lematic because there are no options, as the matron of the English old age home asserted. The people with whom I have worked are indeed concerned about decline, most especially about its relational consequences. As core caregivers, elderly people are worried that diminishing strength makes them less able to attend to others. Equally, they wonder what assistance they might need as their own bodies decline and who might provide it. Thinking in terms of providing and receiving care entails considering possible relationships.

Successful, or at least good, aging is contingent upon interdependence. Such mutuality has moral and temporal aspects, reflected in the notion of "the intergenerational contract." The contract is not a document but an unwritten understanding that parents care for their children until failing strength requires the children to care for them. Moral obligation infuses the reciprocity between parents and children. In many African societies, the reciprocity extends to grandparents, who are heavily engaged in caring for their grandchildren. The logic is one of mutual interdependence over time: those who have given resources, effort, and affection to the younger generations that depended on them should receive the same when they themselves become dependent.

The contrast with the hegemonic "successful aging" paradigm is stark. That discourse locates the cultivation of virtue in practices of self-care in everyday life—practices that are heavily shaped by expert knowledge, technology, and institutionalized control measures. Successful aging is healthy aging, achieved through virtuous care of the body and mind—keeping active, eating properly, monitoring the body for risk of chronic diseases. Desirable interdependence implies different values; it makes a virtue of caring for relationships with those who will provide support when the time comes. The body is a means of social engagement and usefulness to others, not primarily something to be nurtured for its own sake.

Yet like all paradigms, "desired interdependence" is problematic in practice, with different, unequal, and uncertain possibilities. The substance and strength of care relationships are highly varied. Individual differences make the practice of interdependence diverse. Some people have alienated their offspring. Those who did not care well for their children may find that the children feel little sense of obligation to care for them in their old age. This is typically the case for men who drank heavily and never managed to keep a wife or support their children.

Uganda, like all but a few countries in southern Africa, has no national pension system that might mitigate inequalities. Very few people enjoy pensions from employers. So nearly everyone is dependent on family members when they become too weak to work or when they fall sick. The African adage that "people are wealth" holds for those blessed with many devoted children and grandchildren. Those who are truly poor are those with no living adult children and grandchildren of their own, and no siblings, nieces or nephews willing to provide support.

Wealth is also money, of course. Those who had enough resources to give their children education and access to salaried jobs are mostly well cared for as they become old and sickly. Having concerned "working-class" children, that is, children with salaries who are attentive and dutiful, is the ideal. Our university colleagues in Kampala are often preoccupied with bringing their parents from the village to the city for high-standard treatment of hypertension, diabetes, and cancer. They show affection and virtue by facilitating medical examinations, medications, and cataract surgery from private clinics or large hospitals where they have connections. At the opposite end of the spectrum is an old lady who stopped by to chat with her age-mate on her way back from the local public dispensary in a rural area. She recounted how the health worker asked why she was bothering them for the scarce medicines they had in stock. Laughing in the way people sometimes laugh at harshness, she repeated to her friend and me the words of the health worker: "You are old, you should just stay home and wait to die." Without financial support from children, she was relegated to minimal medical care.

Demographic and epidemiological changes make the realization of desired interdependence difficult. In Uganda and other eastern and southern African countries, the AIDS epidemic left many older people without any living children, after they had struggled to care for them through years of mortal sickness. Such bereaved elderly people are dependent on other relatives, or perhaps neighbors, who might or might not offer regular support. At the same time, they are part of a generation likely to live longer and develop chronic health problems.

There are those who invested in education for their children, only to discover that the political economy has changed. Their adult children cannot find work and are not prepared to return to rural life with the hoe; they can hardly support themselves, much less their elderly parents (Roth 2008). The remittances that labor migration promised do not always materialize. As Enid Schatz and Janet Seeley (2015, 9) write: "Although interdependence in old age may be desired and valued, it is a social exchange that individuals are having to reinterpret as actors change, but also as older persons age and have different, likely fewer, resources to offer, while their needs simultaneously increase."

Children should care for their parents, but which children should care? And how? Achieving desired interdependence is not always straightforward. Gender and kinship questions arise. In Uganda, men rarely cook, so that task falls to women, as does nursing care and household duties like laundry. Men are more likely to have access to cash, so they should purchase medicine and other necessary commodities. In a patrilineal, virilocal society, wives live with their husbands' parents, so old people may be dependent on their daughters-in-law. Men should respect their wives' parents, so sons-in-law, as well as sons, may provide cash. All of these are possibilities to hope for; none of them are certain.

In the micropolitics of elder care, there are tensions and disagreements about who has what responsibility. Moreover, not every old person in Africa wants to be dependent, with the uncertainties that entails. Nor are all members of the younger generation willing and able to care for their old parents and grandparents. Just as the paradigm of successful aging is being challenged in practice, if not always in open debate, so is that of desired interdependence.

Contestations, negotiations, criticism, and the development of alternatives will no doubt characterize the practice of desired interdependence in the coming years. But as a paradigm and ideal, the principle itself will surely be upheld for the foreseeable future. There is widespread affirmation of the value of interdependence, and it is commonly considered shameful for family members to neglect old people. Many would say that interdependence is the African way. The Global North, in contrast, is criticized for parking old people in institutions or leaving them to live on their own rather than together with other family members. The individualist model of minding your own body and expecting others to mind theirs does not have traction. Bodies are almost bound to deteriorate at some point; biology is still destiny in Africa as elsewhere. However, bodily failure is not a failure of the person, but an opportunity, or at least an occasion, for interdependent others to care. This African vision, even though imperfectly realized in practice, provides a thought-provoking alternative to the paradigm of individual successful aging.

REFERENCES

Blythe, Ronald. 1979. *The View in Winter: Reflections on Old Age*. London: Penguin.

Rose, Nicholas. 2007. *The Politics of Life Itself: Biomedicine, Power, and Subjectivity in the Twenty-First Century*. Princeton, NJ: Princeton University Press.

Roth, Claudia. 2008. "'Shameful!' The Inverted Intergenerational Contract in Bobo-Dioulasso, Burkina Faso." In *Generations in Africa: Connections and Conflicts*, edited by Erdmute Alber, Sjaak van der Geest, and Susan Reynolds Whyte, 47–69. Münster: LIT Verlag.

Schatz, Enid, and Janet Seeley. 2015. "Gender, Ageing, and Carework in East and Southern Africa: A Review." *Global Public Health: An International Journal for Research, Policy, and Practice* 10 (10): 1185–1200.

Schwartz, Jeremy I., David Guwatudde, Rachel Nugent, and Charles Mondo Kiiza. 2014. "Looking at Non-communicable Diseases in Uganda through a Local Lens: An Analysis Using Locally Derived Data." *Globalization and Health* 10: 77.

NOTES ON CONTRIBUTORS

ABIGAIL T. BROOKS is an assistant professor of sociology and director of the Women's Studies Program at Providence College. Her 2017 book, *The Ways Women Age: Using and Refusing Cosmetic Intervention*, examines North American women's experiences and interpretations of aging in an era of cosmetic surgery.

ELANA D. BUCH is an assistant professor of anthropology at the University of Iowa. Author of several articles, her research as a sociocultural and medical anthropologist examines the intersections between caregiving and power in later life and among disabled adults in the United States.

TONI CALASANTI is a professor of sociology at Virginia Tech and first author of *Gender, Social Inequalities, and Aging* and coeditor of *Age Matters: Re-aligning Feminist Thinking* and *Nobody's Burden: Lessons from the Great Depression on the Struggle for Old-Age Security.*

ANNA I. CORWIN is an assistant professor of anthropology at St. Mary's College of California. Author of several articles, her research examines the intersections among aging, embodiment, well-being, social interaction, and language.

JASON DANELY is a senior lecturer of anthropology at Oxford Brookes University. He is the author of *Aging and Loss: Mourning and Maturity in Contemporary Japan* and coeditor (with Caitrin Lynch) of *Transitions and Transformations: Cultural Perspectives on Aging and the Life Course.*

JUDITH FARQUHAR is Max Palevsky Professor Emeritus of Anthropology and Social Sciences at the University of Chicago. She is the author of *Knowing Practice: The Clinical Encounter of Chinese Medicine*; *Appetites: Food and Sex in Post-Socialist China*; *Ten Thousand Things: Nurturing Life in Contemporary Beijing*; and (as coeditor with Margaret Lock) *Beyond the Body Proper: Reading the Anthropology of Material Life.*

ASTRID PERNILLE JESPERSEN is an associate professor of ethnology, head of the Copenhagen Centre for Health Research in the Humanities, and part of the Center for Healthy Aging at the University of Copenhagen.

NEAL KING is a professor of sociology and of women's and gender studies at Virginia Tech. His books include *Heroes in Hard Times: Cop Action Movies in the U.S.* and (as coeditor with Martha McCaughey) *Reel Knockouts: Violent Women in the Movies.*

SARAH LAMB is a professor of anthropology at Brandeis University and author of *White Saris and Sweet Mangoes: Aging, Gender, and Body in North India*; *Aging and the Indian Diaspora: Cosmopolitan Families in India and Abroad*; and (as coeditor with Diane Mines) *Everyday Life in South Asia.*

ASKE JUUL LASSEN is a postdoctoral fellow at the Saxo Institute, the Copenhagen Centre for Health Research in the Humanities, and the Center for Healthy Aging at the University of Copenhagen. He is the author of several articles examining everyday experiences and state agendas of active aging in Europe.

ANNETTE LEIBING is a professor of medical anthropology on the Faculty of Nursing at the University of Montreal. Her books include *Thinking about Dementia: Culture, Loss, and the Anthropology of Senility* and *The Shadow Side of Fieldwork: Exploring the Blurred Boundaries between Ethnography and Life.*

MEIKA LOE is a professor of sociology and women's studies and director of Women's Studies at Colgate University. She is the author of *Aging Our Way: Lessons for Living from 85 and Beyond*; *The Rise of Viagra: How the Little Blue Pill Changed Sex in America*; and (as coeditor with Kelly Joyce) *Technogenarians: Studying Health and Illness through an Ageing, Science, and Technology Lens.*

JANET McINTOSH is an associate professor of anthropology at Brandeis University and author of *The Edge of Islam: Power, Personhood, and Ethnoreligious Boundaries on the Kenya Coast* and *Unsettled: Denial and Belonging among White Kenyans.*

JESSICA ROBBINS-RUSZKOWSKI is an assistant professor at the Institute of Gerontology and Department of Anthropology at Wayne State University. Author of several articles, she studies how individuals' experiences of aging, health, and illness are part of broader social, cultural, political-economic, and historical processes.

JANELLE S. TAYLOR is a professor of anthropology at the University of Washington. A sociocultural and medical anthropologist, she is the author of *The Public Life of the Fetal Sonogram: Technology, Consumption, and the Politics of Reproduction* and (as coeditor with Linda Layne and Danielle Wozniak) *Consuming Motherhood.*

EMILY WENTZELL is an associate professor of anthropology at the University of Iowa. She is author of *Maturing Masculinities: Aging, Chronic Illness, and Viagra in Mexico* and (as coeditor with Marcia Inhorn) *Medical Anthropology at the Intersections: Histories, Activisms, and Futures.*

SUSAN REYNOLDS WHYTE is a professor of anthropology at the University of Copenhagen and member of the Center for Healthy Aging. She is the author of *Questioning Misfortune: The Pragmatics of Uncertainty in Eastern Uganda*; coauthor (with Sjaak van der Geest and Anita Hardon) of *Social Lives of Medicines*; editor of *Second Chances: Surviving AIDS in Uganda*; coeditor (with Benedicte Ingstad) of *Disability and Culture* and *Disability in Local and Global Worlds*; and coeditor (with Erdmute Alber and Sjaak van der Geest) of *Generations in Africa: Connections and Conflicts*.

IMANI WOODY holds a PhD in human services specializing in nonprofit management. She is the founding director and CEO of Mary's House for Older Adults, and chair of SAGE Metro DC, an organization serving LGBTQ elders.

QICHENG ZHANG is a professor of classical Chinese literature and cultural studies at the Beijing University of Chinese Medicine and the author of many books on the Chinese heritage of life nurturing.

INDEX

Page numbers in italics refer to figures

active aging: *aktywność* ("active-ness," "activity") (Poland), 115, 119, 120, 121; aloneness and, 151–152; Brazil and, 17; China and, 17, 168; decline and, 145, 149, 165; Denmark and, 141–153; dependence and, 143–144, 145, 146; disengagement theory and, 19n23; Europe and, 10, 17, 19n20, 114, 122, 141, 143–144, 145; European Union and, 10, 122, 142, 144; exercise and, 10–11, 150; globalization and, 17; India and, 17; individual agency and, 8, 41; Japan and, 17, 158–159, 162; Katz, Stephen, on, 11, 41–42; loneliness and, 152; Mexico and, 17; motivation technologies and, 145–150; old age and, 145, 148; Poland and, 122–123; social dependence and, 143–144; successful aging and, 8, 34, 104–105, 114, 126, 163, 233, 236, 245; United States and, 234; Universities of the Third Age (UTA) and, 10–11, 113, 114–116; World Health Organization (WHO) and, 143; as youth-centric, 152
activity centers (Denmark), 141, 144–145, 147, 149–150, 151
affordable housing, 227
Africa: aging and, 197, 243; biopolitics and, 244; Botswana, 196–197; colonialism and, 189–190, 191; dependence and, 246–247; Ghana, 71; HIV/AIDS and, 246; individual responsibility and, 247; interdependence and, 186, 188–189, 196–197, 245, 246, 247; intergenerational reciprocity and, 245; social dependence and, 18n12; successful aging paradigm and, 247; Uganda, 243–247; Western views and, 186–187. *See also* Kenya
African Americans, 55, 58, 59, 60, 61, 65, 88, 95. *See also names of individual African Americans*
African Americans (lesbian, gay, and bisexual/LGB), 55–66; African American culture and, 59, 60, 61; age and, 55, 57; ageism and, 56, 58, 62–65; aging and, 57, 65–66; alienation and, 57; church/religious institutions and, 57, 59, 64, 65; coming out and, 58, 62, 63–64, 65; dependence and, 57; discrimination and, 55–56, 57, 58, 61, 62–65; exclusion and, 55–56, 58, 65; gender and, 55, 65, 66; grief/loss and, 57, 59–60, 63; heteronormativity and, 55–56, 57; heterosexism and, 58, 59; homophobia and, 56, 58, 59; invisibility and, 59; isolation and, 57, 58–59, 61–62; multiple identities and, 57–65; personhood and, 65; race and, 55, 64–66; racism and, 56, 58, 64–65, 66; service barriers and, 65–66; sexism and, 58, 64–65; sexual identity and, 57, 59, 60, 61; sexual orientation and, 55, 57, 60, 62, 65; study methodology and, 56–57; successful aging and, 65–66; witch-hunts and, 58. *See also names of individual African Americans*
Agatha, Sister, 103–104
age-grade systems (Japan), 159, 163–164, 165n6, 166n12
age-grade systems (Kenya), 185–186, 187, 190, 191–192, 196
ageism: acceptable terms and, 19n27; African Americans (lesbian, gay, and bisexual/LGB) and, 56, 58, 62–65; agelessness and, 240; bodily aging study and, 30; comfortable aging and, 227; definition of, xi; exposure and, 14; fitness/youth culture and, 42; gender and, xi, 28, 38, 39, 64–65; individual agency and, 29; institutionalized nature of, 29; invisibility and, 63; Kahn, Robert, on, 27; lesbian, gay, and bisexual (LGB) people and, 62–65, 66; North America and, xi, 13; old age and, 38–39; Rowe, John, on, 27; sexism and, 64–65; sexual identity and, 64–65; social inequalities and, 39; stereotypes and, 64, 164; successful aging and, xi, 6, 13, 28, 29, 38–39, 42; United States and, 14, 62–63; value of old age and, 17, 39; welfare and, 143; women and, 62, 64–65
agelessness: ageism and, 240; North America and, 12, 19n24, 231–232; personhood and, 240; successful aging and, xii, 4, 7, 11, 12, 42, 106, 235; United States and, 232, 234
age relations, 28–29
aging: acceptance of, 47, 232, 243; Africa and, 197, 243; African Americans (lesbian, gay, and bisexual/LGB) and, 57, 65–66; aging in place, 219, 222; aging naturally,

aging (*continued*)
　　44, 47–50, 51–52; binary paradigm of, xii;
　　biopolitics and, 16–17, 244; Brazil and, 205,
　　206, 214; Catholic nuns and, 101, 104; class
　　and, xii, 16–17; culture and, xii, 53n7,
　　99; denial and, 224; dependence and,
　　xiii–xiv; double standard of, 42–43, 52n3;
　　ethnographic research and, 123; exclusion
　　and, 123; failure/embarrassment and, xii,
　　16, 27–28, 106, 156, 164; gender and, xii,
　　44; globalization and, xiii–xiv, 196; health
　　and, xiii–xiv; inclusion and, 119; India
　　and, xii, 230–233, 237–240; interdepen-
　　dence and, xiii–xiv, 245; Kenya and, 196,
　　197; lesbian, gay, and bisexual (LGB)
　　people and, 55, 62; lifestyle drugs and,
　　70–71; masculinity and, 72; medicalization
　　of aging, 16–17, 70–71, 73, 74, 79; medicine
　　and, 232; moral responsibilities and, 2,
　　42, 123; Poland and, 117–118; race and,
　　xii, 52n3; religion and, xii; Seiler, Emilie,
　　on, 236; sexuality and, xii, 43, 70–71, 79;
　　stigma and, 38; United States and, xii–xiii,
　　51, 232–233, 237; Viagra and, 68, 70–71;
　　Western views and, 240; White House
　　Conference on Aging, 226; workplaces
　　and, 34; youth and, 99. *See also* active
　　aging; bodily aging; comfortable aging;
　　successful aging; *individual titles of works*
aging in place, 219, 222. *See also* home care
aging naturally, 44, 47–50, 51–52
Aging Our Way (Loe), 218, 221
aging-related industries, 11, 12, 16, 28, 51. *See
　　also* cosmetic anti-aging interventions
Aguzzoli, Nilva de Lourdes, 211
AIDS/HIV, 63, 192–193, 244, 246
aktywność ("active-ness," "activity")
　　(Poland), 115, 119, 120, 121
Alan, 133–134
Alexander-Israel, D., 206
Alison, 47
Allison, Anne, 166n13
allotment gardening (Poland), 113, 119–122
aloneness, 151–152
Alzheimer's Association (Rio de Janeiro), 206
Alzheimer's disease: advanced stages of,
　　209; awareness and, 208–209; caregiv-
　　ers and, 206–208, 211–214, 220; Catholic
　　nuns and, 98, 103–104, 121; desperation
　　and, 208; friendship and, 129, 133; "Giv-
　　ing Alzheimer's Patients Their Way, Even
　　Chocolate" (*New York Times*), 220; hero-
　　ism and, 204–205, 208, 211–214; inde-
　　pendence and, 210, 212; India and, 5–6;
　　interdependence and, 212; life exten-
　　sion and, 127; optimism limits and, 209,
　　212–213; personhood and, 204, 205–206,
　　207–210, 212, 214; pharmaceuticals and,
　　206, 208, 209, 214n4; Poland and, 113–114,
　　121; self-help and, 209; selfhood and,
　　208–209, 209–210, 211; state heroism
　　and, 214; successful aging and, 204–205;
　　Taylor, Richard, on, 209; *The 36-Hour Day*

(Maze and Rabins), 207; United States
　　and, 209. *See also* dementia
Alzheimer's disease (Brazil), 203–214;
　　Alzheimer's Association (Rio de Janeiro),
　　206; awareness and, 208–209; caregiv-
　　ers and, 206–208, 211–214; Center for
　　Alzheimer's Disease and Other Mental
　　Disorders of Aging (CDA) and, 203–204,
　　206–207, 209–210, 211; Dona Eliza and,
　　206–207; "glocal" perspective and, 205,
　　208, 214; grandchildren and, 211–213,
　　214n3, 214n4; heroism and, 204–205,
　　208, 211–214; middle generation and, 213;
　　1990s and, 206, 207; personhood and,
　　204, 205–206, 207–210, 212, 214; shanty-
　　town (*favela*) and, 210–211; social relations
　　and, 211, 214; *The 36-Hour Day* (Maze and
　　Rabins) and, 207; 2005 and, 208. *See also*
　　dementia
American Academy of Anti-Aging Medicine,
　　241n6
Americans. *See* United States
American Society for Aesthetic Plastic
　　Surgery, 42
Amour (film), 15
Andrews, Molly, 29
Anna, Pani, 112–113, 115, 118, 123n1
Anne, 45, 46, 53n5
anti-aging, 11, 16, 30–34, 42
anti-aging industries, 28, 51. *See also* aging-
　　related industries
anti-aging medicine, 12, 42, 241n6. *See also*
　　medicalization of aging
anti-aging products/services, 12, 16, 30,
　　31–34, 41, 42–43, 51, 70. *See also* cosmetic
　　anti-aging interventions; plastic surgery;
　　names of individual products
Arellano, Maria, 85–86, 89, 97n1
Arne, 130
Ashtavakra Gita, 237, 241n8
asramas (life stages) (India), xii, 237–238,
　　241n9. *See also* Hinduism
Astor, 58–59, 61
attractiveness: gender and, 31; successful
　　aging and, 11–12; women and, 16, 32–33, 37,
　　39, 43, 45, 48–49, 50–51, 52, 53n5. *See also*
　　beauty; cosmetic anti-aging interven-
　　tions; youth-beauty imperative
Australia, 10–11

baby boomers (United States), 7, 8, 12. *See
　　also* population aging
Baltes, Paul B., 229n2
Banerjee, Purnima, 5, 230–233, 239, 240
Barb, 37
Bartky, Sandra, 43
beauty, 30, 34, 42, 43, 44, 45, 47, 49. *See also*
　　attractiveness; cosmetic anti-aging inter-
　　ventions; youth-beauty imperative
Beijing (China), 168–170, 171, 172–173, 175–176,
　　176–178, 178–179, 181, 183. *See also* China;
　　yangsheng (nurturing life) (China)
Being Mortal (Gawande), 15, 226

Belltower, 88, 89, 90, 97n1
Bengalis, 19n18, 230, 231–232, 233, 241n1, 242n11, 242n12, 242n13. *See also* India
Berk, Roland, 158
Bernard, Sister Mary, 102–103
Bert, 130, 135
Besnier, Niko, 132
Best Exotic Marigold Hotel, The (film), 15
Bhatia, Vijay, 239
biocitizenship, 7, 11, 18n6
biomedicine, 6–7, 16–17, 244
biopolitics, 3, 6, 12, 16–17, 18n6, 244
bisexuals, 58, 65. *See also* African Americans (lesbian, gay, and bisexual/LGB)
bodily aging, 12, 14, 30–38, 68–69, 70, 75–78, 79, 98, 240, 247. *See also* decline
Bordo, Susan, 42
Boston, 233
Botox, 52n4
Botswana, 196–197; individualism and, 196
Brazil, 17, 205–206, 210–211, 214; globalization and, 205, 208, 214. *See also* Alzheimer's disease (Brazil)
bridewealth (Kenya), 188, 190–191, 198n4
Brijnath, Bianca, 5–6
Britain, 123n2, 189–190. *See also* colonialism
Brooks, Frances, 236–237
Bruce, Barbara, 2–3
Brummel, Beth, 193–194
Buch, Elana, 19n17
Buddhism, 11, 162
Butler, Judith, 165n4

Calasanti, Toni M., 14, 19n32, 29, 30
calligraphy, 180, 181, 182
Canada, 123n2
caregivers, 133–134, 204, 206–208, 211–214, 220, 221–223. *See also* home care
Carol, 133–134
Caroline, 44, 45
Carrie, 35, 37, 38
Catherine, 48
Catholicism, 11
Catholic nuns, 98–109; aging and, 101, 104; Alzheimer's disease and, 98, 103–104, 121; being versus doing and, 105, 108, 229n4; death/dying and, 102, 106, 107; decline and, 103, 106–107, 108; education and, 100–101; health and, 98; independence and, 5, 100, 103–104, 107–108, 108–109; individual agency and, 100, 101–103, 107, 108–109; interdependence and, 104, 107–108; old age and, 102, 104, 106–107, 108; permanent personhood and, 100, 106–107, 108–109; productive activity and, 100, 104–105, 108–109; rehabilitation center (Poland) and, 113–114, 121; research and, 98–100; successful aging and, 5, 98–99, 100, 104, 108–109; terms for, 109n2; vows and, 101–102, 104, 108, 109n2. *See also names of individual nuns*
Cattell, Maria, 197
Celia, 134

Center for Alzheimer's Disease and Other Mental Disorders of Aging (CDA) (Brazil), 203–204, 206–207, 209–210, 211
Centers for Disease Control and Prevention (United States), 9, 55
changshou (longevity) (China), 170, 174. *See also* longevity
Cheryl, 60–61
Chicago, elders in, 85–97. *See also* home care
children, 9–10, 106, 235, 245–246
China, 168–183; active aging and, 17, 168; Chinese backwardness and, 172; Chinese Law Assuring the Rights and Interests of the Aged, 183n1; choral singing and, 179, 181; communism, 168, 171; Daoism, 168, 170, 171, 174–175; elderly and, 62–63; ethnographic research and, 168–170, 173; filial piety and, 169; health and, 181–182; health care and, 171, 174; Japan and, 180–181; longevity and, 170, 173–175, 178–179; neoliberalism and, 168; population aging and, 17, 169, 171, 173; prevention and, 168, 170; reform era and, 171, 172; retirement and, 169, 173, 176; self-care and, 169–170, 171, 173–174; the *Zhuangzi*, 168, 170. *See also yangsheng* (nurturing life) (China)
choral singing (China), 179, 181
Choto Ma, 239
Christiane, 212
Christian missions (Kenya), 191
church/religious institutions, 57, 59, 64, 65. *See also* Catholic nuns
Claire, 44, 45, 46
Clara, 60, 63, 64
Clarisse, 62
class, xii, 16–17, 19n32, 36, 55, 87, 93, 96, 116–119
cognition, 8, 10, 106, 126, 128, 203, 207, 209. *See also* Alzheimer's disease; Alzheimer's disease (Brazil); dementia
Cole, Thomas, 14
colonialism, 28, 186, 189–190, 191–192
comfortable aging, 218–229; ageism and, 227; aging in place and, 219, 222; care acceptance and, 221–223; death/dying and, 220, 224–226; disability and, 220, 224, 228, 229; failure/embarrassment and, 221; home care and, 227; interdependence and, 221–223; limitations/vulnerability and, 219, 220, 221, 223–224, 229; mortality and, 220, 224–226, 228, 229; as new paradigm, 220–221, 228; obstacles and, 227; old age and, 224; oldest old and, 220; prevention and, 221; productive activity and, 219, 220, 221, 228; quality of life and, 219; resources and, 220, 221, 226–227, 229; social relations and, 221, 222–223, 226, 229; structural factors and, 226–227; successful aging and, 219, 220, 221, 228; United States and, 226–227; women and, 220. *See also names of individuals*
Coming into the End Zone (Grumbach), 223
communism (China), 168, 171

Complaints of a Dutiful Daughter (Hoffmann), 210
computer skills, 115–116
Cora, 131–132
Cordial Club (Denmark), 141, 142, 144–145, 150
Corwin, Anna, 5
cosmeceuticals, 31. *See also* anti-aging products/services
cosmetic anti-aging interventions, 31, 32, 42, 43, 44–47, 51–52, 52n4, 205
council of elders. *See* elders' councils (Kenya)
Crawford, Robert, xivn2
Crowley, Chris, 3, 12
Cruikshank, Margaret, 52, 220
Cumming, Elaine, 19n23

Daisy, 147–148, 151
dancing fools (Japan), 160–162, 166n10
DaneAge, 144, 146, 150
Danes. *See* Denmark
Danish Law on Social Service, 146
Daoism (China), 168, 170, 171, 174–175
Darlene, 59
Darryl, 32–33, 34
Davies, Judie, 213
death/dying: Banerjee, Purnima-di and, 231–232; Brooks, Frances, on, 236–237; Catholic nuns and, 102, 106, 107; comfortable aging and, 220, 224–226; failure/embarrassment and, 237, 241; Florence and, 228; Frankl, Viktor, on, 226; Hinduism and, 238, 239; India and, 5, 230–231, 237, 239–240, 242n12; Japan and, 162, 163; Lamb, Sarah, on, 127; medicalization of aging and, 16–17; North America and, 241; United States and, 226, 234, 235–236, 237; vulnerability and, 237; Western views and, 106, 237, 240. *See also* mortality
Debbie, 131
Debra, 45, 46
decline: active aging and, 145, 149, 165; Alzheimer's disease and, 203, 207; Catholic nuns and, 103, 106–107, 108; dementia and, 127; elders (India) and, 239; exclusion and, 106; failure/embarrassment and, 29; friendship and, 127; Japan and, 157, 162, 165; North America and, 2, 241; old age and, xi, 34, 148, 149; prevention (Denmark) and, 145, 148–150; rehabilitation and, 145; senior welfare centers (Japan) and, 162; successful aging and, 3, 17, 41, 98, 159–160, 162, 235; Uganda and, 244–245; United States and, 232–233; Victorian era and, 14; Western views and, 240
dementia, 126–137; caregivers and, 133–134; as clinical syndrome, 127; cognition and, 203; comfort therapy and, 220; decline and, 127; ethnographic research and, 128; exclusion and, 13, 132, 211; friendship and, 127–137; fusional relations and, 212, 213; "Giving Alzheimer's Patients Their Way, Even Chocolate" (*New York Times*), 220;

gossip and, 131–132; grandchildren and, 211–213; moral communities and, 131–132; moral laboratories and, 128–131, 133, 134, 136; optimism limits and, 209; personhood and, 13, 132, 135, 136, 205–206, 209, 210; pharmaceuticals and, 206, 208; prevention and, 204; *seva* (service to elders) (India) and, 5–6; shantytown (*favela*) and, 210–211; sociality and, 126–127, 211; successful aging and, 128, 135–136, 204–205; United States and, 128. *See also* Alzheimer's disease; Alzheimer's disease (Brazil); *names of individuals*
Denial of Aging: Perpetual Youth, Eternal Life, and Other Dangerous Fantasies, The (Gillick), 12
Denmark, 141–153; active aging and, 141–153; activity centers and, 144–145, 147, 149–150, 151; Cordial Club, 141, 142, 144–145, 150; DaneAge, 144, 146, 150; Danish Law on Social Service, 146; dependence and, 146–148, 149; fieldwork and, 144–145; health and, 142, 145–146, 148; home care and, 143, 145, 146, 147, 148–149, 152; independence and, 146, 147, 152, 153; lifestyle diseases and, 148; loneliness and, 150–152; motivation technologies and, 145–150; Nordic Model, 142–143; nursing homes and, 149–150, 152; old age and, 141, 143, 145–146, 152, 153; People's Movement Against Loneliness, 150; policy participation and, 144; population aging and, 143, 152; prevention and, 145, 148–150, 152; preventive home visits (PHVs) and, 148–149; rehabilitation and, 145–148, 149, 152; self-care and, 149, 153; Senior Citizens Councils, 144, 150; welfare and, 142–144, 150, 152–153; Wiedergården, 144–145, 150. *See also names of individual Danes*
dependence: active aging and, 143–144, 145, 146; Africa and, 6, 246–247; African Americans (lesbian, gay, and bisexual/LGB) and, 57; aging and, xiii–xiv; appropriate dependence, 5–6, 238, 239; Brooks, Frances, on, 236–237; Europe and, 146; failure/embarrassment and, 103, 104, 108, 241; India and, 9, 231, 238, 239; Kenya and, 6; Koenig, Dora, on, 4; moral responsibilities and, 103, 104, 106, 118; North America and, 9, 241; old age and, xi; personhood and, 240; rehabilitation (Denmark) and, 146–148, 149; social values and, 11; successful aging paradigm and, 7, 99, 103, 235; United States and, 9–10; values and, 17; Western views and, 188, 240. *See also* independence; interdependence
desired interdependence, 187–189, 243–247. *See also* interdependence
diet, xii–xiii, 2, 7, 31, 32, 34, 41, 43, 45. *See also* food
disability: comfortable aging and, 220, 224, 228, 229; exclusion and, 106; longevity and, 165; social relations and, 150;

successful aging and, 8, 10, 27, 55, 126, 236; "third age" and, 118–119

discrimination, xi, 55–56, 57, 58, 61, 62–65, 115

disease: Daisy and, 148; as failure/embarrassment, xiii, 14–15, 237; Kenya and, 192–193; Poland and, 119; successful aging and, xi, 8, 10, 27, 41, 55, 126, 245. *See also* Alzheimer's disease; Alzheimer's disease (Brazil)

disengagement theory, 19n23

domestic labor, 37–38, 72. *See also* home care

Dona Eliza, 206–207

Donald, 62

Do Not Go Gentle: Successful Aging for Baby Boomers and All Generations (Kownacki), 8

Doris, 60, 61, 62, 63–64

Dorota, 122

Dorothy, 236

double standard of aging, 42–43, 52n3

Dreama, 34

Eastern Europe, 19n20

eldercare, 238, 242n11, 246–247. *See also* caregivers; home care

elderhood (Kenya), 185–197; bridewealth and, 188, 190–191, 198n4; colonialism and, 189–190, 191; elders' councils, 187–188, 189–190, 198n3; female, 192; gerontocracy and, 186, 187, 193–194; *giteo* (attitude toward elders) and, 188, 194; interdependence and, 186; land and, 186, 187, 188, 190, 191, 198n6; market economy and, 190; men and, 190–191, 197; modernity and, 189, 193, 196; "Mzee" honorific and, 189, 193; Orma and, 190; palm wine and, 186, 187, 192; power attrition and, 189–193; rituals and, 185, 186, 187–188, 191, 192, 195; witchcraft and, 185, 186, 192, 197, 198n6; women and, 192, 193, 197, 198n2, 198n4, 198n6; youth and, 186, 188, 190–191, 192–195, 196, 197, 198n6

elders (Chicago), 85–97. *See also* home care

elders (India), 230, 231, 232, 237, 238–240, 242n11. *See also* India

elders' councils (Kenya), 187–188, 189–190, 198n3

elderspeak, 107

Eliza (Dona), 206–207

Elizabeth (aging naturally and), 47, 48–49, 50

Elizabeth (anti-aging and), 33, 37–38

Ellen, 131

embarrassment. *See* failure/embarrassment

Embree, John F., 157

England, 243

English-language instruction, 112, 115–116, 122

erectile dysfunction, 68–79; anti-aging products/services and, 32; bodily aging and, 75–78; health and, 75–76; herbal supplements and, 72–73; masculinity and, 74–79; medicalization of aging and, 70–71, 73, 74, 79; men and, 32, 42, 71–79; Mexico and, 6, 71–79; New Zealand and, 71; Patrick and, 36–37; research methods and, 73–74;

United States and, 71; Viagra, 6, 42, 68–71, 72, 76, 205; women and, 71, 77–78

Erikson, Erik H., 156

Espino, David V., 208

Esther, 129–130

ethnicity, 19n32, 43, 52n3

ethnocentricity, 16, 17

ethnographic research: aging and, 123; China and, 168–170, 173; dementia and, 128; Denmark and, 144–145; gender and, 30–31; home care and, 88–89; India and, 233; Mexico and, 73–74; Poland and, 112; successful aging and, 16, 17; United States and, 233, 241n5; Universities of the Third Age (UTA) and, 113–114

Europe: active aging and, 10, 17, 19n20, 114, 122, 141, 143–144, 145; dependence and, 146; "European Year for Active Ageing and Solidarity between Generations" (2012), 1, 18n2, 114; failure/embarrassment and, 102; independence and, 17; Kenya and, 189–190, 191–192; old age and, 145, 146; personhood and, 206; productive activity and, 10–11; successful aging and, xii, 1, 6, 79, 188; Universities of the Third Age (UTA) and, 123n2; welfare and, 143. *See also* colonialism; *names of individual countries*

European Union, 1, 10, 18n2, 114, 115, 122, 142, 144

"European Year for Active Ageing and Solidarity between Generations" (2012), 1, 18n2, 114

exclusion: African Americans (lesbian, gay, and bisexual/LGB) and, 55–56, 58, 65; aging and, 123; decline and, 106; dementia and, 13, 132, 211; disability and, 106; old age and, 36–37, 113, 122–123; successful aging paradigm and, 6, 13–14; "third age" and, 14; Universities of the Third Age (UTA) and, 116, 119

exemplary friends, 128, 129, 136–137. *See also* friendship

exercise: active aging and, 10–11, 150; fitness culture, 42; gender and, 31, 32; individual agency and, xii–xiii, 2, 7; Japan and, 158–159, 163; Kåre and, 142, 147; *New York Times* and, 8; successful aging and, 2, 15, 35; women and, 43, 45; *yangsheng* (nurturing life) (China) and, 169, 170–171, 175–176, 178, 179–180, 182

facelifts, 32, 42, 52n4, 53n5, 205. *See also* cosmetic anti-aging interventions

Faderman, Lillian, 58

Fadiman, Jeffrey, 194–195

failure/embarrassment: aging and, xii, 16, 27–28, 106, 156, 164; bodily aging and, 247; comfortable aging and, 221; death/dying and, 237, 241; decline and, 29; dependence and, 103, 104, 108, 241; disease as, xiii, 14–15, 237; Dorothy and, 236; Europe and, 102; health and, xivn2, 7; individual

failure/embarrassment (*continued*)
responsibility and, 4, 29, 42; intergenerational reciprocity and, 188; mortality as, xiii; old age and, xi–xii, 5, 14–15, 102, 165, 232, 237; United States and, 102; Western views and, 106, 237. *See also* moral responsibilities
Fair Labor Standards Act (United States), 88, 93
Farquhar, Judith, 174
Featherstone, Mike, 204–205
Feldman, Edna, 234
females, 16, 187, 192, 198n2. *See also* women
femininity, 30, 32–33, 42, 44–47, 52
Ferguson, James, 18n12
Fetzer Institute, 128, 137
fieldwork. *See* ethnographic research
filial piety (China), 169
Finland, 142
fitness culture, 42. *See also* exercise
Florence, 218–220, 221, 223, 224, 226–227, 227–228
food, 31, 90, 179. *See also* diet
foolish vitality (Japan), 157–158, 162, 164–165
fools' dance (Japan), 160–162, 166n10
Formosa, Marvin, 123n2
Foucault, Michael, 171, 244
"fourth age," 14, 19n30, 114, 119, 122, 160, 162, 165n7
Franciscan Sisters of the Sacred Heart, 99, 100–101. *See also* Catholic nuns
Frankl, Viktor, 226
friendship, 126–137; Alzheimer's disease and, 129, 133; decline and, 127; dementia and, 127–137; ethnographic research and, 128; exemplary friends, 128, 129, 136–137; individualism and, 128; moral communities and, 131–132; moral laboratories and, 128–131, 133, 134; successful aging and, 127. *See also* sociality; social relations
Furukawa-san, 154–156, 160

Garcez-Leme, Luiz E., 208
gardens. *See* allotment gardening (Poland)
Gawande, Atul, 15, 226
gay men, 52n3, 58. *See also* African Americans (lesbian, gay, and bisexual/LGB)
gender: African Americans (lesbian, gay, and bisexual/LGB) and, 55, 65, 66; ageism and, xi, 28, 38, 39, 64–65; aging and, xii, 44; allotment gardening (Poland) and, 119; anti-aging and, 30–34; attractiveness and, 31; class and, 36; Cordial Club (Denmark) and, 141, 144; ethnographic research and, 30–31; exercise and, 31, 32; home care and, 93; invisibility and, 36; labor and, 30, 88; loneliness and, 151; marginality and, 36; old age and, 29, 35–39; Poland and, 116–119, 123n4, 123n5; productive labor and, 30, 31; sociality and, 117; successful aging and, 16–17, 19n32, 28, 31–34, 38–39, 43; Uganda and, 246; Universities of the Third Age (UTA) and, 116–119; Wiedergården (Denmark) and, 144;

workplaces and, 36. *See also* females; femininity; males; masculinity; men; women
gender expression, 55
geriatricians/gerontologists, 1, 18n1, 27, 156
gerontocracy (Kenya), 186, 187, 193–194
Gerontological Society of America, 27
Gerontologist, The, 1, 18n1
Ghana, 71
Gillick, Muriel, 12
Giriama (Kenya), 188
giteo (attitude toward elders) (Kenya), 188, 194
"Giving Alzheimer's Patients Their Way, Even Chocolate" (*New York Times*), 220
Glenn, 221, 223, 224, 225, 227
globalization: active aging and, 17; aging and, xiii–xiv, 196; Alzheimer's disease (Brazil) and, 205, 208, 214; beauty and, 42; Botswana and, 196; computer skills and, 115; India and, 239; Kenya and, 186, 189, 193, 196; population aging and, 17; sexuality and, 70; successful aging and, xii, 6, 71; third age and, 205; Universities of the Third Age (UTA) and, 114; *yangsheng* (nurturing life) (China) and, 170
Going Solo: The Extraordinary Rise and Surprising Appeal of Living Alone (Klinenberg), 9
gossip, 131–132
Government Program for the Benefit of Social Activity/Active-ness of Older People (Poland), 114
grandchildren, 211–213, 214n3, 214n4, 245
Greatest Generation, 220, 221
Greenhalgh, Susan, 7
Greg, 31–32, 36
grief/loss, 57, 59–60, 63
Groisman, Daniel, 210
Grumbach, Doris, 223
Guterman, Jacob, 206

Harman, S. M., 206
Harold, 15
Harry, 131, 132
Havighurst, Robert, 1, 27
Hayakawa, 160–162, 163
health: aging and, xiii–xiv; allotment gardening (Poland) and, 120; Catholic nuns and, 98; China and, 174–175, 181–182; Denmark and, 142, 145–146, 148; erectile dysfunction and, 75–76; failure/ embarrassment and, xivn2, 7; Kenya and, 192–193; Mexico and, 73; moral responsibilities and, xivn2, 7; Poland and, 116, 118–119; sociality and, 126, 220–221; successful aging and, 126, 236; Uganda and, 246; Universities of the Third Age (UTA) and, 116–119; World Health Organization, 1, 10, 143; *yangsheng* (nurturing life) (China) and, 174–175, 181–182; Zhu Hong and, 177–178. *See also* diet; exercise
health care, 116, 171, 174, 244
health insurance, 88, 171
healthy aging. *See* active aging; successful aging

Healthy Aging for Dummies (Agin and Perkins), 2, 11
Healthy Aging Program (CDC), 9
HealthyPeople.gov, 55
Helen, 129, 135
Helen, Sister, 107
HelpAge Kenya, 196
HelpAge Uganda, 244
Henry, William, 19n23
herbal supplements, 31, 72–73
heroism, 204–205, 208, 211–214
heterosexuality, 16, 52n3, 55–56, 57, 58, 59
Himcaps, 72
Hinduism, xii, 11, 231, 237–238, 239, 241n2, 241n8, 241n9. *See also* India
HIV/AIDS, 63, 192–193, 244, 246
Hoffmann, Deborah, 210
Holstein, Martha, 42, 51, 224
home care, 88–93; African Americans and, 88; bodily asymmetry and, 92–93, 96; challenging households and, 91–92; class and, 87, 93, 96; comfortable aging and, 227; Denmark and, 143, 145, 146, 147, 148–149, 152; ethnographic research and, 88–89; food and, 90; funding and, 88; gender and, 93; generation and, 87; government policies and, 88, 96; immigrants and, 88; independence and, 19n17, 86, 87, 89–93, 96, 147, 148; as labor, 88, 93; moral relations and, 93–97; personhood and, 87, 89, 90–91, 96; preventive home visits (PHVs) (Denmark), 148–149; race and, 87, 88, 93, 96; Silverman, Eileen, on, 85–86; United States and, 86, 87, 88–93; women as providers of, 87, 88, 96
homophobia, 56, 58, 59, 63–64
Honig im Kopf (*Head Full of Honey*) (film), 211, 213
Honorata, Pani, 112–113, 118, 123n1
humor, 155–156, 157–159, 160, 164, 165n5
Hurd Clarke, Laura, 53n7

I'll See You in My Dreams (film), 15
immigrants, 88
inclusion, 119. *See also* exclusion
independence: Alzheimer's disease and, 210, 212; Botswanan women and, 196–197; Catholic nuns and, 5, 100, 103–104, 107–108, 108–109; Denmark and, 146, 147, 152, 153; Europe and, 17; home care and, 19n17, 86, 87, 89–93, 96, 147, 148; India and, 238–239; Kahn, Robert, on, 9, 87; Kenya and, 197; loneliness and, 152; North America and, 9–10, 17, 107, 210, 212, 231–232; old age and, 14; personhood and, 12, 16, 86–87, 96; rehabilitation (Denmark) and, 147; Rowe, John, on, 9, 87; self-help and, 9; Simic, Andrei, on, 10; successful aging and, 7, 9–10, 12, 16, 17, 86–87, 99–100, 103–104, 163, 233, 235, 236, 244; United States and, 9–10, 86–87, 222, 232, 235, 238–239; World Health Organization (WHO) and, 10; youth and, 87

India, 230–233, 237–240; active aging and, 17; aging and, xii, 230–233, 237–240; aging policies and, 238; Alzheimer's disease and, 5–6; death/dying and, 5, 230–231, 237, 239–240, 242n12; decline and, 239; dependence and, 9, 231, 238, 239; elders and, 230, 231–232, 237, 238–240, 242n11; ethnographic research and, 233; globalization and, 239; Hinduism in, 231, 237–238, 239, 241n2, 241n8, 241n9; independence and, 238–239; interdependence and, xii, 5, 231, 237; intergenerational reciprocity and, 9, 19n18, 231, 235, 238, 242n11; Maintenance and Welfare of Parents and Senior Citizens, 238, 241n10; *maya* (bodily attachments) and, 242n12; medicine and, 239–240; Muslims in, 241n2; National Old Age Pension Scheme, 238; old-age homes/ elder ashrams and, 239; personhood and, 5, 231; religions and, 241n2; resources and, 239; selfhood and, 237; *seva* (service to elders) and, 5–6, 9, 237, 238; sexuality and, 71; successful aging and, 5–6, 232–233. *See also names of individual Indians*
individual agency: active aging and, 8, 41; ageism and, 29; anti-aging products/services and, 41; Beijing (China) and, 178; Catholic nuns and, 100, 101–103, 107, 108–109; exercise and, xii–xiii, 2, 7; Kahn, Robert, on, 8, 27–28; Laliberte Rudman, Debbie, on, 29; limits and, 17–18; neoliberalism and, 7, 17, 28, 29; North America and, 7, 101, 107; old age and, 41, 87, 96–97; personhood and, 12, 86–87; Rowe, John on, 8, 27–28; self-help and, 8; successful aging and, xii, 2–3, 6–9, 27–28, 34–36, 38–39, 41, 99, 158–159; United States and, 8–9, 101; *yangsheng* (nurturing life) (China) and, 178
individualism: anti-aging and, 11; Botswana and, 196; friendship and, 128; Kenya and, 191, 197; North America and, 206, 210, 241, 247; personhood and, 206, 210; successful aging and, 136; United States and, 220; Western views and, 189
individual responsibility: Africa and, 247; failure/embarrassment and, 4, 29, 42; successful aging and, xi, 41–42, 101, 235, 243, 244; United States and, xiii; women and, 44, 45, 46, 51. *See also* individual agency
inequality, 116, 118, 119, 244. *See also* social inequalities
in-home care. *See* home care
interdependence: Africa and, 186, 188–189, 196–197, 245, 246, 247; aging and, xiii–xiv, 245; aging in place and, 222; Alzheimer's disease and, 212; Botswana and, 196–197; Brazil and, 210; Catholic nuns and, 104, 107; comfortable aging and, 221–223; desired interdependence, 187–189, 243–247; India and, xii, 5, 231, 237; Japan and, 159; Kenya and, 186, 188–189, 197; North America and, 241; old age and, 246; social relations and, 245; successful aging

interdepende (*continued*)
    and, 13, 16, 188–189, 243–247; Uganda and,
    246–247; United States and, 10, 106
intergenerational reciprocity, 9, 19n18, 188,
    196, 197, 231, 235, 238, 242nII, 245–247
International Plan of Action on Aging, 196
interpersonal relations, 93. *See also* friend-
    ship; sociality; social relations
invisibility, 36, 37, 41, 44, 45, 48, 50–51, 53n5,
    59, 63
Iris, 151
isolation, 57, 58–59, 61–62

Jake, 33, 34, 36
Janet, 45
Japan, 154–165; active aging and, 17,
    158–159, 162; age-grade systems and,
    159, 163–164, 165n6, 166n12; China and,
    180–181; dancing fools and, 160–162,
    166n10; death/dying and, 162, 163;
    decline and, 157, 162, 165; elderly and,
    62–63; ethnography and, 156–157;
    exercise and, 158–159, 163; foolish vital-
    ity and, 157–158, 162, 164–165; humor
    and, 155–156, 157–159, 160; individual
    institutions and, 163–164; interdepen-
    dence and, 159; KBG84 (Kohama Bāchan
    Gasshōdan/Granny Chorus of Kohama),
    157–158; Koenji Awaodori festival,
    161; life expectancy and, 159, 165nI;
    Long-Term Care Insurance (LTCI) and,
    163–164, 166nII, 166n12; Okinawa, 165n3;
    old age and, 156–158; Old Person's Asso-
    ciation, 159; personhood and, 159; pre-
    vention and, 163–164; Ryōkan and, 157;
    self-care and, 158–159; senior welfare
    centers and, 159, 162, 165; sexuality and,
    71; stoicism/modesty and, 155, 156–157;
    successful aging and, 155–156; *Suye Mura*
    (Embree) and, 157; "third age" and, 159,
    162. *See also names of individual Japanese*
Jefferson, Margee, 90–93, 97nI
Jim, 35, 36
Jim Crow, 58, 65, 95
Joe, 130
Johanna, 221, 226
John, 33
Julia, 46, 51
Jullien, François, 170
Juvaderm, 52n4

Kahn, Robert: ageism and, 27; indepen-
    dence and, 9, 87; individual agency and,
    8, 27–28; productive activity and, 10, 27;
    social inequalities and, 15; sociality and,
    126; *Successful Aging* (Rowe and Kahn), I, 2,
    9, 27–28; "Successful Aging 2.0: Concep-
    tual Expansions for the 21st Century,"
    18n15, 38; successful aging and, 2, 10, 12,
    27–28, 87, 93, 126
Kaplan, Joan and Michael, 13–14
Kåre, 141–142, 147, 151
Karp, David, 213

Katherine, 35
Katz, Stephen, II, 19n32, 41–42
Kaufman, Sharon, 127, 226
KBG84 (Kohama Bāchan Gasshōdan/Granny
    Chorus of Kohama), 157–158
Kenya, 185–197; age-grade systems and,
    185–186, 187, 190, 191–192, 196; aging
    and, 196, 197; bridewealth and, 188,
    190–191, 198n4; Britain and, 189–190;
    Christian missions and, 191; colonialism
    and, 186, 189–190, 191–192; Constitution,
    197; dependence and, 6; disease and,
    192–193; elders' councils and, 187–188,
    189–190, 198n3; ethnolinguistic groups
    and, 187; Europe and, 189–190, 191–192;
    females and, 187, 198n2; Giriama, 188;
    giteo (attitude toward elders) and, 188,
    194; globalization and, 186, 189, 193, 196;
    health and, 192–193; HelpAge Kenya, 196;
    independence and, 197; individualism
    and, 191, 197; interdependence and, 186,
    188–189, 197; International Plan of Action
    on Aging and, 196; labor and, 190, 194,
    195; life expectancy and, 192–193; market
    economy and, 190, 191, 194; men and,
    187–188, 189, 190–191, 195, 197; Meru, 185,
    186, 187, 188, 191, 194–195, 198nI, 198n3;
    Mijikenda, 185, 186, 187–188, 190, 191, 192,
    194–195, 198n6; Mipoho and, 185, 187;
    Orma, 190; politicians and, 193, 195, 198n3;
    population aging and, 192–193; Samia, 197;
    successful aging and, 6, 186–187, 188–189,
    195, 196; Tiriki and, 195; traditional heal-
    ing and, 191; welfare and, 196; Western
    views and, 189, 196; "Whispers" (Mutahi),
    189; women and, 190, 191, 192, 193, 195, 197;
    youth and, 186, 188, 190–191, 192–195, 196,
    197, 198n6. *See also* elderhood (Kenya)
Kessler, Eva-Marie, 209
Kisser, 149
Kleinman, Arthur, 8–9
Kleinman, Elaine and Maurice, 5
Klinenberg, Eric, 9
Koenig, Dora, 3–5, 18n7
Koenji Awaodori festival (Japan), *161*
Kolkata (India), 5, 233
Kownacki, Richard, 8

labor: aging and, 36; domestic labor, 37–38,
    72; Fair Labor Standards Act (United
    States), 88, 93; gender and, 30, 88; Kenya
    and, 190, 194, 195; men and, 30, 34, 36, 38,
    43, 72, 190; Mexico and, 72; old age and,
    39; productive labor, 30, 31; Uganda and,
    246; women and, 30, 37–38, 72, 88, 190.
    See also home care; workplaces
LaLanne, Jack, II–I2
Laliberte Rudman, Debbie, 29
Lamb, Sarah, 4–5, 13, 16, 29, 52nI, 99, 127,
    134, 157
Lambert, H. E., 191–192
land, 120, 186, 187, 188, 190, 191, 198n6
Landry, Roger, 15

Lassen, Aske Juul, 141, 144, 150
Laura, 51, 53n7
Lawrence, Marie, 234
Learning to Be Old (Cruikshank), 220
Lech, 120
Leme, Mariana D., 208
lesbian, gay, and bisexual (LGB) people, 52n3, 55, 58, 62–65, 66. *See also* African Americans (lesbian, gay, and bisexual/LGB)
Let Evening Come (Morrison), 225
life expectancy, 159, 165n1, 192–193. *See also* longevity; population aging
lifestyle diseases, 148, 192–193
lifestyle drugs, 68–71. *See also* pharmaceuticals; Viagra
Li Jianmin, 179–181, 182–183
Lindemann, Hilde, 132
Lisbeth, 151
Little, Kim, 95–96
Liv, 130, 135
Live Long, Die Short: A Guide to Authentic Health and Successful Aging (Landry), 15
Live Young Forever (LaLanne), 11–12
living alone, 9–10, 239. *See also* home care
Living in the Labyrinth (McGowin), 204
Livingston, Julie, 196
Lodge, Henry, 3, 8, 12, 232
loneliness, 150–152
longevity, 98, 165, 170, 173–175, 178–179, 226, 234, 244. *See also* population aging
long-term care insurance, 28, 163–164, 166n11, 166n12
Loretta, 94
Lorraine, 131, 132

MacArthur Foundation, 1, 27
machismo, 72
Maggie, 32, 34
Maintenance and Welfare of Parents and Senior Citizens (India), 238, 241n10
males, 187–188, 189, 192. *See also* masculinity; men
Mandy, 94
Margaret, 221, 223, 224, 225, 227
market economy (Kenya), 190, 191, 194
Marta, 121–122
Mary (comfortable aging and), 221
Mary (cosmetic anti-aging and), 45, 46
Mary (gender/aging and), 34, 36, 37
masculinity, 6, 30, 36, 68, 72, 74–79
Mattingly, Cheryl, 129, 136
Maude, 134
Maura, 129–130
McDormand, Frances, 99
McFadden, John and Susan, 128
McGowin, Diana, 204, 214n1
McIntosh, Janet, 6, 11, 243–244
Medicaid, 88
medicalization of aging, 16–17, 70–71, 73, 74, 79. *See also* anti-aging medicine
medicine: aging and, 232; anti-aging and, 12, 42, 241n6; *Being Mortal* (Gawande) and, 15; biopolitics and, 244; India and,

239–240; mortality and, 15; old age and, 39; *Ordinary Medicine* (Kaufman), 226; *The Politics of Life Itself: Biomedicine, Power, and Subjectivity in the Twenty-first Century* (Rose), 6–7; successful aging and, xi, 16, 41; Uganda and, 246; United States and, 239–240. *See also* biomedicine
Mehlman, Maxwell J., 31
Melissa, 45
men: anti-aging products/services and, 16, 31–34, 42; body image and, 52n3; double standard of aging and, 42–43, 52n3; erectile dysfunction and, 32, 42, 71–79; Kenya and, 187–188, 189, 190–191, 195, 197; labor and, 30, 34, 36, 38, 43, 72, 190; loneliness and, 151; Mexico and, 6, 71–79; old age and, 38; pharmaceuticals and, 42; Poland and, 116–119, 123n4, 123n5; sexuality and, 30, 37; sociality and, 117; successful aging and, 31–34, 38; Uganda and, 246; Universities of the Third Age (UTA) and, 116–119; workplaces and, 30, 34, 35, 36, 38. *See also* African Americans (lesbian, gay, and bisexual/LGB); erectile dysfunction; gender; males; masculinity; Viagra
menopause, 50
Meru (Kenya), 185, 186, 187, 188, 191, 194–195, 198n1, 198n3
Mexican Social Security System (Instituto Mexicano del Seguro Social/IMSS), 73
Mexico, 68–79; active aging and, 17; erectile dysfunction and, 6, 71–79; men and, 6, 71–79; pharmaceuticals and, 72–73; research methods and, 73–74; sexuality and, 68, 69, 71–79; Viagra and, 68–69; women and, 71–72
Meyers, Hattie, 93–95, 96
M-force, 72–73
Mia, 51
middle age, 30, 31–34, 35
Mijikenda (Kenya), 185, 186, 187–188, 190, 191, 192, 194–195, 198n6
Mike, 32, 33–34, 36
minorities, 55, 88. *See also* African Americans; African Americans (lesbian, gay, and bisexual/LGB); race
Mipoho (Kenya), 185, 187
modernity, 6, 16–17, 186, 189, 193, 196
moral communities, 131–132
moral laboratories, 128–131, 133, 134, 136
moral personhood, 244
moral relations, 93–97
moral responsibilities: aging and, 2, 42, 123; dependence and, 103, 104, 106, 118; health and, xivn2, 7; Victorian era and, 14; women and, 53n7. *See also* failure/embarrassment; individual agency; individual responsibility
Morgan, Lynn, 132
Morrison, Mary C., 225
mortality: biopolitics and, 244; Brooks, Frances, on, 236–237; comfortable aging and, 220, 221, 224–226, 228, 229; Dora and, 5; as failure/embarrassment, xiii; medicine

mortality (*continued*)
  and, 15; North America and, 241; personhood and, 240; successful aging paradigm
  and, 235. *See also* death/dying
motherhood, 49–50
motivation technologies, 145–150
Murphy, Maureen, 89
Muslims, 241n2
Myerhoff, Barbara, 164

Nancy, 47–48
Naomi, 129, 135
National Old Age Pension Scheme (India), 238
National Studies (China), 170
natural aging. *See* aging naturally
neoliberalism, 7, 17, 28, 29, 99–100, 108, 158,
  164, 168, 204
Newman, Marjorie, 234
New York Times, 8, 11, 99, 220, 234, 236
New Zealand, 71
Nina, 47, 50
Njuri Ncheke (elders' council) (Kenya), 187,
  198n3
"No, You Can't Just Dodder" (Fountain), 11
Noella, Sister, 103–104
Nora, 35
Nordic Model (Denmark), 142–143
North America: ageism and, xi, 13; agelessness
  and, 12, 19n24, 231–232; anti-aging and, 16;
  death/dying and, 241; decline and, 2, 241;
  dependence and, 9, 241; independence and,
  9–10, 17, 107, 210, 212, 231–232; individual
  agency and, 7, 101, 107; individualism and,
  206, 210, 241, 247; interdependence and,
  241; living alone and, 9–10; mortality and,
  241; old age and, xi, xiv, 243; permanent
  personhood and, 4–5, 18n24, 106, 107,
  231–232; personhood and, 206, 210, 231–232,
  240; productive activity and, 10–11, 107;
  successful aging and, xii, 2, 4–5, 6, 17, 29, 43,
  52n1, 100, 126; *The Ways Women Age: Using
  and Refusing Cosmetic Intervention* (Brooks),
  52n4. *See also* Mexico; United States
Norway, 142
Number Our Days (Myerhoff), 164
nuns. *See* Catholic nuns
nursing homes, 88, 106, 143, 149–150, 152
nurturing life. *See* *yangsheng* (nurturing life)
  (China)

Ogola, George, 189
old age, 34–39; acceptance of, 243; active
  aging and, 145, 148; ageism and, 38–39;
  aloneness and, 151–152; Catholic nuns and,
  102, 104, 106–107, 108; class and, 36; Cole,
  Thomas, on, 14; comfortable aging and,
  224; decline and, xi, 34, 148, 149; Denmark
  and, 141, 143, 145–146, 152, 153; dependence and, xi; devaluation of, 28, 35,
  42; Europe and, 145, 146; exclusion and,
  36–37, 113, 122–123; failure/embarrassment
  and, xi–xii, 5, 14–15, 102, 165, 232, 237;
  foolish vitality and, 157–158; gender and,

29, 35–39; Hinduism and, xii, 237–238;
  independence and, 14; individual agency
  and, 41, 87, 96–97; interdependence and,
  246; Japan and, 156–158, 162; labor and,
  39; life stages and, 29, 39; masculinity
  and, 36; medicine and, 39; men and, 38;
  Nordic Model (Denmark) and, 143; North
  America and, xi, xiv, 243; oldest old and,
  165n2, 220, 225, 226; Poland and, 117–118,
  122–123; psychosocial crisis and, 156;
  resources and, 28, 245–246; sexuality and,
  37; sociality and, 87, 96–97; stigma and,
  28, 41; successful aging and, 35, 41; Uganda
  and, 245–246; United States and, 28; Universities of the Third Age (UTA) and, 114,
  116; value of, 17, 39; Victorian era and, 14;
  welfare and, 143, 153; Western views and,
  17–18, 240; women and, 38; young old and,
  165n2. *See also* "fourth age"; "third age"
Older Americans Act (United States), 88
oldest old, 157, 165n2, 220, 225, 226
Old Person's Association (Japan), 159
100 Days to Successful Aging (Bruce), 2–3
Ordinary Medicine (Kaufman), 226
Orma (Kenya), 190
Otto, Lene, 148

palm wine (Kenya), 186, 187, 192
Pani, 123n1. *See also* Anna, Pani; Honorata, Pani
Patrick, 36–37
Paz, Octavio, 72
pensions, 10, 28, 143, 152, 238, 245
People's Movement Against Loneliness
  (Denmark), 150
Perlane, 52n4
permanent personhood, 4–5, 7, 11–12, 18n24,
  99, 100, 106–107, 108–109, 134, 231–232
personal responsibility. *See* individual
  agency; individual responsibility
personhood: African Americans (lesbian, gay,
  and bisexual/LGB) and, 65; agelessness
  and, 240; Alzheimer's disease and, 204,
  205–206, 207–210, 212, 214; Botswana and,
  196; Brazil and, 205–206, 210; Catholic nuns
  and, 100; cross-cultural perspectives of, 5;
  dementia and, 13, 132, 135, 136, 205–206,
  209, 210; dependence and, 240; Europe and,
  206; gossip and, 132; home care and, 87, 89,
  90–91, 96; independence and, 12, 16, 86–87,
  96; India and, 5, 231; individual agency and,
  12, 86–87; individualism and, 206, 210; as
  intersubjective, 196; Japan and, 159; moral
  personhood, 244; mortality and, 240; North
  America and, 206, 210, 231–232, 240; as
  relational, 86, 132, 136, 210; successful aging
  and, xii, 6, 16–17, 100; as term, 18n11; United
  States and, 8; Western views and, 189, 240.
  See also permanent personhood
personhood movement, 204, 205, 209, 214
Peter, 130, 135
Pfeiffer, Eric, 9
pharmaceuticals, 31, 42, 68, 72–73, 78, 79,
  206, 208, 209, 214n4. *See also* anti-aging

products/services; erectile dysfunction; Viagra

plastic surgery, 32, 42, 52n4, 53n5, 205. *See also* cosmetic anti-aging interventions

Plusmore, 88, 89, 93–94, 95, 97n1

Poland, 112–123; active aging and, 122–123; aging and, 117–118; *aktywność* ("active-ness," "activity") and, 115, 119, 120, 121; allotment gardening and, 113, 119–122; Alzheimer's disease and, 113–114, 121; Catholic nuns and, 113–114; class and, 118; computer skills and, 115–116; disease and, 119; elder-care institutions and, 121; elder discrimination and, 115; English-language instruction and, 115–116; European Union and, 115; gender and, 116–119, 123n4, 123n5; Government Program for the Benefit of Social Activity/Active-ness of Older People, 114; health and, 116, 118–119; health care and, 116; inequality and, 116, 118; land and, 120; men and, 116–119, 123n4, 123n5; old age and, 117–118, 122–123; Polish Union of Allotment Gardeners, 119–120; Poznań, 113; rehabilitation centers and, 113–114, 121–122; socialism and, 115–116, 119, 120–121; sociality and, 113–114, 122–123; "third age" and, 122; women and, 116–119, 123n4, 123n5; Wrocław, 112, 113, 115, 116, 117, 121. *See also* Universities of the Third Age (UTA); *names of individual Poles*

Polish Union of Allotment Gardeners, 119–120. *See also* allotment gardening (Poland)

politicians (Kenya), 193, 195, 198n3

Politics of Life Itself: Biomedicine, Power, and Subjectivity in the Twenty-first Century, The (Rose), 6–7

population aging: baby boomers, 7, 8, 12; Brazil and, 17, 205; China and, 17, 169, 171, 173; Denmark and, 143, 152; globalization and, 17; Kenya and, 192–193; successful aging and, 1, 12; United States and, 7, 55

Powersex, 72

Poznań (Poland), 113

prevention, 145, 148–150, 152, 163–164, 168, 170, 204, 221

preventive home visits (PHVs) (Denmark), 148–149

productive activity: Australia and, 10–11; biocitizenship and, 11; Catholic nuns and, 100, 104–105, 108–109; comfortable aging and, 219, 220, 221, 228; Europe and, 10–11; Kahn, Robert, on, 10, 27; Lawrence, Marie, on, 234; North America and, 10–11, 107; Rowe, John, on, 10, 27; successful aging and, 7, 10–11, 27, 55, 93, 99–100, 104–105, 234, 235; United States and, xiii; Western views and, 99–100; White House Conference on Aging and, 226; World Health Organization (WHO) and, 10

productive labor, 30, 31

Propetia, 42

psychosocial crisis, 156

Qicheng, Zhang, 175

race: African Americans (lesbian, gay, and bisexual/LGB) and, 55, 64–66; aging and, xii, 43, 52n3; home care and, 87, 88, 93, 96; successful aging and, 16–17, 19n32, 38, 55

"Racing toward Immortality (Or at Least Your 150th Birthday)" (*New York Times*), 236

racism, xi, 56, 58, 64–65, 66

Rebecca, 47, 49, 50

reform era (China), 171, 172

Regina, Sister, 105

rehabilitation (Denmark), 145–148, 149, 152

rehabilitation centers (Poland), 113–114, 121–122

religion. *See* Catholic nuns; *names of individual religions*

religious institutions/church. *See* church/religious institutions

research, 3, 98–100. *See also* ethnographic research

resources, 11, 28, 220, 221, 226–227, 229, 233, 239, 245–246

retirement, 10–11, 28, 143–144, 169, 173, 176

Rio de Janeiro, 203, 206, 210. *See also* Center for Alzheimer's Disease and Other Mental Disorders of Aging (CDA) (Brazil)

rituals (Kenya), 185, 186, 187–188, 191, 192, 195

Robbins, John, 237

Rose, 58

Rose, Nikolas, 6–7, 243, 244

Rosenthal, Alice, 234

Rowe, Betty, 234

Rowe, John: ageism and, 27; independence and, 9, 87; individual agency and, 8, 27–28; productive activity and, 10, 27; social inequalities and, 15; sociality and, 126; *Successful Aging* (Rowe and Kahn), 1, 2, 9, 27–28; "Successful Aging 2.0: Conceptual Expansions for the 21st Century," 18n15, 38; successful aging and, 2, 10, 12, 27–28, 87, 93, 126

Russia, 120

Ruth, 221, 224–225

Ryle, Gilbert, 161

Ryōkan, 157, 159

Samia (Kenya), 197

Sampson, George, 95–96

Sarah, 48, 49

Sarkar, Narayan, 238

Schatz, Enid, 246

Schwender, Clemens, 209

Seeley, Janet, 246

Seiler, Emilie, 236

self-care, 10, 149, 153, 158–159, 169–170, 171, 173–174, 245. *See also* independence; individual agency; individual responsibility

self-help, 1–2, 8, 9, 170, 173–174, 209

selfhood, 90, 91, 208–209, 209–210, 211, 237.
  See also personhood
self-value, 44, 45–46, 48, 53n5
Senior Citizens Councils (Denmark), 144, 150
senior welfare centers (Japan), 159, 162, 165
seva (service to elders) (India), 5–6, 9, 237,
  238
sexism, xi, 58, 64–65
sexual identity, 57, 59, 60, 61, 64–65
sexuality: aging and, xii, 43, 70–71, 79; anti-
  aging products/services and, 42; double
  standard of aging and, 42–43; Ghana and,
  71; globalization and, 70; India and, 71;
  Japan and, 71; Kenya and, 187; lifestyle
  drugs and, 70–71; masculinity and, 77,
  78; men and, 30, 37; Mexico and, 68, *69*,
  71–79; old age and, 37; successful aging
  and, 16–17, 19n32, 28, 78; Sweden and,
  71; Viagra and, 68; Western views and,
  70; women and, 37, 42–43, 44, 48, 49–50,
  50–51; youth and, 68, 70, 74–75, 76–77.
  See also African Americans (lesbian, gay,
  and bisexual/LGB); erectile dysfunction;
  heterosexuality
sexual orientation, 38, 43, 52n3, 55, 57, 60,
  62, 65
Seymour, 221, 223, 225
Shana, 221–222, 224, 225
shantytown (*favela*) (Brazil), 210–211
Shelly, 37
Shirley, 235–236
Shneidman, Edwin, 223
Silverman, Eileen, 85–86, 87, 97n1
Simic, Andrei, 10
Sloterdijk, Peter, 204–205, 212
Snowdon, David, 99
social dependence, 18n12, 143–144. *See also*
  interdependence
social inequalities, 15–16, 19n32, 29, 38, 39,
  96, 118. *See also* class; ethnicity; gender;
  race; sexuality
socialism, 115–116, 119, 120–121, 168, 172
sociality: allotment gardening (Poland) and,
  122; Alzheimer's disease and, 211; Chica-
  goan elders and, 93–97; cognition and,
  126, 128; Cordial Club (Denmark) and, 141;
  dementia and, 126–127, 211; gender and,
  117; health and, 126, 220–221; Kahn, Robert, on, 126; men and, 117; old age and, 87,
  96–97; Poland and, 113–114, 122–123; Rowe,
  John, on, 126; successful aging and, 16,
  126–127, 136; Universities of the Third Age
  (UTA) and, 113, 117, 122; women and, 117
social relations, 120, 150, 211, 214, 220–221,
  222–223, 226, 229, 245
socioeconomic status, 15, 38. *See also* class;
  inequality; social inequalities
Sontag, Susan, 42–43, 52n3
spirituality, 162, 177, 182–183, 238. *See also*
  names of individual religions
Stemmer, Ellen and Max, 233, 235
stereotypes, 16, 50–51, 64, 70, 72, 119, 143,
  158, 164

Still Alice (film), 15
"Student abandons everything and becomes
  the 'father' of his grandmother with
  Alzheimer's" (Plena), 211, 214n3
Study of Aging in America (MacArthur Foundation), 1, 27
successful aging: active aging and, 8, 34,
  104–105, 114, 126, 163, 236, 245; African
  Americans (lesbian, gay, and bisexual/
  LGB) and, 65–66; ageism and, 28, 29,
  38–39; agelessness and, xii, 4, 7, 11, 12,
  42, 106, 235; Alzheimer's disease and,
  204–205; anti-aging and, 41, 42; attractiveness and, 11–12; binary paradigm of,
  113; bodily aging and, 30–38, 70, 79, 98;
  Catholic nuns and, 5, 98–99, 100, 104;
  class and, 55; cognition and, 8, 10, 126,
  128; colonialism and, 28; comfortable
  aging and, 219, 220, 221, 228; as contemporary obsession, xiii, 6, 9; counter
  discourses and, 15; cross-culturally, 114,
  237; cultural critiques of, 13–16; decline
  and, 3, 17, 41, 159–160, 162; definitions
  of, 55; dementia and, 128, 135–136,
  204–205; disability and, 8, 10, 27, 55,
  126, 236; disease and, xi, 8, 10, 27, 41,
  55, 126, 245; ethnocentricity and, 16,
  17; ethnographic research and, 16, 17;
  Europe and, 1, 6, 79, 188; exercise and,
  2, 15, 35; foolish vitality and, 164–165;
  "fourth age" and, 162; friendship and,
  127; gender and, 16–17, 19n32, 28, 31–34,
  38–39, 43; geriatricians/gerontologists
  and, 156; globalization and, xii, 6, 71;
  Havighurst, Robert, on, 1, 27; health and,
  126, 236; heroism and, 204–205; humor
  and, 157–159, 160, 164, 165n5; independence and, 12, 16, 17, 86–87, 99–100, 163,
  235, 236, 244; India and, 5–6, 232–233;
  individual agency and, 2–3, 6–9, 27–28,
  34–36, 38–39, 41, 158–159; individualism and, 136; individual responsibility
  and, xi, 41–42, 101, 235, 243, 244; individual versus institutions and, 163–164;
  interdependence and, 13, 16, 188–189,
  243–247; interpersonal relations and, 93;
  invisibility and, 41; Japan and, 155–156;
  Kahn, Robert, on, 2, 10, 12, 27–28, 87, 93,
  126; Katz, Stephen, on, 11, 19n32, 41–42;
  Kenya and, 6, 186–187, 188–189, 195, 196;
  Lamb, Sarah, on, 4–5, 13, 16, 29, 52n1, 99,
  127, 134; medicine and, xi, 16, 41; men
  and, 31–34, 38; middle age and, 30, 35;
  neoliberalism and, 99–100, 108, 158, 164,
  204; North America and, 2, 4–5, 6, 17, 29,
  43, 52n1, 100, 126; as obsession, xiii; old
  age and, 35, 41; personhood and, 4–5, 6,
  11–12, 16–17, 134; pharmaceuticals and,
  68, 78, 79; population aging and, 1, 12;
  productive activity and, 10–11, 27, 55, 93,
  99–100, 234, 235; race and, 16–17, 19n32,
  38, 55; research and, 98–99; resources
  and, 233; Rowe, John, on, 2, 10, 12, 27–28,

87, 93, 126; self-care and, 158–159, 245; self-help and, 1–2, 8, 9; senior welfare centers (Japan) and, 159, 162; sexuality and, 16–17, 19n32, 28, 78; sexual orientation and, 38, 55; social factors and, 38; social inequalities and, 15–16, 19n32, 29, 38, 39; sociality and, 16, 126–127, 136; as term, 1; United States and, 8–9, 41, 43, 44, 51, 55, 79, 100, 188, 226, 232–233, 233–235; Universities of the Third Age (UTA) and, 114; voices and, 3, 16, 20n34, 39; Western views and, 5, 17–18, 99–100, 188; White House Conference on Aging and, 226; women and, 31–34, 38, 39, 43–52; youth and, 42, 70, 79, 188. *See also* successful aging paradigm; *individual titles of works*

Successful Aging (Rowe and Kahn), 1, 2, 9, 27–28

"Successful Aging 2.0: Conceptual Expansions for the 21st Century" (Rowe and Kahn), 18n15, 38

successful aging movement, xi, xiii, 3, 6–12, 13–16, 52n1, 169, 233, 240

successful aging paradigm: active aging and, 104–105; Africa and, 247; ageism and, 6, 13, 38–39, 42; agelessness and, xii, 7, 106; assumptions and, 3; as binary, xii; Catholic nuns and, 99, 100, 104, 108–109; critical examination of, 243; decline and, 98, 235; dependence and, 7, 99, 103, 235; Europe and, xii; exclusion and, 6, 13–14; gender and, 38–39; globalization and, xii; independence and, 7, 9–10, 99, 103–104; individual agency and, xii, 2, 7, 38–39, 41, 99; inspiration and, 6; Koenig, Dora, on, 4–5; mortality and, 235; neoliberalism and, 108, 158; North America and, xii; permanent personhood and, 7, 99, 100, 106–107; personhood and, xii; productive activity and, 7, 99, 100, 104–105; related labels and, 1; as social-cultural phenomenon, xii; social inequalities and, 19n32, 38; Uganda and, 245; United States and, 233

Sue, 33

Suye Mura (Embree), 157

Sweden, 71, 142

Tagore, Rabindranath, 240, 242n13

Taylor, Charles, 129

Taylor, Janelle, 13, 210

Taylor, Richard, 209

technogenarians, 223

Ten Thousand Things (Farquhar and Zhang), 168, 183n2

Teresa, 131

Thea, 130

"third age," 14, 19n30, 114, 118–119, 122, 159, 162, 165n7, 205. *See also* Universities of the Third Age (UTA)

36-Hour Day, The (Maze and Rabins), 207

Thomas, Samuel, 186, 188, 191, 194, 195

Tiriki (Kenya), 195

Tom, 34

Townsend, Peter, 143–144

traditional healing (Kenya), 191

Traphagan, John W., 159, 166n6

Twigg, Julia, 13

Uganda, 243–247

Uganda Health Sector Strategic Plan, 244

U.N. Department of Social and Economic Affairs, 196

United States: active aging and the, 234; ageism and the, 14, 62–63; agelessness and the, 232, 234; aging and the, xii–xiii, 51, 232–233, 237; Alzheimer's disease and the, 209; American Academy of Anti-Aging Medicine, 241n6; American myth, 8–9; American Society for Aesthetic Plastic Surgery, 42; baby boomers and the, 7, 8, 12; children and the, 9–10; comfortable aging and the, 226–227; death/dying and the, 226, 234, 235–236, 237; decline and the, 232–233; dementia and the, 128; dependence and the, 9–10; "elderspeak" and the, 107; erectile dysfunction and the, 71; ethnographic research and the, 233, 241n5; failure/embarrassment and the, 102; home care and the, 86, 87, 88–93; independence and the, 9–10, 86–87, 222, 232, 235, 238–239; indigenous American communities, 106; individual agency and the, 8–9, 101; individualism and the, 220; individual responsibility and the, xiii; interdependence and the, 10, 106; intergenerational reciprocity and the, 235; longevity and the, 234; medicine and the, 239–240; nursing homes and the, 106; old age and the, 28; old-age dependency ratio, 7; oldest old and the, 220; permanent personhood and the, 232; personhood and the, 8; population aging and the, 7, 55; productive activity and the, xiii; Study of Aging in America (MacArthur Foundation), 1, 27; successful aging and the, 8–9, 41, 43, 44, 51, 55, 79, 100, 188, 232–233, 233–235; Viagra and the, 68; women and the, 43, 44, 51

Universities of the Third Age (UTA), 112–122; active aging and, 10–11, 113, 114–116; *aktywność* ("active-ness," "activity") (Poland) and, 115; allotment gardening (Poland) and, 113, 119–122; Britain and, 123n2; Canada and, 123n2; class and, 116–119; computer skills and, 115–116; definition of, 112; English-language instruction and, 115–116, 122; ethnographic research and, 113–114; Europe and, 123n2; exclusion and, 116, 119; gender and, 116–119; globalization and, 114; Government Program for the Benefit of Social Activity/Active-ness of Older People (Poland), 114; health and, 116–119; inequality and, 116, 119; men and,

Universities of the Third Age (UTA) (*continued*) 116–119; old age and, 114, 116; origins of, 19n22, 114, 123n2; socialism and, 115–116; sociality and, 113, 117, 122; successful aging and, 114; women and, 116–119

Valter, 149, 151
Vellas, Pierre, 123n2
Viagra, 6, 42, 68–71, 72, 76, 205. *See also* erectile dysfunction
Victorian morality, 14
vows (Catholic nuns), 101–102, 104, 108, 109n2

Wahome, Mutahi, 189
Walter, 59
Warren, 61, 62–63
Washington, Grace, 90–93, 97n1
Washington, Hattie, 89
Ways Women Age: Using and Refusing Cosmetic Intervention, The (Brooks), 52n4
welfare, 142–144, 150, 152–153, 158, 196
Wendell, Susan, 47
Wendy, 45
Wentzell, Emily, 6
Western views: Africa and, 186–187; death/dying and, 106, 237, 240; dependence and, 188; failure/embarrassment and, 106, 237; individualism and, 189; Kenya and, 189, 196; neoliberalism and, 99–100; old age and, 17–18, 240; personhood and, 189; productive activity and, 99–100; sexuality and, 70; successful aging and, 5, 99–100. *See also* Europe; North America; United States
"Whispers" (Mutahi), 189
White, Betty, 164
White House Conference on Aging, 226
Whyte, Susan, 18n12
Wiedergården (Denmark), 144–145, 150
Wilen, S. B., 206
Winning Strategies for Successful Aging (Pfeiffer), 9
Winters, Barbara, 234
witchcraft (Kenya), 185, 186, 192, 197, 198n6
women: ageism and, 62, 64–65; aging naturally and, 44, 47–50, 51–52; anti-aging products/services and, 16, 31–34, 42–43, 51; attractiveness and, 16, 32–33, 37, 39, 43, 45, 48–49, 50–51, 52, 53n5; beauty and, 30, 34, 43, 44, 47, 49; Botswana and, 196–197; comfortable aging and, 220; cosmetic anti-aging interventions and, 32, 43, 44–47, 51; cultural pressure and, 53n7; double standard of aging and, 42–43, 52n3; eldercare and, 242n11, 246; elderhood (Kenya) and, 192, 193, 197, 198n2, 198n4, 198n6; erectile dysfunction and, 71, 77–78; exercise and, 43, 45; Hinduism and, 24n9; home care and, 87, 88, 96; individual responsibility and, 44, 45, 46, 51; invisibility and, 37, 44, 45, 48, 50–51, 53n5; Kenya and, 190, 191, 192, 193, 195, 197; labor and, 30, 37–38,

72, 88, 190; loneliness and, 151; menopause and, 50; Mexico and, 71–72; moral responsibilities and, 53n7; motherhood and, 49–50; old age and, 38; Poland and, 116–119, 123n4, 123n5; self-value and, 44, 45–46, 48, 53n5; sexism and, 58; sexuality and, 37, 42–43, 44, 48, 49–50, 50–51; sociality and, 117; successful aging and, 31–34, 38, 39, 43–52; Uganda and, 246; Universities of the Third Age (UTA) and, 116–119; *The Ways Women Age: Using and Refusing Cosmetic Intervention* (Brooks), 52n4; youth-beauty imperative and, 45, 52n3. *See also* African Americans (lesbian, gay, and bisexual/LGB); females; femininity; gender
workplaces, 30, 34, 35, 36, 38, 39, 45, 58, 72
World Health Organization (WHO), 1, 10, 143
Wrocław (Poland), 112, 113, 115, 116, 117, 121

yangsheng (nurturing life) (China), 168–183; Beijing and, 171, 172–173, 175–176, 183; calligraphy and, 182; Daoism and, 174–175; exercise and, 169, 170–171, 175–176, 178, 179–180, 182; food and, 179; globalization and, 170; health and, 174–175, 181–182; health care and, 171, 174; individual agency and, 178; Li Jianmin and, 179–181, 182–183; National Studies and, 170; older people and, 173; prevention and, 170; public benefit and, 178–179; retirees and, 176; self-help and, 170, 173–174; successful aging movement and, 169; as term, 168, 170; youth and, 181; the *Zhuangzi* and, 168, 170; Zhu Hong and, 176–178, 182–183
Younger Next Year: Live Strong, Fit, and Sexy—Until You're 80 and Beyond (Crowley and Lodge), 3, 8, 232
"Young woman changes her routine in order to dedicate herself to her grandmother with Alzheimer's—The disease changed the lives of granny and grandchild who even sleep together in the same bed" (Globo.com), 212, 214n3
youth: active aging and, 152; ageism and, 42; aging and, 99; allotment gardening (Poland) and, 120; Brazil and, 205; children, 9–10, 106, 235, 245–246; grandchildren, 211–213, 214n3, 214n4, 245; independence and, 87; Kenya and, 186, 188, 190–191, 192–195, 196, 197, 198n6; resources and, 28; sexuality and, 68, 70, 74–75, 76–77; successful aging and, 42, 70, 79, 188; yangsheng (nurturing life) (China) and, 181. *See also* intergenerational reciprocity
youth-beauty imperative, 43, 45, 48–49, 50–51, 52, 52n3, 70, 79, 99. *See also* attractiveness; beauty
youth-centrism, 42, 44

Zbyszek, 120–121
Zhuangzi, the, 168, 170
Zhu Hong, 176–178, 182–183

Printed in the United States
By Bookmasters